Diabetes
SOURCEBOOK

Sixth Edition

Health Reference Series

Sixth Edition

Diabetes
SOURCEBOOK

Basic Consumer Health Information about Type 1 and Type 2 Diabetes, Gestational Diabetes, and Other Types of Diabetes and Prediabetes, with Details about Medical, Dietary, and Lifestyle Disease Management Issues, Including Blood Glucose Monitoring, Weight Control, Oral Diabetes Medications, and Insulin

Along with Facts about the Most Common Complications of Diabetes and Their Prevention, Financial Assistance through Insurance, Current Research in Diabetes Care, Tips for People following a Diabetic Diet, a Glossary of Related Terms, and a Directory of Resources for Further Help and Information

OMNIGRAPHICS

155 W. Congress, Suite 200 Detroit, MI 48226

Bibliographic Note
Because this page cannot legibly accommodate all the copyright notices, the Bibliographic Note portion of the Preface constitutes an extension of the copyright notice.

* * *

Omnigraphics, Inc.
Editorial Services provided by Omnigraphics, Inc.,
a division of Relevant Information, Inc.

Keith Jones, *Managing Editor*

* * *

Copyright © 2016 Relevant Information, Inc.
ISBN 978-0-7808-1454-7
E-ISBN 978-0-7808-1453-0

Library of Congress Cataloging-in-Publication Data

Names: Omnigraphics, Inc.

Title: Diabetes sourcebook : basic consumer health information about type 1 and type 2 diabetes, gestational diabetes, and other types of diabetes and prediabetes, with details about medical, dietary, and lifestyle disease management issues, including blood glucose monitoring, meal planning, weight control, oral diabetes medications, and insulin; along with facts about the most common complications of diabetes and their prevention, current research in diabetes care, tips for people following a diabetic diet, a glossary of related terms, and a directory of resources for further help and information.

Description: Sixth edition. | Detroit, MI : Omnigraphics, Inc., [2016] | Series: Health reference series | Includes bibliographical references and index. | Description based on print version record and CIP data provided by publisher; resource not viewed.

Identifiers: LCCN 2015042779 (print) | LCCN 2015042283 (ebook) | ISBN 9780780814530 (ebook) | ISBN 9780780814547 (hardcover : alk. paper)

Subjects: LCSH: Diabetes--Popular works.

Classification: LCC RC660.4 (print) | LCC RC660.4 .D56 2016 (ebook) | DDC 616.4/62--dc23

LC record available at http://lccn.loc.gov/2015042779

Electronic or mechanical reproduction, including photography, recording, or any other information storage and retrieval system for the purpose of resale is strictly prohibited without permission in writing from the publisher.

The information in this publication was compiled from the sources cited and from other sources considered reliable. While every possible effort has been made to ensure reliability, the publisher will not assume liability for damages caused by inaccuracies in the data, and makes no warranty, express or implied, on the accuracy of the information contained herein.

This book is printed on acid-free paper meeting the ANSI Z39.48 Standard. The infinity symbol that appears above indicates that the paper in this book meets that standard.

Printed in the United States

Table of Contents

Preface xi

Part I: Diabetes – An Overview

Chapter 1—Introduction to Diabetes.. 3
        Section 1.1—What Is Diabetes?........................... 4
        Section 1.2—Why Is Diabetes a Problem? 6

Chapter 2—Type 1 Diabetes.. 9

Chapter 3—Prediabetes... 13

Chapter 4—Insulin Resistance.. 17

Chapter 5—Type 2 Diabetes.. 27

Chapter 6—Gestational Diabetes.. 29

Chapter 7—Causes of Diabetes... 33

Chapter 8—Prevalence of Diabetes in United States 45

Chapter 9—FAQs on Diabetes 47

Part II: Risks, Prevention, and Diagnosis of Diabetes

Chapter 10—Will Diabetes Be Part of Your Story? 55

Chapter 11—Am I at Risk for Type 2 Diabetes?......................... 61

Chapter 12—Women at High Risk for Diabetes 67
    Section 12.1—Women and Risk of Type 2 Diabetes......................... 68
    Section 12.2—Am I at Risk for Gestational Diabetes?..................... 71

Chapter 13—Family History – A Potential Risk Factor for Diabetes 75

Chapter 14—Saving Yourself – Role of the Individual in Helping Prevent Diabetes................ 79
    Section 14.1—The Power to Prevent Diabetes and Saving Yourself 80
    Section 14.2—Keep Your Diabetes under Control.......................... 85

Chapter 15—How Staying Healthy Can Help in the Prevention of Diabetes 97
    Section 15.1—Keep Your Mouth Healthy 98
    Section 15.2—Keep Your Teeth Healthy......... 102
    Section 15.3—Keep Your Kidneys Healthy..... 104
    Section 15.4—Keep Your Heart and Blood Vessels Healthy 111
    Section 15.5—Keep Your Feet Healthy........... 115
    Section 15.6—Keep Your Eyes Healthy 117

Chapter 16—Diabetes Prevention – Questions for Your Doctor 123

Chapter 17—Team Care Approach for Diabetes Management 125

Chapter 18—Tips to Prevent Type 2 Diabetes......................... 129

Chapter 19—Diagnosis of Diabetes 133

Chapter 20—Blood Sugar Number 141
    Section 20.1—Blood Sugar Test...................... 142
    Section 20.2—FAQs on Blood Sugar Test and Blood Glucose Monitoring Devices.................... 144

Chapter 21—The A1C Test and Diabetes................................. 149

Part III: Medications and Diabetes Care

Chapter 22—Diabetes Treatment 159
Chapter 23—Diabetes Medications 161
        Section 23.1—Diabetes Medications –
                An Overview 162
        Section 23.2—Managing Diabetes
                Medications 166
        Section 23.3—Women and Diabetes
                Medications 169
Chapter 24—Insulin and Its Role in Diabetes
               Treatment 177
Chapter 25—Diabetes and Adult Vaccines 185
Chapter 26—Diabetes Treatment Fraud 189
Chapter 27—New Diabetes Drugs – Tresiba and
               Ryzodeg 70/30 193

Part IV: Dietary and Other Lifestyle Issues Important for Diabetes Control

Chapter 28—Eat Right! 197
        Section 28.1—Eat Healthy Food 198
        Section 28.2—Carbohydrate Counting 204
        Section 28.3—Diabetes and Dietary
                Supplements 210
Chapter 29—Smoking and Diabetes 217
Chapter 30—Weight Management and Diabetes 219
        Section 30.1—Diabetic Patients and
                Weight Concerns 220
        Section 30.2—Helping Your Child Manage
                Weight 223
Chapter 31—Physical Activity and Diabetes 227

Part V: Complications of Diabetes and Co-Occurring Disorders

Chapter 32—Complications Associated with Diabetes 235
Chapter 33—Diabetes-Related Bone Disease 239

Chapter 34—Diabetes-Related Eye Diseases............................ 243

Chapter 35—Diabetes-Related Foot Problems......................... 251

Chapter 36—Diabetes and the Flu 259

Chapter 37—Diabetes and Gastroparesis 263

Chapter 38—Diabetes, Heart Disease, and Stroke.................. 267

Chapter 39—Diabetes and Hepatitis B 271

Chapter 40—Diabetic Kidney Disease.. 273

Chapter 41—Diabetes-Related Mouth Problems 279

Chapter 42—Diabetes-Related Nerve Damage........................ 283

Chapter 43—Diabetes and Polycystic Ovary Syndrome........... 291

Chapter 44—Diabetes and Proteinuria 293

Part VI: Diabetes in Specific Populations

Chapter 45—Diabetes in Children and Adolescents................. 299

Chapter 46—Diabetes and Women 303

Chapter 47—Diabetes and Pregnancy....................................... 307

    Section 47.1—Diabetes and Pregnancy
                      Preparation 308

    Section 47.2—Gestational Diabetes and
                      Pregnancy.................................. 315

Chapter 48—Diabetes in the Elderly.. 319

Chapter 49—Diabetes in Minority Groups................................. 323

Part VII: Living with Diabetes

Chapter 50—Take Care of Your Diabetes Each Day 329

Chapter 51—Monitor Your Diabetes 335

Chapter 52—Be Active! 347

Chapter 53—Stay Healthy! 351

Chapter 54—Managing Diabetes during Sick Days	355
Chapter 55—Managing Your Diabetes during Special Times	359
Chapter 56—Managing Your Diabetes during the Holidays	365
Chapter 57—Diabetes and Employee Rights	369

Part VIII: Research and Clinical Trials on Diabetes

Chapter 58—Ongoing Research in Diabetes Care	385
Section 58.1—Research on Diabetes at CDC	386
Section 58.2—Research on Diabetes at NIDDK	388
Section 58.3—Pancreatic Islet Transplantation	390
Section 58.4—Stem Cell Research	396
Chapter 59—Targeted Drug Development: Why Is Diabetes Lagging Behind?	401
Chapter 60—Clinical Trials and Their Role in Diabetes Treatment	409

Part IX: Additional Help and Information

Chapter 61—Financial Help for Diabetes Care	421
Chapter 62—Recipes for People with Diabetes and Their Families	429
Chapter 63—Glossary of Terms Related to Diabetes	445
Chapter 64—Directory of Diabetes-Related Resources	453
Index	**461**

Preface

About This Book

Diabetes is a chronic disorder characterized by high levels of blood sugar. It can lead to a host of complications, including heart disease, stroke, high blood pressure, blindness, kidney disease, nervous system disease, and limb amputation. Although many of the complications of diabetes occur over long periods of time, poorly controlled blood glucose levels can also result in acute medical emergencies, such as seizures or coma or even death.

The number of people with diabetes in the United States is growing. According to the 2014 publication from the Center for Disease Control and Prevention, 29.1 million children and adults in the United States are living with diabetes. Among people aged twenty and older, 208,000 people have been diagnosed with diabetes (type 1 or type 2). Furthermore, an estimated 86 million adults aged 20 years and older have prediabetes. Despite its prevalence, many Americans are unaware of the basic facts about diabetes and the progress being made in the fight against it. For example, new forms of treatment are being developed making it easier to manage, and work on pancreatic islet transplantation and an artificial pancreas offer hope for an eventual cure.

Diabetes Sourcebook, Sixth Edition, provides basic consumer information about the different types of diabetes and how they are diagnosed. It discusses strategies for controlling diabetes and managing daily life challenges. It includes information about the complications of diabetes and their prevention and offers guidelines for recognizing and treating diabetic emergencies. The book concludes with updated information regarding the most recent research in diabetes care, a glossary of related terms, and a list of resources for additional help and information.

How to Use This Book

This book is divided into parts and chapters. Parts focus on broad areas of interest. Chapters are devoted to single topics within a part.

Part One: Diabetes – An Overview gives an introduction to prediabetes and diabetes. It also offers details on various types of diabetes, causes, and its prevalence in the United States. The part ends with FAQs on diabetes.

Part Two: Risks, Prevention, and Diagnosis of Diabetes describes various risk factors and prevention strategies related to diabetes. The role that you can play as an individual, as part of a family, and adopting a healthy lifestyle to prevent diabetes is discussed in detail. The part concludes with information on the various diagnostic tests available for checking diabetes.

Part Three: Medications and Diabetes Care offers an overview of diabetes treatment, medicines, and vaccines. It also describes the role of insulin in diabetes treatment, including the different types and methods used to administer insulin.

Part Four: Dietary and Other Lifestyle Issues Important for Diabetes Control describes the components of the diabetic diet and the types of meal planning that can be used to control blood glucose levels. It explains the importance of physical activity and weight management and offers tips for handling the challenges diabetics face in daily life.

Part Five: Complications of Diabetes and Co-Occurring Disorders provides facts about the impact diabetes can have on the bones, eyes, feet, cardiovascular system, kidneys, mouth, and elsewhere in the body. It describes the symptoms of these complications and discusses ways to prevent their occurrence. It also describes disorders that often accompany diabetes and offers suggestions for their prevention and treatment

Part Six: Diabetes in Specific Populations discusses the particular challenges of managing diabetes among pregnant women, the elderly, and children. It also discusses about risk factors, tests and health tips that women with diabetes need to be aware of during and post pregnancy.

Part Seven: Living with Diabetes provides useful information on how to manage and monitor your diabetes everyday and health tips to enable diabetics stay healthy and active. It also offers suggestions for overcoming such challenges as managing diabetes while coping with illness and celebrating special occasions.

Part Eight: Research and Clinical Trials on Diabetes Care describes current research in the management and prevention of diabetes. It discusses emerging stem cell research related to diabetes, and provides information on clinical trials currently being conducted.

Part Nine: Additional Help and Information includes a glossary of terms related to diabetes, recipes for diabetics and their families, information about sources of financial assistance, and a directory of other resources for additional help and support.

Bibliographic Note

This volume contains documents and excerpts from publications issued by the following U.S. government agencies: Centers for Disease Control and Prevention (CDC); ClinicalTrials.gov; Genetics Home Reference (NLM); National Center for Complementary and Alternative Medicine (NCCIH); National Center for Chronic Disease Prevention and Health Promotion (NCCDPHP); National Center for Complementary and Integrative Health (NCCIH); National Institute on Aging (NIA); National Diabetes Education Program (NDEP); National Diabetes Information Clearinghouse (NDIC); National Institute of Arthritis and Musculoskeletal and Skin Diseases (NIAMS); National Institutes of Health (NIH); National Institute of Child Health and Human Development (NICHD); National Institute for Diabetes and Digestive and Kidney Diseases (NIDDK); National Eye Institute (NEI); National Women's Health Information Center (OWH); Office of Disease Prevention and Health Promotion (ODPHP); Office of Minority Health (OMH); Office on Women's Health in the Department of Health and Human Services (OWH); U.S. Department of Health and Human Services (HHS); U.S. Equal Employment Opportunity Commission (EEOC); and U.S. Food and Drug Administration (FDA).

About the Health Reference Series

The *Health Reference Series* is designed to provide basic medical information for patients, families, caregivers, and the general public. Each volume takes a particular topic and provides comprehensive coverage. This is especially important for people who may be dealing with a newly diagnosed disease or a chronic disorder in themselves or in a family member. People looking for preventive guidance, information about disease warning signs, medical statistics, and risk factors for health problems will also find answers to their questions in the *Health Reference Series*. The *Series*, however, is not intended to serve as a tool for diagnosing illness, in prescribing treatments, or as a substitute for the physician/patient relationship. All people concerned about medical symptoms or the possibility of disease are encouraged to seek professional care from an appropriate health care provider.

A Note about Spelling and Style

Health Reference Series editors use *Stedman's Medical Dictionary* as an authority for questions related to the spelling of medical terms and the *Chicago Manual of Style* for questions related to grammatical structures, punctuation, and other editorial concerns. Consistent adherence is not always possible, however, because the individual volumes within the *Series* include many documents from a wide variety of different producers, and the editor's primary goal is to present material from each source as accurately as is possible. This sometimes means that information in different chapters or sections may follow other guidelines and alternate spelling authorities.

Our Advisory Board

We would like to thank the following board members for providing initial guidance to the development of this series:

- Dr. Lynda Baker, Associate Professor of Library and Information Science, Wayne State University, Detroit, MI
- Nancy Bulgarelli, William Beaumont Hospital Library, Royal Oak, MI
- Karen Imarisio, Bloomfield Township Public Library, Bloomfield Township, MI
- Karen Morgan, Mardigian Library, University of Michigan-Dearborn, Dearborn, MI
- Rosemary Orlando, St. Clair Shores Public Library, St. Clair Shores, MI

Health Reference Series *Update Policy*

The inaugural book in the *Health Reference Series* was the first edition of *Cancer Sourcebook* published in 1989. Since then, the *Series* has been enthusiastically received by librarians and in the medical community. In order to maintain the standard of providing high-quality health information for the layperson the editorial staff at Omnigraphics felt it was necessary to implement a policy of updating volumes when warranted.

Medical researchers have been making tremendous strides, and it is the purpose of the *Health Reference Series* to stay current with the most recent advances. Each decision to update a volume is made on an individual basis. Some of the considerations include how much new information is available and the feedback we receive from people who use the books. If there is a topic you would like to see added to the update list, or an area of medical concern you feel has not been adequately addressed, please write to:

Managing Editor
Health Reference Series
Omnigraphics, Inc.
155 W. Congress, Suite 200
Detroit, MI 48226

Part One

Diabetes – An Overview

Chapter 1

Introduction to Diabetes

Chapter Contents

Section 1.1—What Is Diabetes? 4
Section 1.2—Why Is Diabetes a Problem? 6

Section 1.1

What Is Diabetes?

Text in this section is excerpted from "Diabetes," National Institute on Aging (NIA), National Institutes of Health (NIH), August 2014.

Too Much Glucose in the Blood

Diabetes means your blood glucose (often called blood sugar) is too high. Your blood always has some glucose in it because your body needs glucose for energy to keep you going. But too much glucose in the blood isn't good for your health.

Glucose comes from the food you eat and is also made in your liver and muscles. Your blood carries the glucose to all of the cells in your body. Insulin is a chemical (a hormone) made by the pancreas. The pancreas releases insulin into the blood. Insulin helps the glucose from food get into your cells.

If your body does not make enough insulin or if the insulin doesn't work the way it should, glucose can't get into your cells. It stays in your blood instead. Your blood glucose level then gets too high, causing prediabetes or diabetes.

Types of Diabetes

There are three main kinds of diabetes: type 1, type 2, and gestational diabetes. The result of type 1 and type 2 diabetes is the same: glucose builds up in the blood, while the cells are starved of energy. Over the years, high blood glucose damages nerves and blood vessels, oftentimes leading to complications such as heart disease, stroke, blindness, kidney disease, nerve problems, gum infections, and amputation.

Type 1 Diabetes

Type 1 diabetes, which used to be called juvenile diabetes or insulin-dependent diabetes, develops most often in young people. However, type 1 diabetes can also develop in adults. With this form of diabetes, your body no longer makes insulin or doesn't make enough insulin because

Introduction to Diabetes

your immune system has attacked and destroyed the insulin-producing cells. About 5 to 10 percent of people with diabetes have type 1 diabetes.

To survive, people with type 1 diabetes must have insulin delivered by injection or a pump.

Type 2 Diabetes

Type 2 diabetes, which used to be called adult-onset diabetes or non insulin-dependent diabetes, is the most common form of diabetes. Although people can develop type 2 diabetes at any age—even during childhood—type 2 diabetes develops most often in middle-aged and older people.

Type 2 diabetes usually begins with insulin resistance—a condition that occurs when fat, muscle, and liver cells do not use insulin to carry glucose into the body's cells to use for energy. As a result, the body needs more insulin to help glucose enter cells. At first, the pancreas keeps up with the added demand by making more insulin. Over time, the pancreas doesn't make enough insulin when blood sugar levels increase, such as after meals. If your pancreas can no longer make enough insulin, you will need to treat your type 2 diabetes.

Gestational Diabetes

Some women develop gestational diabetes during the late stages of pregnancy. Gestational diabetes is caused by the hormones of pregnancy or a shortage of insulin. Although this form of diabetes usually goes away after the baby is born, a woman who has had it and her child are more likely to develop diabetes later in life.

Signs of Diabetes

Many people with diabetes experience one or more symptoms, including extreme thirst or hunger, a frequent need to urinate and/or fatigue. Some lose weight without trying. Additional signs include sores that heal slowly, dry, itchy skin, loss of feeling or tingling in the feet and blurry eyesight. Some people with diabetes, however, have no symptoms at all.

How Many Have Diabetes?

Nearly 29 million Americans age 20 or older (12.3 percent of all people in this age group) have diabetes, according to 2014 estimates from the Centers for Disease Control and Prevention (CDC). About 1.9 million people aged 20 years or older were newly diagnosed with diabetes in 2010 alone. People can get diabetes at any age, but the risk increases as we get older. In 2014, over 11 million older adults living in the United States—nearly 26 percent of people 65 or older—had diabetes.

If Diabetes Is Not Managed

Diabetes is a very serious disease. Over time, diabetes that is not well managed causes serious damage to the eyes, kidneys, nerves, heart, gums and teeth. If you have diabetes, you are more likely than people without diabetes to have heart disease or a stroke. People with diabetes also tend to develop heart disease or stroke at an earlier age than others.

The best way to protect yourself from the serious complications of diabetes is to manage your blood glucose, blood pressure and cholesterol and to avoid smoking. It is not always easy, but people who make an ongoing effort to manage their diabetes can greatly improve their overall health.

Section 1.2

Why Is Diabetes a Problem?

Text in this section is excerpted from "Diabetes," Centers for Disease Control and Prevention (CDC), June 24, 2015.

What's the problem?

Most of the food we eat is turned into glucose (sugar) for our bodies to use for energy. Insulin helps glucose into our body cells. When you have diabetes, your body either doesn't make enough insulin or can't use its own insulin very well. The most common, types of diabetes include type 2, type 1, and gestational (occurs during pregnancy). Type 2 affects 90–95% of people with diabetes and usually appears after age 40. Type 1 affects 5–10% of those with diabetes and most often appears

Introduction to Diabetes

in childhood or teen years. People with type 1 diabetes need insulin to survive. Gestational diabetes affects 2.5–4% of pregnant women.

People with diabetes may have some or none of the following symptoms: frequent urination, excessive thirst, unexplained weight loss, extreme hunger, blurry vision, tingling or numbness in hands or feet, recurring fatigue, very dry skin, slow-healing sores, or more infections than usual.

If not well managed, diabetes can seriously impact a person's quality of life. Complications, many of which are preventable, include the following: heart disease, stroke, blindness, kidney failure, foot or leg amputations, nerve damage, and complications of pregnancy.

Who's at risk?

About 17 million people in the United States, or 6.2% of the population, have diabetes. About one-third of these don't know they have it. Risk factors for type 1 diabetes include autoimmune disease, genetic predisposition, and environmental factors. Prediabetes is a new term for a condition that people get before they are diagnosed with diabetes.

People who develop diabetes don't go from normal blood glucose numbers directly to type 2 diabetes. Almost all go through a phase called impaired glucose tolerance or impaired fasting glucose, conditions in which the blood glucose level is elevated but is not high enough to be classified as diabetes.

Type 2 diabetes is more likely to develop in people who are older, are obese, have a family history of diabetes, have a prior history of gestational diabetes (5–10% of women with gestational diabetes are found to have type 2 diabetes after pregnancy), are physically inactive, and belong to a certain racial or ethnic group. African-Americans, Hispanic/Latino Americans, American Indians, Alaska Natives, and some Asian-Americans and Pacific Islanders are at particularly high risk for type 2 diabetes. Type 2 diabetes was previously called adult-onset diabetes but is increasingly being diagnosed in children and adolescents.

Can it be prevented?

Research studies in the United States and abroad have found that lifestyle changes can prevent or delay the onset of type 2 diabetes among high-risk adults. Currently, there are no known methods to prevent type 1 diabetes. However, several clinical trials are currently in progress.

People with diabetes must develop a life-long commitment to regular medical care and diabetes self-management. Treatment for diabetes is aimed at keeping blood glucose near normal levels at all times. To do that, people with diabetes must balance three important things: what they eat and drink, how much physical activity they do, and what diabetes medicines they take (if their doctor has prescribed diabetes pills or insulin). People with diabetes often learn to check their blood glucose levels at home with a glucometer as part of diabetes self-management. In addition, controlling blood pressure is very important for people with high blood pressure and diabetes.

Treatment must be individualized and address medical, emotional, cultural, and lifestyle issues. Potential barriers to treatment and preventive services include lack of financial resources, linguistic barriers, limited access to transportation, lack of physical activity because of unsafe neighborhoods, and lack of healthy food choices. Communities can overcome some of these barriers by using community health workers (other titles include: promotores de salud, lay health advisors, outreach workers, and peer educators) to serve as bridges between community members and health care systems. Community health workers communicate and model healthy lifestyle choices in culturally and linguistically appropriate ways.

Chapter 2

Type 1 Diabetes

What is type 1 diabetes?

Type 1 diabetes is a disorder characterized by abnormally high blood sugar levels. In this form of diabetes, specialized cells in the pancreas called beta cells stop producing insulin. Insulin controls how much glucose (a type of sugar) is passed from the blood into cells for conversion to energy. Lack of insulin results in the inability to use glucose for energy or to control the amount of sugar in the blood.

Type 1 diabetes can occur at any age; however, it usually develops by early adulthood, most often starting in adolescence. The first signs and symptoms of the disorder are caused by high blood sugar and may include frequent urination (polyuria), excessive thirst (polydipsia), fatigue, blurred vision, tingling or loss of feeling in the hands and feet, and weight loss. These symptoms may recur during the course of the disorder if blood sugar is not well controlled by insulin replacement therapy. Improper control can also cause blood sugar levels to become too low (hypoglycemia). This may occur when the body's needs change, such as during exercise or if eating is delayed. Hypoglycemia can cause headache, dizziness, hunger, shaking, sweating, weakness, and agitation.

Uncontrolled type 1 diabetes can lead to a life-threatening complication called diabetic ketoacidosis. Without insulin, cells cannot

---

Text in this chapter is excerpted from "Type 1 Diabetes," Genetics Home Reference, National Institutes of Health (NIH), October 5, 2015; and text from "Your Guide to Diabetes: Type 1 and Type 2," National Institute of Diabetes and Kidney Diseases (NIDDK), National Institutes of Health (NIH), February 12, 2014.

take in glucose. A lack of glucose in cells prompts the liver to try to compensate by releasing more glucose into the blood, and blood sugar can become extremely high. The cells, unable to use the glucose in the blood for energy, respond by using fats instead. Breaking down fats to obtain energy produces waste products called ketones, which can build up to toxic levels in people with type 1 diabetes, resulting in diabetic ketoacidosis. Affected individuals may begin breathing rapidly; develop a fruity odor in the breath; and experience nausea, vomiting, facial flushing, stomach pain, and dryness of the mouth (xerostomia). In severe cases, diabetic ketoacidosis can lead to coma and death.

Over many years, the chronic high blood sugar associated with diabetes may cause damage to blood vessels and nerves, leading to complications affecting many organs and tissues. The retina, which is the light-sensitive tissue at the back of the eye, can be damaged (diabetic retinopathy), leading to vision loss and eventual blindness. Kidney damage (diabetic nephropathy) may also occur and can lead to kidney failure and end-stage renal disease (ESRD). Pain, tingling, and loss of normal sensation (diabetic neuropathy) often occur, especially in the feet. Impaired circulation and absence of the normal sensations that prompt reaction to injury can result in permanent damage to the feet; in severe cases, the damage can lead to amputation. People with type 1 diabetes are also at increased risk of heart attacks, strokes, and problems with urinary and sexual function.

How common is type 1 diabetes?

Type 1 diabetes occurs in 10 to 20 per 100,000 people per year in the U.S. By age 18, approximately 1 in 300 people in the U.S. develop type 1 diabetes. The disorder occurs with similar frequencies in Europe, the United Kingdom, Canada, and New Zealand. Type 1 diabetes occurs much less frequently in Asia and South America, with reported incidences as low as 1 in 1 million per year. For unknown reasons, during the past 20 years the worldwide incidence of type 1 diabetes has been increasing by 2 to 5 percent each year.

Type 1 diabetes accounts for 5 to 10 percent of cases of diabetes worldwide. Most people with diabetes have type 2 diabetes, in which the body continues to produce insulin but becomes less able to use it.

What genes are related to type 1 diabetes?

The causes of type 1 diabetes are unknown, although several risk factors have been identified. The risk of developing type 1 diabetes

Type 1 Diabetes

is increased by certain variants of the *HLA-DQA1*, *HLA-DQB1*, and *HLA-DRB1* genes. These genes provide instructions for making proteins that play a critical role in the immune system. The *HLA-DQA1*, *HLA-DQB1*, and *HLA-DRB1* genes belong to a family of genes called the human leukocyte antigen (HLA) complex. The HLA complex helps the immune system distinguish the body's own proteins from proteins made by foreign invaders such as viruses and bacteria.

Type 1 diabetes is generally considered to be an autoimmune disorder. Autoimmune disorders occur when the immune system attacks the body's own tissues and organs. For unknown reasons, in people with type 1 diabetes the immune system damages the insulin-producing beta cells in the pancreas. Damage to these cells impairs insulin production and leads to the signs and symptoms of type 1 diabetes.

HLA genes, including *HLA-DQA1*, *HLA-DQB1*, and *HLA-DRB1*, have many variations, and individuals have a certain combination of these variations, called a haplotype. Certain HLA haplotypes are associated with a higher risk of developing type 1 diabetes, with particular combinations of *HLA-DQA1*, *HLA-DQB1*, and *HLA-DRB1* gene variations resulting in the highest risk. These haplotypes seem to increase the risk of an inappropriate immune response to beta cells. However, these variants are also found in the general population, and only about 5 percent of individuals with the gene variants develop type 1 diabetes. HLA variations account for approximately 40 percent of the genetic risk for the condition.

Other HLA variations appear to be protective against the disease. Additional contributors, such as environmental factors and variations in other genes, are also thought to influence the development of this complex disorder.

How do people inherit type 1 diabetes?

A predisposition to develop type 1 diabetes is passed through generations in families, but the inheritance pattern is unknown.

What other names do people use for type 1 diabetes?

- Autoimmune diabetes
- Diabetes mellitus, insulin-dependent
- Diabetes mellitus type 1
- Diabetes mellitus, type 1

- Insulin-dependent diabetes mellitus
- Juvenile diabetes
- Juvenile-onset diabetes
- Juvenile-onset diabetes mellitus
- T1D
- Type 1 diabetes mellitus

Treatment for type 1 diabetes includes:

- Taking shots, also called injections, of insulin
- Sometimes taking medicines by mouth
- Making healthy food choices
- Being physically active
- Controlling your blood pressure levels. Blood pressure is the force of blood flow inside your blood vessels
- Controlling your cholesterol levels. Cholesterol is a type of fat in your body's cells, in your blood, and in many foods

Chapter 3

Prediabetes

What is prediabetes?

Prediabetes means the amount of glucose, also called sugar, in your blood is higher than normal but not high enough to be called diabetes. Glucose is a form of sugar your body uses for energy. Too much glucose in your blood can damage your body over time. If you have prediabetes, also called impaired fasting glucose (IFG) or impaired glucose tolerance (IGT), you are more likely to develop type 2 diabetes, heart disease, and stroke.

Who should be tested for prediabetes?

If you are 45 years old or older, your doctor may recommend that you be tested for prediabetes, especially if you are overweight. Being overweight is a key contributor, along with inactivity, to prediabetes. If your body mass index (BMI) is higher than 25, you are overweight. BMI is a measure of your weight relative to your height. If you're not sure if you are overweight, ask your doctor.

Even if you are younger than 45, consider getting tested for prediabetes if you are overweight and:

- are physically inactive
- have a parent, brother, or sister with diabetes

Text in this chapter is excerpted from "Prediabetes What You Need to Know," National Diabetes Information Clearinghouse (NDIC), July 2012; and text from "Diabetes," National Institute on Aging (NIA), National Institutes of Health (NIH), August 2014.

- have high blood pressure or high cholesterol-blood fat
- have abnormal levels of high-density lipoprotein (HDL), or good, cholesterol or triglycerides—another type of blood fat
- had gestational diabetes—diabetes that develops only during pregnancy—or gave birth to a baby weighing more than 9 pounds
- are African American, Alaska Native, American Indian, Asian American, Hispanic/Latino, or Pacific Islander American
- have polycystic ovary syndrome, also called PCOS
- have a dark, velvety rash around your neck or armpits
- have blood vessel problems affecting your heart, brain, or legs.

If your test results are normal, you should be retested in 3 years. If you have prediabetes, ask your doctor if you should be tested again in 1 year.

How do I know if I have prediabetes?

Most people with prediabetes don't have any symptoms. Your doctor can test your blood to find out if your blood glucose levels are higher than normal.

Prediabetes : Am I at risk?

1 in 3 U.S. adults has prediabetes. Most don't know it. Are you at risk?

You may have prediabetes and be at risk for type 2 diabetes if you:

- Are 45 years of age or older
- Are overweight
- Have a family history of type 2 diabetes
- Have high blood pressure
- Are physically active fewer than three times per week
- Ever had diabetes while pregnant (gestational diabetes) or gave birth to a baby that weighed more than 9 pounds

Prediabetes

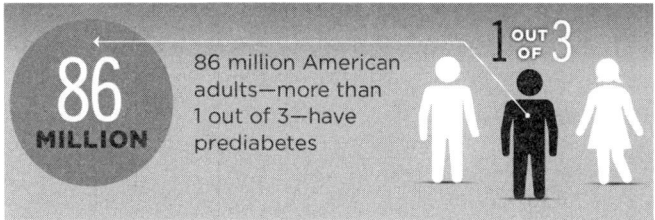

Figure 3.1. *Prediabetes ratio among the U.S. Adults*

Prediabetes can lead to serious health problems

If you have prediabetes and don't lose weight or increase your physical activity, you could develop type 2 diabetes within five years.

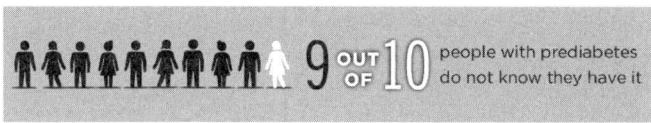

Figure 3.2. *Knowledge about prediabetes among U.S. Adults*

Type 2 diabetes is a serious condition that can lead to health issues such as:

- Heart attack,
- Stroke, blindness,
- Kidney failure,
- loss of toes, feet or legs.

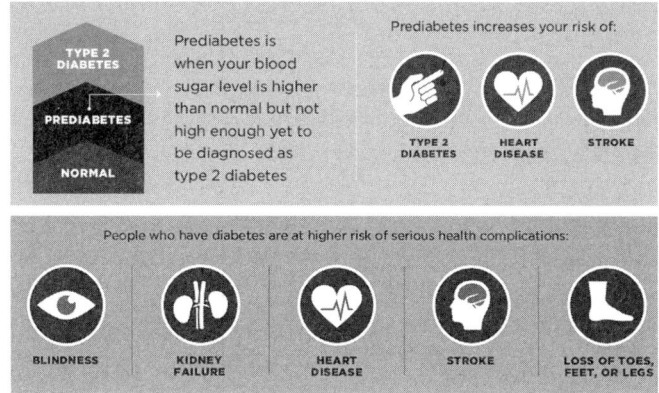

Figure 3.3. *Risks of Prediabetes*

Chapter 4

Insulin Resistance

What is insulin resistance?

Insulin resistance is a condition in which the body produces insulin but does not use it effectively. When people have insulin resistance, glucose builds up in the blood instead of being absorbed by the cells, leading to type 2 diabetes or prediabetes.

Most people with insulin resistance don't know they have it for many years—until they develop type 2 diabetes, a serious, lifelong disease. The good news is that if people learn they have insulin resistance early on, they can often prevent or delay diabetes by making changes to their lifestyle.

Insulin resistance can lead to a variety of serious health disorders.

What happens with insulin resistance?

In insulin resistance, muscle, fat, and liver cells do not respond properly to insulin and thus cannot easily absorb glucose from the bloodstream. As a result, the body needs higher levels of insulin to help glucose enter cells.

The beta cells in the pancreas try to keep up with this increased demand for insulin by producing more. As long as the beta cells are

---

Text in this chapter is excerpted from "Insulin Resistance and Prediabetes," National Institute of Diabetes and Digestive and Kidney Diseases (NIDDK), National Institutes of Health (NIH), June 2014.

able to produce enough insulin to overcome the insulin resistance, blood glucose levels stay in the healthy range.

Over time, insulin resistance can lead to type 2 diabetes and prediabetes because the beta cells fail to keep up with the body's increased need for insulin. Without enough insulin, excess glucose builds up in the bloodstream, leading to diabetes, prediabetes, and other serious health disorders.

What causes insulin resistance?

Although the exact causes of insulin resistance are not completely understood, scientists think the major contributors to insulin resistance are excess weight and physical inactivity.

Other Causes

Other causes of insulin resistance may include ethnicity; certain diseases; hormones; steroid use; some medications; older age; sleep problems, especially sleep apnea; and cigarette smoking.

Does sleep matter?

Yes. Studies show that untreated sleep problems, especially sleep apnea, can increase the risk of obesity, insulin resistance, and type 2 diabetes. Night shift workers may also be at increased risk for these problems. Sleep apnea is a common disorder in which a person's breathing is interrupted during sleep. People may often move out of deep sleep and into light sleep when their breathing pauses or becomes shallow. This results in poor sleep quality that causes problem sleepiness, or excessive tiredness, during the day.

Many people aren't aware of their symptoms and aren't diagnosed. People who think they might have sleep problems should talk with their health care provider.

How does insulin resistance relate to type 2 diabetes and prediabetes?

Insulin resistance increases the risk of developing type 2 diabetes and prediabetes. Prediabetes usually occurs in people who already have insulin resistance. Although insulin resistance alone does not cause type 2 diabetes, it often sets the stage for the disease by placing a high demand on the insulin-producing beta cells. In prediabetes, the

Insulin Resistance

beta cells can no longer produce enough insulin to overcome insulin resistance, causing blood glucose levels to rise above the normal range.

Once a person has prediabetes, continued loss of beta cell function usually leads to type 2 diabetes. People with type 2 diabetes have high blood glucose. Over time, high blood glucose damages nerves and blood vessels, leading to complications such as heart disease, stroke, blindness, kidney failure, and lower-limb amputations.

Studies have shown that most people with prediabetes develop type 2 diabetes within 10 years, unless they change their lifestyle. Lifestyle changes include losing 5 to 7 percent of their body weight—10 to 14 pounds for people who weigh 200 pounds—by making changes in their diet and level of physical activity.

What are the symptoms of insulin resistance and prediabetes?

Insulin resistance and prediabetes usually have no symptoms. People may have one or both conditions for several years without knowing they have them. Even without symptoms, health care providers can identify people at high risk by their physical characteristics, also known as risk factors.

People with a severe form of insulin resistance may have dark patches of skin, usually on the back of the neck. Sometimes people have a dark ring around their neck. Dark patches may also appear on elbows, knees, knuckles, and armpits. This condition is called acanthosis nigricans.

What is metabolic syndrome?

Metabolic syndrome, also called insulin resistance syndrome, is a group of traits and medical conditions linked to overweight and obesity that puts people at risk for both CVD and type 2 diabetes. Metabolic syndrome is defined as the presence of any three of the following:

- Large waist size—waist measurement of 40 inches or more for men and 35 inches or more for women

- High triglycerides in the blood—triglyceride level of 150 milligrams per deciliter (mg/dL) or above, or taking medication for elevated triglyceride level

- Abnormal levels of cholesterol in the blood—HDL, or good, cholesterol level below 40 mg/dL for men and below 50 mg/dL for women, or taking medication for low HDL

- High blood pressure—blood pressure level of 130/85 or above, or taking medication for elevated blood pressure
- Higher than normal blood glucose levels—fasting blood glucose level of 100 mg/dL or above, or taking medication for elevated blood glucose

In addition to type 2 diabetes, metabolic syndrome has been linked to the following health disorders:

- Obesity
- CVD
- PCOS
- Nonalcoholic fatty liver disease
- Chronic kidney disease

However, not everyone with these disorders has insulin resistance, and some people may have insulin resistance without getting these disorders.

People who are obese or who have metabolic syndrome, insulin resistance, type 2 diabetes, or prediabetes often also have low-level inflammation throughout the body and blood clotting defects that increase the risk of developing blood clots in the arteries. These conditions contribute to increased risk for CVD.

How are insulin resistance and prediabetes diagnosed?

Health care providers use blood tests to determine whether a person has prediabetes, but they do not usually test specifically for insulin resistance. Insulin resistance can be assessed by measuring the level of insulin in the blood.

However, the test that most accurately measures insulin resistance, called the euglycemic clamp, is too costly and complicated to be used in most health care providers' offices. The clamp is a research tool used by scientists to learn more about glucose metabolism. Research has shown that if blood tests indicate prediabetes, insulin resistance most likely is present.

Blood Tests for Prediabetes

All blood tests involve drawing blood at a health care provider's office or commercial facility and sending the sample to a lab for analysis. Lab analysis of blood is needed to ensure test results are accurate.

Insulin Resistance

Glucose measuring devices used in a health care provider's office, such as finger-stick devices, are not accurate enough for diagnosis but may be used as a quick indicator of high blood glucose.

Prediabetes can be detected with one of the following blood tests:
- the A1C test
- the fasting plasma glucose (FPG) test
- the oral glucose tolerance test (OGTT)

Understanding Test Results

A blood test indicating prediabetes means that insulin resistance has progressed to the point where the beta cells in the pancreas can no longer compensate and a person's blood glucose levels are rising toward type 2 diabetes. The higher the test results, the greater the risk of type 2 diabetes. The level of risk also depends on an individual's other risk factors.

Test numbers

For example, people with an A1C below 5.7 percent may still be at risk for diabetes if they have a family history of type 2 diabetes or have gained excess weight around the waist. People with an A1C above 6.0 percent should be considered at very high risk of developing diabetes. A level of 6.5 percent or above means a person has diabetes.

Follow up

People whose test results indicate they have prediabetes may be retested in 1 year and should consider making lifestyle changes to reduce their risk of developing type 2 diabetes.

Varying results

Although all these tests can be used to test for prediabetes, in some people one test will indicate a diagnosis of prediabetes or diabetes when another test does not. People with differing test results may be in an early stage of the disease, where blood glucose levels have not risen high enough to show on every test.

Health care providers repeat laboratory tests to confirm test results. Diabetes develops over time, so even with variations in test results, health care providers can tell when overall blood glucose levels are becoming too high.

Can insulin resistance and prediabetes be reversed?

Yes. Physical activity and weight loss help the body respond better to insulin. The Diabetes Prevention Program (DPP) was a federally funded study of 3,234 people at high risk for diabetes.

The DPP and other large studies proved that people with prediabetes can often prevent or delay diabetes if they lose a modest amount of weight by cutting fat and calorie intake and increasing physical activity—for example, walking 30 minutes a day, 5 days a week.

People at High Risk for Diabetes

DPP study participants were overweight and had prediabetes. Many had family members with type 2 diabetes. Prediabetes, obesity, and a family history of diabetes are strong risk factors for type 2 diabetes. About half of the DPP participants were from minority groups with high rates of diabetes, including African Americans, Alaska Natives, American Indians, Asian Americans, Hispanics/Latinos, and Pacific Islander Americans.

DPP participants also included others at high risk for developing type 2 diabetes, such as women with a history of gestational diabetes and people ages 60 and older.

Approaches to Preventing Diabetes

The DPP tested three approaches to preventing diabetes:

- **Making lifestyle changes**. People in the lifestyle change group exercised, usually by walking 5 days a week for about 30 minutes a day, and lowered their intake of fat and calories.
- **Taking the diabetes medication metformin**. Those who took metformin also received information about physical activity and diet.
- **Receiving education about diabetes**. The third group only received information about physical activity and diet and took a placebo—a pill without medication in it.

People in the lifestyle change group showed the best outcomes. However people who took metformin also benefited. The results showed that by losing an average of 15 pounds in the first year of the study, people in the lifestyle change group reduced their risk of developing type 2 diabetes by 58 percent over 3 years.

Lifestyle change was even more effective in those ages 60 and older. People in this group reduced their risk by 71 percent.

People in the metformin group also benefited, reducing their risk by 31 percent.

Lasting Results

The Diabetes Prevention Program Outcomes Study (DPPOS) has shown that the benefits of weight loss and metformin last for at least 10 years. The DPPOS has continued to follow most DPP participants since the DPP ended in 2001. The DPPOS showed that 10 years after enrolling in the DPP:

- People in the lifestyle change group reduced their risk for developing diabetes by 34 percent
- Those in the lifestyle change group ages 60 or older had even greater benefit, reducing their risk of developing diabetes by 49 percent
- Participants in the lifestyle change group also had fewer heart and blood vessel disease risk factors, including lower blood pressure and triglyceride levels, even though they took fewer medications to control their heart disease risk
- Those in the metformin group reduced their risk of developing diabetes by 18 percent

Even though controlling weight with lifestyle changes is challenging, it produces long-term health rewards by lowering the risk for type 2 diabetes, lowering blood glucose levels, and reducing other heart disease risk factors.

What steps can help reverse insulin resistance and prediabetes?

By losing weight and being more physically active, people can reverse insulin resistance and prediabetes, thus preventing or delaying type 2 diabetes. People can decrease their risk by:

- eating a healthy diet and reaching and maintaining a healthy weight
- increasing physical activity
- not smoking
- taking medication

Eating, Diet, and Nutrition

Adopting healthy eating habits can help people lose a modest amount of weight and reverse insulin resistance. Experts encourage people to slowly adopt healthy eating habits that they can maintain, rather than trying extreme weight-loss solutions. People may need to get help from a dietitian or join a weight-loss program for support.

In general, people should lose weight by choosing healthy foods, controlling portions, eating less fat, and increasing physical activity. People are better able to lose weight and keep it off when they learn how to adapt their favorite foods to a healthy eating plan.

The DASH (Dietary Approaches to Stop Hypertension) eating plan, developed by the NIH, has been shown to be effective in decreasing insulin resistance when combined with weight loss and physical activity.

Dietary Supplements

Vitamin D studies show a link between people's ability to maintain healthy blood glucose levels and having enough vitamin D in their blood. However, studies to determine the proper vitamin D levels for preventing diabetes are ongoing; no special recommendations have been made about vitamin D levels or supplements for people with prediabetes.

Currently, the Institute of Medicine (IOM), the agency that recommends supplementation levels based on current science, provides the following guidelines for daily vitamin D intake:

- People ages 1 to 70 years may require 600 International Units (IUs).
- People ages 71 and older may require as much as 800 IUs.

The IOM also recommended that no more than 4,000 IUs of vitamin D be taken per day.

To help ensure coordinated and safe care, people should discuss use of complementary and alternative medicine practices, including the use of dietary supplements, with their health care provider.

Physical Activity

Regular physical activity tackles several risk factors at once. Regular physical activity helps the body use insulin properly.

Regular physical activity also helps a person:

- lose weight
- control blood glucose levels

Insulin Resistance

- control blood pressure
- control cholesterol levels

People in the DPP who were physically active for 30 minutes a day, 5 days a week, reduced their risk of type 2 diabetes. Many chose brisk walking as their physical activity.

Most people should aim for at least 30 minutes of exercise most days of the week. For best results, people should do both aerobic activities, which use large muscle groups and make the heart beat faster, and muscle strengthening activities.

Aerobic activities include brisk walking, climbing stairs, swimming, dancing, and other activities that increase the heart rate.

Muscle strengthening activities include lifting weights and doing sit-ups or push-ups.

People who haven't been physically active recently should talk with their health care provider about which activities are best for them and have a checkup before starting an exercise program.

Not Smoking

Those who smoke should quit. A health care provider can help people find ways to quit smoking. Studies show that people who get help have a better chance of quitting.

Medication

The medication metformin is recommended for treatment of some individuals at very high risk of developing type 2 diabetes. In the DPP, metformin was shown to be most effective in preventing or delaying the development of type 2 diabetes in younger, heavier people with prediabetes. In general, metformin is recommend for those who are younger than age 60 and have:

- combined IGT and IFG
- A1C above 6 percent
- low HDL cholesterol
- elevated triglycerides
- a parent or sibling with diabetes
- a BMI of at least 35

Metformin also lowers the risk of diabetes in women who have had gestational diabetes. People at high risk should ask their health care provider if they should take metformin to prevent type 2 diabetes.

Several medications have been shown to reduce type 2 diabetes risk to varying degrees, but the only medication recommended by the ADA for type 2 diabetes prevention is metformin. Other medications that have delayed diabetes have side effects or haven't shown long-lasting benefits. No medication, including metformin, is approved by the U.S. Food and Drug Administration to treat insulin resistance or prediabetes or to prevent type 2 diabetes.

Chapter 5

Type 2 Diabetes

What is type 2 diabetes?

Type 2 diabetes is the most common type of diabetes. Type 2 diabetes occurs because the body doesn't use the hormone insulin properly. Insulin helps your body absorb glucose and use it for energy. If your body doesn't make enough insulin or doesn't use insulin properly, you have a condition called insulin resistance. Insulin resistance requires the body to produce higher levels of insulin. Over time, the body cannot keep up with the demand for extra insulin and type 2 diabetes develops.

You are more likely to get type 2 diabetes if you:

- are age 45 or older
- are overweight
- are physically inactive
- have a parent, brother, or sister with diabetes
- have high blood pressure or high cholesterol—blood fat
- have abnormal levels of HDL, or good, cholesterol or triglycerides—another type of blood fat

---

Text in this chapter is excerpted from "Type 2 Diabetes – What You Need to Know," National Diabetes Information Clearinghouse (NDIC), July 2012; and text from "Your Guide to Diabetes: Type 1 and Type 2," National Institute of Diabetes and Kidney Diseases (NIDDK), National Institutes of Health (NIH), February 12, 2014.

- had gestational diabetes—diabetes that develops only during pregnancy—or gave birth to a baby weighing more than 9 pounds
- have prediabetes—meaning your blood glucose levels are higher than normal but not high enough to be called diabetes
- are African American, Alaska Native, American Indian, Asian American, Hispanic/Latino, or Pacific Islander American
- have polycystic ovary syndrome, also called PCOS
- have a dark, velvety rash around your neck or armpits
- have blood vessel problems affecting your heart, brain, or legs

Type 2 diabetes usually begins with insulin resistance—a condition that occurs when fat, muscle, and liver cells do not use insulin to carry glucose into the body's cells to use for energy. As a result, the body needs more insulin to help glucose enter cells. At first, the pancreas keeps up with the added demand by making more insulin. Over time, the pancreas doesn't make enough insulin when blood sugar levels increase, such as after meals. If your pancreas can no longer make enough insulin, you will need to treat your type 2 diabetes.

Treatment for type 2 diabetes includes:

- using diabetes medicines
- making healthy food choices
- being physically active
- controlling your blood pressure levels
- controlling your cholesterol levels

Chapter 6

Gestational Diabetes

What is gestational diabetes?

Gestational diabetes is a type of diabetes that develops only during pregnancy. Diabetes means your blood glucose, also called blood sugar, is too high. Your body uses glucose for energy. Too much glucose in your blood is not good for you or your baby.

Gestational diabetes is usually diagnosed during late pregnancy. If you are diagnosed with diabetes earlier in your pregnancy, you may have had diabetes before you became pregnant.

Treating gestational diabetes can help both you and your baby stay healthy. You can protect your baby and yourself by taking action right away to control your blood glucose levels.

If you have gestational diabetes, a health care team will likely be part of your care. In addition to your obstetrician-gynecologist, or OB/GYN—the doctor who will deliver your baby—your team might include a doctor who treats diabetes, a diabetes educator, and a dietitian to help you plan meals.

You will probably be tested for gestational diabetes between weeks 24 and 28 of your pregnancy.

If you have a higher chance of getting gestational diabetes, your doctor may test for diabetes during the first visit after you become

---

Text in this chapter is excerpted from "What I Need to Know about Gestational Diabetes," National Institute of Diabetes and Kidney Diseases (NIDDK), National Institutes of Health (NIH), August 2013.

pregnant. If your blood glucose level is above normal at that time, you may be diagnosed with diabetes rather than gestational diabetes.

> **What are my chances of getting gestational diabetes?**
>
> Your chances of getting gestational diabetes are higher if you
> - are overweight
> - have had gestational diabetes before
> - have given birth to a baby weighing more than 9 pounds
> - have a parent, brother, or sister with type 2 diabetes
> - have prediabetes, meaning your blood glucose levels are higher than normal yet not high enough for a diagnosis of diabetes
> - are African American, American Indian, Asian American, Hispanic/Latina, or Pacific Islander American have a hormonal disorder called polycystic ovary syndrome, also known as PCOS

When will I be tested for gestational diabetes?

You will probably be tested for gestational diabetes between weeks 24 and 28 of your pregnancy.

If you have a higher chance of getting gestational diabetes, your doctor may test for diabetes during the first visit after you become pregnant. If your blood glucose level is above normal at that time, you may be diagnosed with diabetes rather than gestational diabetes.

How will gestational diabetes affect my baby?

If you have high blood glucose levels because your gestational diabetes is not under control, your baby will also have high blood glucose. Your baby's pancreas will have to make extra insulin to control the high blood glucose. The extra glucose in your baby's blood is stored as fat.

Untreated or uncontrolled gestational diabetes can cause problems for your baby, such as:

- being born with a larger than normal body—a condition called macrosomia—which can make delivery difficult and more dangerous for your baby

- having low blood glucose, also called hypoglycemia, right after birth
- having breathing problems, a condition called respiratory distress syndrome
- having a higher chance of dying before or soon after birth

Your baby also might be born with jaundice. Jaundice is more common in newborns of mothers who had diabetes during their pregnancy. With jaundice, the skin and whites of the eyes turn yellow. Jaundice usually goes away, but your baby may need to be placed under special lights to help. Making sure your baby gets plenty of milk from breastfeeding will also help the jaundice go away.

Your baby will be more likely to become overweight and develop type 2 diabetes as he or she grows up.

How will gestational diabetes affect me?

Gestational diabetes may increase your chances of:

- having high blood pressure and too much protein in the urine, a condition called preeclampsia
- having surgery—called a cesarean section or c-section—to deliver your baby because your baby may be large
- becoming depressed
- developing type 2 diabetes and the problems that can come with this disease

Preeclampsia

Preeclampsia occurs during the second half of pregnancy. If not treated, preeclampsia can cause problems for you and your baby that could cause death. The only cure for preeclampsia is to give birth. If you develop preeclampsia late in your pregnancy, you may need to have a cesarean section to deliver your baby early. If you develop preeclampsia earlier, you may need bed rest and medicines, or you may have to be hospitalized to allow your baby to develop as much as possible before delivery.

Depression

Depression can make you too tired to manage your diabetes and care for your baby. If during or after your pregnancy you feel anxious, sad, or unable to cope with the changes you are facing, talk with your health care team. Depression can be treated. Your health care team may suggest ways you can get support and help to feel better. Remember, in order to take care of your baby, you must first take care of yourself.

Checkups

Keep up with your checkups. "Feeling fine" does not mean you should skip any appointments. Women with gestational diabetes often have no symptoms. Your health care team will be on the lookout for any problems from gestational diabetes.

After Giving Birth

Your diabetes will probably go away after your baby is born. However, even if your diabetes goes away after the birth, you:

- may have gestational diabetes if you get pregnant again
- will be more likely to have type 2 diabetes later in your life

Chapter 7

Causes of Diabetes

What causes Type 1 diabetes?

Type 1 diabetes is caused by a lack of insulin due to the destruction of insulin-producing beta cells in the pancreas. In type 1 diabetes—an autoimmune disease—the body's immune system attacks and destroys the beta cells. Normally, the immune system protects the body from infection by identifying and destroying bacteria, viruses, and other potentially harmful foreign substances. But in autoimmune diseases, the immune system attacks the body's own cells. In type 1 diabetes, beta cell destruction may take place over several years, but symptoms of the disease usually develop over a short period of time.

Type 1 diabetes typically occurs in children and young adults, though it can appear at any age. In the past, type 1 diabetes was called juvenile diabetes or insulin-dependent diabetes mellitus.

Latent autoimmune diabetes in adults (LADA) may be a slowly developing kind of type 1 diabetes. Diagnosis usually occurs after age 30. In LADA, as in type 1 diabetes, the body's immune system destroys the beta cells. At the time of diagnosis, people with LADA may still produce their own insulin, but eventually most will need insulin shots or an insulin pump to control blood glucose levels.

Text in this chapter is excerpted from "Causes of Diabetes," National Institute of Diabetes and Digestive and Kidney Diseases (NIDDK), National Institutes of Health (NIH), June 2014.

Genetic Susceptibility

Heredity plays an important part in determining who is likely to develop type 1 diabetes. Genes are passed down from biological parent to child. Genes carry instructions for making proteins that are needed for the body's cells to function. Many genes, as well as interactions among genes, are thought to influence susceptibility to and protection from type 1 diabetes. The key genes may vary in different population groups. Variations in genes that affect more than 1 percent of a population group are called gene variants.

Certain gene variants that carry instructions for making proteins called human leukocyte antigens (HLAs) on white blood cells are linked to the risk of developing type 1 diabetes. The proteins produced by HLA genes help determine whether the immune system recognizes a cell as part of the body or as foreign material. Some combinations of HLA gene variants predict that a person will be at higher risk for type 1 diabetes, while other combinations are protective or have no effect on risk.

While HLA genes are the major risk genes for type 1 diabetes, many additional risk genes or gene regions have been found. Not only can these genes help identify people at risk for type 1 diabetes, but they also provide important clues to help scientists better understand how the disease develops and identify potential targets for therapy and prevention.

Genetic testing can show what types of HLA genes a person carries and can reveal other genes linked to diabetes. However, most genetic testing is done in a research setting and is not yet available to individuals. Scientists are studying how the results of genetic testing can be used to improve type 1 diabetes prevention or treatment.

Autoimmune Destruction of Beta Cells

In type 1 diabetes, white blood cells called T cells attack and destroy beta cells. The process begins well before diabetes symptoms appear and continues after diagnosis. Often, type 1 diabetes is not diagnosed until most beta cells have already been destroyed. At this point, a person needs daily insulin treatment to survive. Finding ways to modify or stop this autoimmune process and preserve beta cell function is a major focus of current scientific research.

Recent research suggests insulin itself may be a key trigger of the immune attack on beta cells. The immune systems of people who are susceptible to developing type 1 diabetes respond to insulin as if it were a foreign substance, or antigen. To combat antigens, the body makes proteins called antibodies. Antibodies to insulin and other proteins produced by beta cells are found in people with type 1 diabetes. Researchers test for these antibodies to help identify people at increased risk of developing the disease. Testing the types and levels of antibodies in the blood can help determine whether a person has type 1 diabetes, LADA, or another type of diabetes.

Environmental Factors

Environmental factors, such as foods, viruses, and toxins, may play a role in the development of type 1 diabetes, but the exact nature of their role has not been determined. Some theories suggest that environmental factors trigger the autoimmune destruction of beta cells in people with a genetic susceptibility to diabetes. Other theories suggest that environmental factors play an ongoing role in diabetes, even after diagnosis.

Viruses and infections. A virus cannot cause diabetes on its own, but people are sometimes diagnosed with type 1 diabetes during or after a viral infection, suggesting a link between the two. Also, the onset of type 1 diabetes occurs more frequently during the winter when viral infections are more common.

Viruses possibly associated with type 1 diabetes include coxsackievirus B, cytomegalovirus, adenovirus, rubella, and mumps. Scientists have described several ways these viruses may damage or destroy beta cells or possibly trigger an autoimmune response in susceptible people. For example, anti-islet antibodies have been found in patients with congenital rubella syndrome, and cytomegalovirus has been associated with significant beta cell damage and acute pancreatitis—inflammation of the pancreas. Scientists are trying to identify a virus that can cause type 1 diabetes so that a vaccine might be developed to prevent the disease.

Infant feeding practices. Some studies have suggested that dietary factors may raise or lower the risk of developing type 1 diabetes. For example, breastfed infants and infants receiving vitamin D supplements may have a reduced risk of developing type 1 diabetes, while early exposure to cow's milk and cereal proteins may increase risk. More research is needed to clarify how infant nutrition affects the risk for type 1 diabetes.

What causes Type 2 diabetes?

Type 2 diabetes—the most common form of diabetes—is caused by a combination of factors, including insulin resistance, a condition in which the body's muscle, fat, and liver cells do not use insulin effectively. Type 2 diabetes develops when the body can no longer produce enough insulin to compensate for the impaired ability to use insulin. Symptoms of type 2 diabetes may develop gradually and can be subtle; some people with type 2 diabetes remain undiagnosed for years.

Type 2 diabetes develops most often in middle-aged and older people who are also overweight or obese. The disease, once rare in youth, is becoming more common in overweight and obese children and adolescents. Scientists think genetic susceptibility and environmental factors are the most likely triggers of type 2 diabetes.

Genetic Susceptibility

Genes play a significant part in susceptibility to type 2 diabetes. Having certain genes or combinations of genes may increase or decrease a person's risk for developing the disease. The role of genes is suggested by the high rate of type 2 diabetes in families and identical twins and wide variations in diabetes prevalence by ethnicity. Type 2 diabetes occurs more frequently in African Americans, Alaska Natives, American Indians, Hispanics/Latinos, and some Asian Americans, Native Hawaiians, and Pacific Islander Americans than it does in non-Hispanic whites.

Recent studies have combined genetic data from large numbers of people, accelerating the pace of gene discovery. Though scientists have now identified many gene variants that increase susceptibility to type 2 diabetes, the majority have yet to be discovered. The known genes appear to affect insulin production rather than insulin resistance. Researchers are working to identify additional gene variants and to learn how they interact with one another and with environmental factors to cause diabetes.

Studies have shown that variants of the *TCF7L2* gene increase susceptibility to type 2 diabetes. For people who inherit two copies of the variants, the risk of developing type 2 diabetes is about 80 percent higher than for those who do not carry the gene variant. However, even in those with the variant, diet and physical activity leading to weight loss help delay diabetes, according to the Diabetes Prevention Program (DPP), a major clinical trial involving people at high risk.

Genes can also increase the risk of diabetes by increasing a person's tendency to become overweight or obese. One theory, known

Causes of Diabetes

as the "thrifty gene" hypothesis, suggests certain genes increase the efficiency of metabolism to extract energy from food and store the energy for later use. This survival trait was advantageous for populations whose food supplies were scarce or unpredictable and could help keep people alive during famine. In modern times, however, when high-calorie foods are plentiful, such a trait can promote obesity and type 2 diabetes.

Obesity and Physical Inactivity

Physical inactivity and obesity are strongly associated with the development of type 2 diabetes. People who are genetically susceptible to type 2 diabetes are more vulnerable when these risk factors are present.

An imbalance between caloric intake and physical activity can lead to obesity, which causes insulin resistance and is common in people with type 2 diabetes. Central obesity, in which a person has excess abdominal fat, is a major risk factor not only for insulin resistance and type 2 diabetes but also for heart and blood vessel disease, also called cardiovascular disease (CVD). This excess "belly fat" produces hormones and other substances that can cause harmful, chronic effects in the body such as damage to blood vessels.

The DPP and other studies show that millions of people can lower their risk for type 2 diabetes by making lifestyle changes and losing weight. The DPP proved that people with prediabetes—at high risk of developing type 2 diabetes—could sharply lower their risk by losing weight through regular physical activity and a diet low in fat and calories. In 2009, a follow-up study of DPP participants—the Diabetes Prevention Program Outcomes Study (DPPOS)—showed that the benefits of weight loss lasted for at least 10 years after the original study began.

Insulin Resistance

Insulin resistance is a common condition in people who are overweight or obese, have excess abdominal fat, and are not physically active. Muscle, fat, and liver cells stop responding properly to insulin, forcing the pancreas to compensate by producing extra insulin. As long as beta cells are able to produce enough insulin, blood glucose levels stay in the normal range. But when insulin production falters because of beta cell dysfunction, glucose levels rise, leading to prediabetes or diabetes.

Abnormal Glucose Production by the Liver

In some people with diabetes, an abnormal increase in glucose production by the liver also contributes to high blood glucose levels. Normally, the pancreas releases the hormone glucagon when blood glucose and insulin levels are low. Glucagon stimulates the liver to produce glucose and release it into the bloodstream. But when blood glucose and insulin levels are high after a meal, glucagon levels drop, and the liver stores excess glucose for later, when it is needed. For reasons not completely understood, in many people with diabetes, glucagon levels stay higher than needed. High glucagon levels cause the liver to produce unneeded glucose, which contributes to high blood glucose levels. Metformin, the most commonly used drug to treat type 2 diabetes, reduces glucose production by the liver.

The Roles of Insulin and Glucagon in Normal Blood Glucose Regulation

A healthy person's body keeps blood glucose levels in a normal range through several complex mechanisms. Insulin and glucagon, two hormones made in the pancreas, help regulate blood glucose levels:

- Insulin, made by beta cells, lowers elevated blood glucose levels.
- Glucagon, made by alpha cells, raises low blood glucose levels.

When blood glucose levels rise after a meal, the pancreas releases insulin into the blood.

- Insulin helps muscle, fat, and liver cells absorb glucose from the bloodstream, lowering blood glucose levels.
- Insulin stimulates the liver and muscle tissue to store excess glucose. The stored form of glucose is called glycogen.
- Insulin also lowers blood glucose levels by reducing glucose production in the liver.

When blood glucose levels drop overnight or due to a skipped meal or heavy exercise, the pancreas releases glucagon into the blood.

- Glucagon signals the liver and muscle tissue to break down glycogen into glucose, which enters the bloodstream and raises blood glucose levels.
- If the body needs more glucose, glucagon stimulates the liver to make glucose from amino acids.

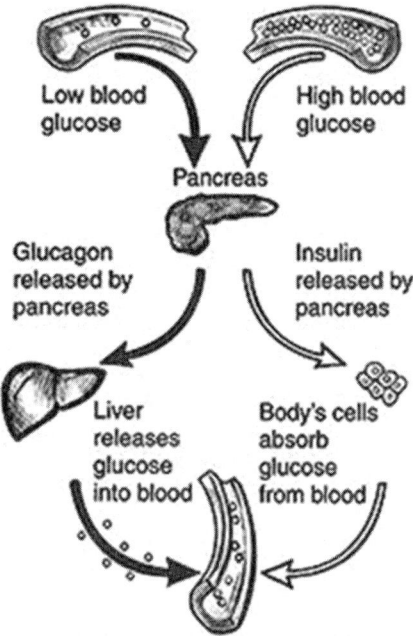

Figure 7.1. *Insulin and glucagon help regulate blood glucose levels.*

Metabolic Syndrome

Metabolic syndrome, also called insulin resistance syndrome, refers to a group of conditions common in people with insulin resistance, including:

- higher than normal blood glucose levels
- increased waist size due to excess abdominal fat
- high blood pressure
- abnormal levels of cholesterol and triglycerides in the blood

People with metabolic syndrome have an increased risk of developing type 2 diabetes and CVD. Many studies have found that lifestyle changes, such as being physically active and losing excess weight, are the best ways to reverse metabolic syndrome, improve the body's response to insulin, and reduce risk for type 2 diabetes and CVD.

Cell Signaling and Regulation

Cells communicate through a complex network of molecular signaling pathways. For example, on cell surfaces, insulin receptor molecules capture, or bind, insulin molecules circulating in the bloodstream. This interaction between insulin and its receptor prompts the biochemical signals that enable the cells to absorb glucose from the blood and use it for energy.

Problems in cell signaling systems can set off a chain reaction that leads to diabetes or other diseases. Many studies have focused on how insulin signals cells to communicate and regulate action. Researchers have identified proteins and pathways that transmit the insulin signal and have mapped interactions between insulin and body tissues, including the way insulin helps the liver control blood glucose levels. Researchers have also found that key signals also come from fat cells, which produce substances that cause inflammation and insulin resistance.

This work holds the key to combating insulin resistance and diabetes. As scientists learn more about cell signaling systems involved in glucose regulation, they will have more opportunities to develop effective treatments.

Beta Cell Dysfunction

Scientists think beta cell dysfunction is a key contributor to type 2 diabetes. Beta cell impairment can cause inadequate or abnormal patterns of insulin release. Also, beta cells may be damaged by high blood glucose itself, a condition called glucose toxicity.

Scientists have not determined the causes of beta cell dysfunction in most cases. Single gene defects lead to specific forms of diabetes called maturity-onset diabetes of the young (MODY). The genes involved regulate insulin production in the beta cells. Although these forms of diabetes are rare, they provide clues as to how beta cell function may be affected by key regulatory factors. Other gene variants are involved in determining the number and function of beta cells. But these variants account for only a small percentage of type 2 diabetes cases. Malnutrition early in life is also being investigated as a cause of beta cell dysfunction. The metabolic environment of the developing fetus may also create a predisposition for diabetes later in life.

Risk Factors for Type 2 Diabetes

People who develop type 2 diabetes are more likely to have the following characteristics:

- Age 45 or older
- Overweight or obese

Causes of Diabetes

- Physically inactive
- Parent or sibling with diabetes
- Family background that is african american, alaska native, american indian, asian american, hispanic/latino, or pacific islander american
- History of giving birth to a baby weighing more than 9 pounds
- History of gestational diabetes
- High blood pressure—140/90 or above—or being treated for high blood pressure
- High-density lipoprotein (hdl), or good, cholesterol below 35 milligrams per deciliter (mg/dl), or a triglyceride level above 250 mg/dl
- Polycystic ovary syndrome, also called PCOS
- Predieteacosis nigricans, a condition associated with insulin resistance, characterized by a dark, velvety rash around the neck or armpits
- History of CVD

The American Diabetes Association (ADA) recommends that testing to detect prediabetes and type 2 diabetes be considered in adults who are overweight or obese and have one or more additional risk factors for diabetes. In adults without these risk factors, testing should begin at age 45.

What causes gestational diabetes?

Scientists believe gestational diabetes is caused by the hormonal changes and metabolic demands of pregnancy together with genetic and environmental factors.

Insulin Resistance and Beta Cell Dysfunction

Hormones produced by the placenta and other pregnancy-related factors contribute to insulin resistance, which occurs in all women during late pregnancy. Insulin resistance increases the amount of insulin needed to control blood glucose levels. If the pancreas can't produce enough insulin due to beta cell dysfunction, gestational diabetes occurs.

As with type 2 diabetes, excess weight is linked to gestational diabetes. Overweight or obese women are at particularly high risk for gestational diabetes because they start pregnancy with a higher need for insulin due to insulin resistance. Excessive weight gain during pregnancy may also increase risk.

Family History

Having a family history of diabetes is also a risk factor for gestational diabetes, suggesting that genes play a role in its development. Genetics may also explain why the disorder occurs more frequently in African Americans, American Indians, and Hispanics/Latinos. Many gene variants or combinations of variants may increase a woman's risk for developing gestational diabetes. Studies have found several gene variants associated with gestational diabetes, but these variants account for only a small fraction of women with gestational diabetes.

Future Risk of Type 2 Diabetes

Because a woman's hormones usually return to normal levels soon after giving birth, gestational diabetes disappears in most women after delivery. However, women who have gestational diabetes are more likely to develop gestational diabetes with future pregnancies and develop type 2 diabetes. Women with gestational diabetes should be tested for persistent diabetes 6 to 12 weeks after delivery and at least every 3 years thereafter.

Also, exposure to high glucose levels during gestation increases a child's risk for becoming overweight or obese and for developing type 2 diabetes later on. The result may be a cycle of diabetes affecting multiple generations in a family. For both mother and child, maintaining a healthy body weight and being physically active may help prevent type 2 diabetes.

Other Causes of Diabetes

Genetic Mutations

Some relatively uncommon forms of diabetes known as monogenic diabetes are caused by mutations, or changes, in a single gene. These mutations are usually inherited, but sometimes the gene mutation occurs spontaneously. Most of these gene mutations cause diabetes by reducing beta cells' ability to produce insulin.

The most common types of monogenic diabetes are neonatal diabetes mellitus (NDM) and MODY. NDM occurs in the first 6 months

Causes of Diabetes

of life. MODY is usually found during adolescence or early adulthood but sometimes is not diagnosed until later in life.

Other rare genetic mutations can cause diabetes by damaging the quality of insulin the body produces or by causing abnormalities in insulin receptors.

Genetic Diseases

Diabetes occurs in people with Down syndrome, Klinefelter syndrome, and Turner syndrome at higher rates than the general population. Scientists are investigating whether genes that may predispose people to genetic syndromes also predispose them to diabetes.

The genetic disorders cystic fibrosis and hemochromatosis are linked to diabetes. Cystic fibrosis produces abnormally thick mucus, which blocks the pancreas. The risk of diabetes increases with age in people with cystic fibrosis. Hemochromatosis causes the body to store too much iron. If the disorder is not treated, iron can build up in and damage the pancreas and other organs.

Damage to or Removal of the Pancreas

Pancreatitis, cancer, and trauma can all harm the pancreatic beta cells or impair insulin production, thus causing diabetes. If the damaged pancreas is removed, diabetes will occur due to the loss of the beta cells.

Endocrine Diseases

Endocrine diseases affect organs that produce hormones. Cushing's syndrome and acromegaly are examples of hormonal disorders that can cause prediabetes and diabetes by inducing insulin resistance. Cushing's syndrome is marked by excessive production of cortisol—sometimes called the "stress hormone." Acromegaly occurs when the body produces too much growth hormone. Glucagonoma, a rare tumor of the pancreas, can also cause diabetes. The tumor causes the body to produce too much glucagon. Hyperthyroidism, a disorder that occurs when the thyroid gland produces too much thyroid hormone, can also cause elevated blood glucose levels.

Autoimmune Disorders

Rare disorders characterized by antibodies that disrupt insulin action can lead to diabetes. This kind of diabetes is often associated with other autoimmune disorders such as lupus erythematosus.

Another rare autoimmune disorder called stiff-man syndrome is associated with antibodies that attack the beta cells, similar to type 1 diabetes.

Medications and Chemical Toxins

Some medications, such as nicotinic acid and certain types of diuretics, anti-seizure drugs, psychiatric drugs, and drugs to treat human immunodeficiency virus (HIV), can impair beta cells or disrupt insulin action. Pentamidine, a drug prescribed to treat a type of pneumonia, can increase the risk of pancreatitis, beta cell damage, and diabetes. Also, glucocorticoids—steroid hormones that are chemically similar to naturally produced cortisol—may impair insulin action. Glucocorticoids are used to treat inflammatory illnesses such as rheumatoid arthritis, asthma, lupus, and ulcerative colitis.

Many chemical toxins can damage or destroy beta cells in animals, but only a few have been linked to diabetes in humans. For example, dioxin—a contaminant of the herbicide Agent Orange, used during the Vietnam War—may be linked to the development of type 2 diabetes. In 2000, based on a report from the Institute of Medicine, the U.S. Department of Veterans Affairs (VA) added diabetes to the list of conditions for which Vietnam veterans are eligible for disability compensation. Also, a chemical in a rat poison no longer in use has been shown to cause diabetes if ingested. Some studies suggest a high intake of nitrogen-containing chemicals such as nitrates and nitrites might increase the risk of diabetes. Arsenic has also been studied for possible links to diabetes.

Lipodystrophy

Lipodystrophy is a condition in which fat tissue is lost or redistributed in the body. The condition is associated with insulin resistance and type 2 diabetes.

Chapter 8

Prevalence of Diabetes in United States

More than 29 million people in the United States have diabetes, up from the previous estimate of 26 million in 2010, according to the Centers for Disease Control and Prevention. One in four people with diabetes doesn't know he or she has it.

Another 86 million adults—more than one in three U.S. adults – have prediabetes, where their blood sugar levels are higher than normal but not high enough to be classified as type 2 diabetes. Without weight loss and moderate physical activity, 15 percent to 30 percent of people with prediabetes will develop type 2 diabetes within five years.

Key findings from the National Diabetes Statistics Report, 2014 (based on health data from 2012), include:

- 29 million people in the United States (9.3 percent) have diabetes.

- 1.7 million people aged 20 years or older were newly diagnosed with diabetes in 2012.

- Non-Hispanic black, Hispanic, and American Indian/Alaska Native adults are about twice as likely to have diagnosed diabetes as non-Hispanic white adults.

Text in this chapter is excerpted from "Diabetes Latest," National Center for Chronic Disease Prevention and Health Promotion (NCCDPHP), Center for Disease Control and Prevention (CDC), June 17, 2014.

Diabetes Sourcebook, Sixth Edition

- 208,000 people younger than 20 years have been diagnosed with diabetes (type 1 or type 2).
- 86 million adults aged 20 years and older have prediabetes.
- The percentage of U.S. adults with prediabetes is similar for non-Hispanic whites (35 percent), non-Hispanic blacks (39 percent), and Hispanics (38 percent).

Diabetes is a serious disease that can be managed through physical activity, diet, and appropriate use of insulin and oral medications to lower blood sugar levels. Another important part of diabetes management is reducing other cardiovascular disease risk factors, such as high blood pressure, high cholesterol and tobacco use.

People with diabetes are at increased risk of serious health complications including vision loss, heart disease, stroke, kidney failure, amputation of toes, feet or legs, and premature death.

In 2012, diabetes and its related complications accounted for $245 billion in total medical costs and lost work and wages. This figure is up from $174 billion in 2007.

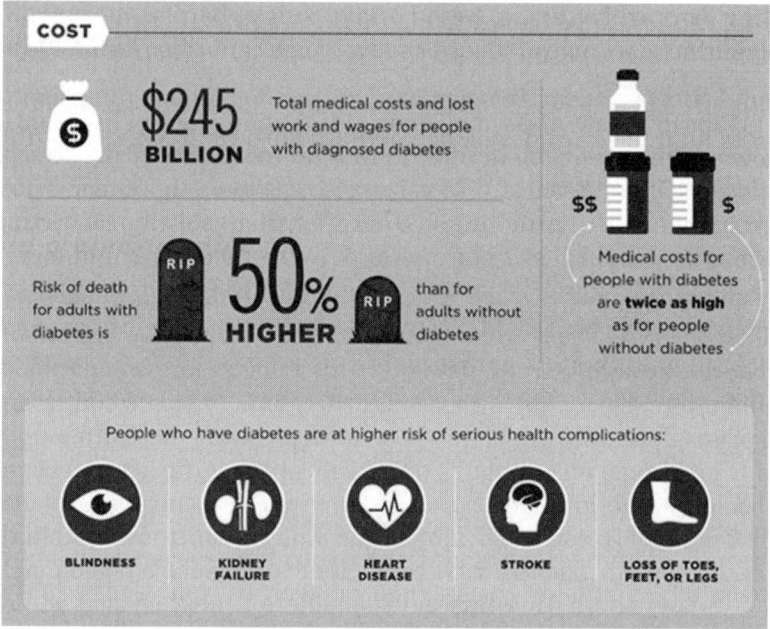

Figure 8.1. *Risks associated with diabetes*

Chapter 9

FAQs on Diabetes

What is diabetes?

Diabetes means your blood glucose (often called blood sugar) is too high. Your blood always has some glucose in it because your body needs glucose for energy to keep you going. But too much glucose in the blood isn't good for your health.

Glucose comes from the food you eat and is also made in your liver and muscles. Your blood carries the glucose to all of the cells in your body. Insulin is a chemical (a hormone) made by the pancreas. The pancreas releases insulin into the blood. Insulin helps the glucose from food get into your cells.

If your body does not make enough insulin or if the insulin doesn't work the way it should, glucose can't get into your cells. It stays in your blood instead. Your blood glucose level then gets too high, causing prediabetes or diabetes.

Text in this chapter is excerpted from "Frequently Asked Questions," National Institute on Aging (NIA), National Institutes of Health (NIH), August 2014.

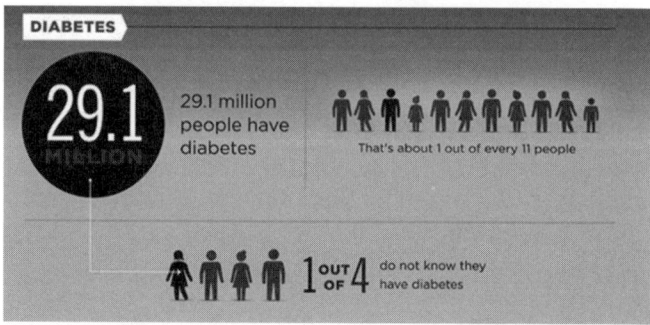

Figure 9.1. *People suffering from diabetes in United States*

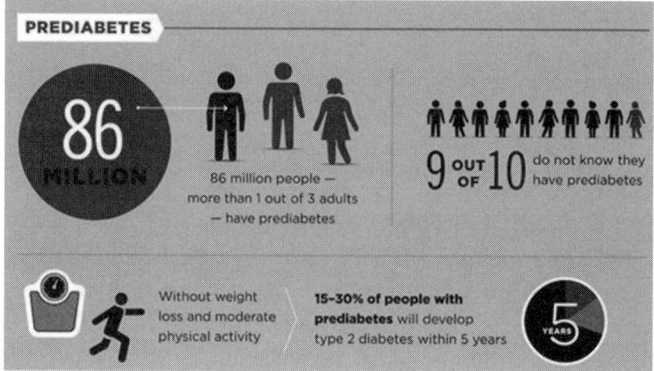

Figure 9.2. *People suffering from prediabetes in United States*

What is the difference between type 1 and type 2 diabetes?

Type 1 diabetes, which used to be called juvenile diabetes or insulin-dependent diabetes, develops most often in young people. However, type 1 diabetes can also develop in adults. With this form of diabetes, your body no longer makes insulin or doesn't make enough insulin because your immune system has attacked and destroyed the insulin-producing cells. About 5 to 10 percent of people with diabetes have type 1 diabetes.

To survive, people with type 1 diabetes must have insulin delivered by injection or a pump.

Type 2 diabetes, which used to be called adult-onset diabetes or non insulin-dependent diabetes, is the most common form of diabetes.

FAQs on Diabetes

Although people can develop type 2 diabetes at any age—even during childhood—type 2 diabetes develops most often in middle-aged and older people.

Type 2 diabetes usually begins with insulin resistance—a condition that occurs when fat, muscle, and liver cells do not use insulin to carry glucose into the body's cells to use for energy. As a result, the body needs more insulin to help glucose enter cells. At first, the pancreas keeps up with the added demand by making more insulin. Over time, the pancreas doesn't make enough insulin when blood sugar levels increase, such as after meals. If your pancreas can no longer make enough insulin, you will need to treat your type 2 diabetes.

How many people have diabetes?

Nearly 29 million Americans age 20 or older (12.3 percent of all people in this age group) have diabetes, according to 2014 estimates from the Centers for Disease Control and Prevention (CDC). About 1.9 million people aged 20 years or older were newly diagnosed with diabetes in 2010 alone. People can get diabetes at any age, but the risk increases as we get older. In 2014, over 11 million older adults living in the United States—nearly 26 percent of people 65 or older—had diabetes.

If I have diabetes, should I avoid all sweets and sugars?

If you have diabetes you should limit the amount of fats and sweets you eat. These foods have calories, but not much nutrition. Some contain saturated fats and cholesterol that increase your risk of heart disease. Limiting these foods will help you lose weight and keep your blood glucose and blood fats under control.

It is okay to have sweets once in a while. Try having sugar-free popsicles, diet soda, fat-free ice cream or frozen yogurt, or sugar-free hot cocoa mix to satisfy a "sweet tooth." Remember, fat-free and low sugar foods still have calories. Talk with your diabetes educator about how to fit sweets into your meal plan.

Who should be tested for diabetes?

Because type 2 diabetes is more common in older people, anyone who is 45 or older should consider getting tested. If you are 45 or older and overweight, getting tested is strongly recommended. If you are younger than 45, overweight, and have one or more risk factors, you also should talk with your doctor about being tested.

What are the ABCs of diabetes?

Heart disease and stroke are the leading causes of death for people with diabetes. Controlling the ABCs of diabetes—your blood glucose, your blood pressure, and your cholesterol, as well as stopping smoking—can help prevent these and other complications from diabetes.

- A is for the A1C test
- B is for Blood pressure
- C is for Cholesterol.
- **The A1C test (A-one-C)** shows you what your blood glucose has been over the last three months. Your health care provider does this test to see what your blood glucose level is most of the time. This test should be done at least twice a year for all people with diabetes and for some people more often as needed. For many people with diabetes, an A1C test result of under 7 percent usually means that their diabetes treatment is working well and their blood glucose is under control.
- **B is for Blood pressure**. The goal for most people is 140/90 but may be different for you. High blood pressure makes your heart work too hard. It can cause heart attack, stroke, and kidney disease. Your blood pressure should be checked at every doctor visit. Talk with your health care provider about your blood pressure goal.
- **C is for Cholesterol**. The LDL goal for most people is less than 100. Low density lipoprotein, or LDL-cholesterol, is the bad cholesterol that builds up in your blood vessels. It causes the vessels to narrow and harden, which can lead to a heart attack. Your doctor should check your LDL at least once a year. Talk with your health care provider about your cholesterol goal.

Ask your health care team:

- What your A1C, blood pressure, and cholesterol numbers are.
- What your abcs should be.
- What you can do to reach your target.

FAQs on Diabetes

Does Medicare help pay for services and supplies for people with diabetes?

Medicare helps pay for certain services and supplies for people with diabetes who have Medicare Part B. All require a doctor's prescription. The diabetes-related services and supplies that are covered include,

- blood sugar monitor and supplies
- an A1C test, which is a lab test that measures how well your blood glucose has been controlled over the past 3 months.
- dilated eye examinations to check for diabetic eye diseases
- glaucoma screening
- flu and pneumonia shots
- diabetes self-management training
- medical nutrition therapy services.

Part Two

Risks, Prevention, and Diagnosis of Diabetes

Chapter 10

Will Diabetes Be Part of Your Story?

Know your risk for diabetes and see if it could be a part of your story.

Everyone has a story complete with the heritage we're given and choices that we make, such as having curly hair, being tall, or loving the outdoors. Our stories are full of memories.

We watch our parents and grandparents deal with health challenges; we savor familiar family meals and remember playing outside on a summer day. Then we become adults and have many responsibilities, including caring for our own health and the health of our families.

Most people's story likely includes themselves, or a family member, or a friend dealing with the burden of diabetes. Is diabetes part of your story?

This chapter includes excerpts from "Will Diabetes Be Part of Your Story?" Centers for Disease Control and Prevention (CDC), November 3, 2014; and text from "Alzheimer's Disease: Unraveling the Mystery," National Institutes on Aging (NIA), January 22, 2015.

What You Should Know

You are at increased risk for developing diabetes if you:

- Are 45 years of age or older.
- Are overweight.
- Have a parent with diabetes.
- Have a sister or brother with diabetes.
- Have a family background that is African-American, Hispanic/Latino, American-Indian, Asian-American, or Pacific-Islander.
- Had diabetes while pregnant (gestational diabetes), or gave birth to a baby weighing 9 pounds or more.
- Are physically active less than three times a week.

Is it You?

- 2 out of every 5 Americans are expected to develop type 2 diabetes during their lifetime.
- More than 29 million Americans have diabetes; 1 in 4 doesn't know.
- 86 million adults – more than 1 in 3 U.S. adults—have prediabetes, where their blood sugar levels are higher than normal but not high enough to be classified as type 2 diabetes.
- More than 1 in 2 Hispanic men and women (over 50%) non-Hispanic black women are predicted to develop diabetes, reports a major study of over 1 million U.S. adults between 1985 and 2011.
- While new cases of diagnosed diabetes may be levelling off, some groups continue to see an increased burden of type 2 diabetes. Now is the time to double down to prevent or delay type 2 diabetes.

Diabetes Risk Factors

There are many factors that increase your risk for diabetes. To find out about your risk, note each item on this list that applies to you.

Will Diabetes Be Part of Your Story?

- I am 45 years of age or older.
- The At-Risk Weight Chart shows my current weight puts me at risk.
- I have a parent, brother, or sister with diabetes.
- My family background is African American, Hispanic/Latino, American Indian, Asian American or Pacific Islander.
- I have had diabetes while I was pregnant (this is called gestational diabetes) or I gave birth to a baby weighing 9 pounds or more.
- I have been told that my blood glucose (blood sugar) levels are higher than normal.
- My blood pressure is 140/90 or higher, or I have been told that I have high blood pressure.
- My cholesterol (lipid) levels are not normal. My HDL cholesterol ("good" cholesterol) is less than 35 or my triglyceride level is higher than 250.
- I am fairly inactive. I am physically active less than three times a week.
- I have been told that I have polycystic ovary syndrome (PCOS).
- The skin around my neck or in my armpits appears dirty no matter how much I scrub it. The skin appears dark, thick and velvety. This is called acanthosis nigricans.
- I have been told that I have blood vessel problems affecting my heart, brain, or legs.

If you have any of the items above, be sure to talk with your health care team about your risk for diabetes and whether you should be tested.

At-Risk Weight Charts

Find your height in the correct chart. If your weight is equal to or greater than the weight listed, you are at increased risk for type 2 diabetes.

If you are not asian american or pacific islander at risk bmi ≥ 25

Table 10.1. At-Risk Weight Charts

Height	Weight
4'10"	119
4'11"	124
5'0"	128
5'1"	132
5'2"	136
5'3"	141
5'4"	145
5'5"	150
5'6"	155
5'7"	159
5'8"	164
5'9"	169
5'10"	174
5'11"	179
6'0"	184
6'1"	189
6'2"	194
6'3"	200
6'4"	205

If you are asian american at risk bmi ≥ 23

Table 10.2. At-Risk Weight Charts

Height	Weight
4'10"	110
4'11"	114
5'0"	118
5'1"	122
5'2"	126
5'3"	130
5'4"	134
5'5"	138
5'6"	142

Will Diabetes Be Part of Your Story?

Table 10.2. Continued

Height	Weight
5'7"	146
5'8"	151
5'9"	155
5'10"	160
5'11"	165
6'0"	169
6'1"	174
6'2"	179
6'3"	184
6'4"	189

If you are pacific islander at risk bmi ≥ 26

Table 10.3. At-Risk Weight Charts

Height	Weight
4'10"	124
4'11"	128
5'0"	133
5'1"	137
5'2"	142
5'3"	146
5'4"	151
5'5"	156
5'6"	161
5'7"	166
5'8"	171
5'9"	176
5'10"	181
5'11"	186
6'0"	191
6'1"	197
6'2"	202
6'3"	208
6'4"	213

Know Your Blood Glucose Numbers

Table 10.4. Know your Blood Glucose Numbers

	Fasting Blood Glucose Test	2-Hour Oral Glucose Tolerance Test
Normal	Below 100	Below 140
Prediabetes	100-125	140-199
Diabetes	126 or above	200 or above

Chapter 11

Am I at Risk for Type 2 Diabetes?

What are the signs and symptoms of type 2 diabetes?

The signs and symptoms of type 2 diabetes can be so mild that you might not even notice them. Nearly 7 million people in the United States have type 2 diabetes and don't know they have the disease. Many have no signs or symptoms. Some people have symptoms but do not suspect diabetes.

Symptoms include:

- increased thirst
- increased hunger
- fatigue
- increased urination, especially at night
- unexplained weight loss

Text in this chapter is excerpted from "Am I at Risk for Type 2 Diabetes? Taking Steps to Lower Your Risk of Getting Diabetes," National Institute of Diabetes and Digestive and Kidney Diseases (NIDDK), National Institutes of Health (NIH), June 2012.

- blurred vision
- numbness or tingling in the feet or hands
- sores that do not heal

Many people do not find out they have the disease until they have diabetes problems, such as blurred vision or heart trouble. If you find out early that you have diabetes, you can get treatment to prevent damage to your body.

What factors increase my risk for type 2 diabetes?

To find out your risk for type 2 diabetes, check each item that applies to you.

- I am age 45 or older.
- I am overweight or obese.
- I have a parent, brother, or sister with diabetes.
- My family background is African American, Alaska Native, American Indian, Asian American, Hispanic/Latino, or Pacific Islander American.
- I have had gestational diabetes.
- I gave birth to at least one baby weighing more than 9 pounds.
- My blood pressure is 140/90 or higher, or I have been told that I have high blood pressure.
- My cholesterol levels are higher than normal. My HDL, or good, cholesterol is below 35, or my triglyceride level is above 250.
- I am fairly inactive.
- I have polycystic ovary syndrome, also called PCOS.
- On previous testing, I had prediabetes—an A1C level of 5.7 to 6.4 percent, impaired fasting glucose (IFG), or impaired glucose tolerance (IGT).
- I have other clinical conditions associated with insulin resistance, such as a condition called acanthosis nigricans, characterized by a dark, velvety rash around my neck or armpits.
- I have a history of cardiovascular disease.

The more items you checked, the higher your risk.

Am I at Risk for Type 2 Diabetes?

Does sleep matter?

Yes. Studies show that untreated sleep problems, especially sleep apnea, can increase the risk of type 2 diabetes. Sleep apnea is a common disorder in which you have pauses in breathing or shallow breaths while you sleep. Most people who have sleep apnea don't know they have it and it often goes undiagnosed. Night shift workers who have problems with sleepiness may also be at increased risk for obesity and type 2 diabetes.

If you think you might have sleep problems, ask your doctor for help.

How can I reduce my risk for type 2 diabetes?

You can do a lot to reduce your risk of getting type 2 diabetes. Being more physically active, reducing fat and calorie intake, and losing a little weight can help you lower your chances of developing type 2 diabetes. Taking the diabetes medicine metformin can also reduce risk, particularly in younger and heavier people with prediabetes and women who have had gestational diabetes. Lowering blood pressure and cholesterol levels also helps you stay healthy.

If you are overweight, then take these steps:

- Reach and maintain a reasonable body weight. Even a 10 or 15 pound weight loss makes a big difference.
- Make wise food choices most of the time.
- Be physically active every day.

If you are fairly inactive, then take this step:

- Be physically active every day.

If your blood pressure is too high, then take these steps:

- Reach and maintain a reasonable body weight.
- Make wise food choices most of the time.
- Reduce your sodium and alcohol intake.
- Be physically active every day.

- Talk with your doctor about whether you need medicine to control your blood pressure.

If your cholesterol or triglyceride levels are too high, then take these steps:

- Make wise food choices most of the time.
- Be physically active every day.
- Talk with your doctor about whether you need medicine to control your cholesterol levels.

Making Changes to Lower My Risk

Making big changes in your life is hard, especially if you are faced with more than one change. You can make it easier by taking these steps:

- Make a plan to change behavior.
- Decide exactly what you will do and give yourself a time frame.
- Plan what you need to get ready.
- Track your goals and activity on a food and activity tracker.
- Think about what might prevent you from reaching your goals.
- Find family and friends who will support and encourage you.
- Decide how you will reward yourself—a shopping trip, movie tickets, an afternoon in the park—when you do what you have planned.

Be Physically Active Every Day

Regular physical activity tackles several risk factors at once. Activity helps you lose weight; keeps your blood glucose, blood pressure, and cholesterol under control; and helps your body use insulin. People in the DPP who were physically active for 30 minutes a day, 5 days a week, reduced their risk of type 2 diabetes. Many chose brisk walking as their physical activity.

If you are not fairly active, you should start slowly. First, talk with your doctor about what kinds of physical activity are safe for you. Make a plan to increase your activity level toward the goal of being active at least 30 minutes a day most days of the week. You can increase your level of physical activity in two main ways:

Am I at Risk for Type 2 Diabetes?

1. Start an exercise program.
2. Increase your daily activity.

Start an exercise program. Pick exercises that suit you. Find a friend to walk with you or join an exercise class that will help you keep going.

- Do aerobic activities, which use your large muscles to make your heart beat faster. The large muscles are those of the upper and lower arms; upper and lower legs; and those that control head, shoulder, and hip movements.
- Do activities to strengthen muscles and bone, such as lifting weights or sit-ups, two to three times a week. Find help—such as a video or a class—to learn how to do these exercises properly.

Increase your daily activity. Choose activities you enjoy. You can work extra activity into your daily routine by doing the following:

- Increase daily activity by decreasing time spent watching TV or at the computer. Set up a reminder on your computer to take an activity break.
- Take the stairs rather than an elevator or escalator.
- Park at the far end of the parking lot and walk.
- Get off the bus a few stops early and walk the rest of the way.
- Walk or bicycle whenever you can.

Take Your Prescribed Medicines

Some people need medicine to help control their blood pressure or cholesterol levels. If you do, take your medicines as directed. Ask your doctor if you should take metformin to prevent type 2 diabetes. Metformin is a medicine that makes insulin work better and can reduce the risk of type 2 diabetes.

Chapter 12

Women at High Risk for Diabetes

Chapter Contents

Section 12.1—Women and Risk of Type 2 Diabetes.................... 68
Section 12.2—Am I at Risk for Gestational Diabetes? 71

Section 12.1

Women and Risk of Type 2 Diabetes

Text in this section is excerpted from "Am I at Risk for Type 2 Diabetes? Taking Steps to Lower Your Risk of Getting Diabetes," National Center for Chronic Disease Prevention and Health Promotion (NCCDPHP), July 2013.

Why should women care about diabetes?

- Diabetes is a group of diseases marked by high levels of blood glucose resulting from defects in insulin production, insulin action, or both. Diabetes can lead to serious complications and premature death.
- The most common forms of diabetes are as follows:
  - Type 1 diabetes accounts for about 5% of all diagnosed cases of diabetes. Type 1 is usually diagnosed in children and young adults, although it can occur at any time. People with type 1 diabetes must use insulin from an injection or a pump to manage their diabetes.
  - Type 2 diabetes accounts for about 95% of all cases diagnosed in adults. Several studies have shown that healthy eating, regular physical activity, and weight loss used with medication if prescribed, can help control complications from type 2 diabetes or can prevent or delay the onset of type 2 diabetes.
  - Gestational diabetes is diagnosed in 2%–10% of pregnant women. Gestational diabetes can cause health problems during pregnancy for both the child and mother. Children whose mothers had gestational diabetes have an increased risk of developing obesity and type 2 diabetes. Although gestational diabetes often goes away after pregnancy, about half of all women who have gestational diabetes get type 2 diabetes later in life.

Women at High Risk for Diabetes

- It is estimated that 12 million women aged 20 years and older have diabetes, and approximately 27 million have prediabetes.

How can women tell if they are at high risk for diabetes?

Women are at high risk for diabetes if they:

- Are overweight (body mass index of 25 kg/m2 or greater) and have one or more additional risk factors, such as:
- Low physical activity (less than 150 minutes of moderate intensity activity, such as walking, per week).
- Family history of type 2 diabetes.
- High-risk race/ethnicity (African American, American Indian or Alaska Native, Asian American, Hispanic or Latino, Native Hawaiian or Pacific Islander).
- Had a baby weighing 9 pounds or more or were diagnosed with gestational diabetes.
- High blood pressure (140/90 mmhg or higher).
- High cholesterol (240 mg/dL or higher).
- History of polycystic ovarian syndrome, a health problem that can affect a woman's hormones, menstrual cycle, and ability to have children.
- Clinical conditions associated with insulin resistance, such as severe obesity, or the development of dark, thick skin in body folds and creases (a condition which is called 'acanthosis nigricans').
- History of cardiovascular disease.
- Have prediabetes.

How well are women at high risk for diabetes doing?

A study of women at high risk for diabetes indicated that:

Physical Activity

- Only 1 of 4 women at high risk for diabetes reported that they exercised 150 minutes of moderate-intensity activity (such as walking) per week.

- No evidence was found that women at high risk for diabetes of different races/ethnicities, educational attainment, or household income differed in how likely they were to be physically active for 150 minutes per week.

Healthy Eating

- 90% of obese Mexican American women with high cholesterol reported that they were advised by their health care provider to eat fewer high-fat or high cholesterol foods; only 78% of non-Hispanic whites were given the same advice.
- There were no significant differences by education among obese women who were given advice about eating fewer high-fat or high-cholesterol foods.
- Only 76% of obese women with middle income (200%–399% of Federal Poverty Level [FPL]) reported that they received advice to eat fewer high-fat or high cholesterol foods; 82% of high income (400% or more FPL) obese women reporting that they received this advice.

Weight Loss

- Only 50% of non-Hispanic black and Mexican American women at high risk for diabetes reported trying to lose weight in the past 12 months compared to 60% of non-Hispanic white women at high risk for diabetes.
- Women at high risk for diabetes with a high school education (57%) or less (47%) were less likely than women at high risk for diabetes with more than a high school education (63%) to report that they tried to lose weight in the past 12 months.
- 1 of 2 women at high risk for diabetes who were near poor (100%–199% FPL) or poor (<100% FPL) reported trying to lose weight in the past 12 months; whereas 1of 3 women from high income families reported trying to lose weight in the past 12 months.

Section 12.2

Am I at Risk for Gestational Diabetes?

Text in this section is excerpted from "Am I at Risk for Gestational Diabetes?" National Institute of Child Health and Human Development (NICHD), National Institutes of Health (NIH), June 2012.

Why do some women get gestational diabetes?

Usually, the body breaks down much of the food you eat into a type of sugar, called glucose. Because glucose moves from the stomach into the blood, some people use the term "blood sugar" instead of "glucose." Your body makes a hormone called insulin that moves glucose out of the blood and into the cells of the body. In women with gestational diabetes, the glucose can't get into the cells, so the amount of glucose in the blood gets higher and higher. This is called high blood sugar or diabetes.

How will I know if I have gestational diabetes?

Based on your risk level and other factors, your health care provider first will give you a glucose screening test (also called a 1-hour post glucola [PG] test or a glucose challenge test). For this test, you will drink a sugar liquid and then have a blood test an hour later. (In most cases, the test uses only a few drops of blood and is usually not painful.) If your blood sugar level is normal after an hour, you probably don't have gestational diabetes. If you are tested early in pregnancy, your health care provider is likely to screen you again when you are between 24 weeks and 28 weeks pregnant.

If your blood sugar level is high after an hour, your health care provider will give you an oral glucose tolerance test (OGTT) to determine if you have gestational diabetes or another problem.

For the OGTT, you will need to fast (not eat or drink anything but water) for 8 to 12 hours before the test. When you arrive, you'll have a blood test to measure your blood sugar level, and then you'll drink a sugar liquid. Your blood will be tested after 1 hour, 2 hours, and 3 hours. (In most cases, the test uses only a few drops of blood and is usually not painful.)

If your blood sugar is high for one of these measurements, you probably don't have gestational diabetes, but your body might be having trouble keeping blood sugar levels balanced. Your health care provider will suggest ways to help keep your levels balanced, such as making changes in what you eat.

If your blood sugar is high for two or more of these measurements, then you have gestational diabetes. Your health care provider will work with you to create a treatment plan that meets your needs and health history.

What does gestational diabetes mean for me?
During Pregnancy

Most women with gestational diabetes have healthy pregnancies and healthy babies because they control their blood sugar levels. Women with gestational diabetes are at higher risk for possible problems, including high blood pressure; preeclampsia (a sudden, dangerous increase in blood pressure); pregnancy loss during the last 4 weeks to 8 weeks; early/preterm labor and delivery; and surgery to deliver the baby (cesarean section, or C-section) and its related risks (such as infection).

Keeping blood sugar levels under control and following the treatment plan outlined by your health care provider are the best ways to improve pregnancy outcomes for women with gestational diabetes.

After Pregnancy

Women who have had gestational diabetes are at greater risk for developing type 2 diabetes during their lifetime. If you had gestational diabetes, your health care provider will test you for diabetes 6 weeks after you give birth to measure your blood sugar level. If the first test is negative, your health care provider will test you every year for diabetes.

Eating a healthy diet, getting regular physical activity, maintaining a healthy weight, and taking certain medications can help prevent and control type 2 diabetes.

What does gestational diabetes mean for my baby?
During and Right after Birth

Most women with gestational diabetes have healthy pregnancies and healthy babies because they control their blood sugar levels.

Babies whose mothers had gestational diabetes are at higher risk for certain health problems, including being large bodied, which can cause problems and injuries during delivery; low blood sugar at birth; early/preterm birth; jaundice (yellowish color of the skin and white parts of the eye); breathing problems; and low levels of certain minerals in the blood.

Keeping blood sugar levels under control is the best way to improve outcomes for babies whose mothers have gestational diabetes.

Later in Life

Babies whose mothers had gestational diabetes are at higher risk for certain health problems as they get older. Some of these problems include overweight and obesity; problems with glucose and/or insulin, such as glucose intolerance and insulin resistance; and type 2 diabetes.

Eating a healthy diet, getting regular physical activity, maintaining a healthy weight, and taking certain medications can help prevent and control type 2 diabetes.

What should I do if I have gestational diabetes?

If you have gestational diabetes, your health care provider will work with you to create a treatment plan that will help keep the condition under control throughout your pregnancy. Most treatment plans include keeping your blood sugar levels within the normal range, eating a healthy diet as outlined by a health care provider, doing regular physical activity, and maintaining a healthy weight. Some women also need to take insulin as part of their treatment plan.

More and more women with gestational diabetes have healthy pregnancies and healthy babies because they follow their treatment plans and control their blood sugar levels.

Chapter 13

Family History – A Potential Risk Factor for Diabetes

Health Problems That May Run in Families

Common health problems that can run in a family include:

- Alzheimer's disease / dementia
- arthritis
- asthma
- blood clots
- cancer
- depression
- diabetes
- heart disease
- high cholesterol
- high blood pressure
- pregnancy losses and birth defects
- stroke.

Clues to Your Disease Risk

Creating a family health history helps you know about diseases and disease risks. It can also show the way a disease occurs in a family. For example, you may find that a family member had a certain disease

---

This chapter includes excerpts from "Creating a Family Health History," National Institute of Health (NIH), May 2015; and text from "Family History," Center for Diseases Control and Prevention (CDC), March 6, 2013.

at an earlier age than usual (10 to 20 years before most people get it). That can increase other family members' risk.

Risk also goes up if a relative has a disease that usually does not affect a certain gender, for example, breast cancer in a man. Certain combinations of diseases within a family—such as breast and ovarian cancer, or heart disease and diabetes—also increase the chance of developing those diseases.

Diabetes is:

Common, especially among Hispanics or Latinos

- Diabetes occurs when the level of sugar in your blood remains too high.

Serious

- Diabetes is linked to heart disease, kidney problems, stroke, blindness, lower leg amputations, and other health problems.

Controllable

- If you have diabetes, ask your doctor about:
- eating healthier and becoming more active,
- controlling the level of sugar and fat in your blood,
- controlling your blood pressure, and
- getting regular exams of your eyes, feet, kidneys, and hemoglobin A1C.

You're more likely to get diabetes if:

- You have family members with diabetes
- You have poor eating habits
- You are obese or inactive

What you can do:

Know your family health history

Find out if you have relatives with diabetes and at what age they found out about their disease.

Family History – A Potential Risk Factor for Diabetes

Talk with your doctor

- Tell your doctor about your family health history of diabetes.
- Ask your doctor about your other risk factors for diabetes.
- Ask your doctor about possible ways to reduce your risk of diabetes.

Chapter 14

Saving Yourself — Role of the Individual in Helping Prevent Diabetes

Chapter Contents

Section 14.1—The Power to Prevent Diabetes and
 Saving Yourself 80
Section 14.2—Keep Your Diabetes under Control 85

Section 14.1

The Power to Prevent Diabetes and Saving Yourself

Text in this section is excerpted from "We Have the Power to Prevent Diabetes," National Diabetes Education Program (NDEP), July 1, 2014; and text from "It's Not Too Late to Prevent Type 2 Diabetes," National Diabetes Education Program (NDEP), December 1, 2013.

Get Started

Here are some powerful steps you can take to get started today:

- **Move More.** Get up, get out, and get moving. Walk, dance, bike ride, swim, or play ball with your friends or family. It doesn't matter what you do as long as you enjoy it. Try different things to keep it fun.

- **Make Healthy Food Choices.** Focus on eating less. Eat fiber-rich fruits and vegetables each day. Choose whole grain foods such as whole wheat bread and crackers, oatmeal, brown rice, and cereals. Cut down on fatty and fried foods. You still can have foods you enjoy, just eat smaller servings. Choose water to drink.

- **Take off Some Weight.** Once you start eating less and moving more, you will lose weight. By losing just 10 pounds, you can cut your chances of getting diabetes.

- **Set Goals You Can Meet.** Start by making small changes. Try being active for 15 minutes a day this week. Then each week add 5 minutes until you build up to at least 30 minutes 5 days a week. Try to cut 150 calories out of your diet each day (that's one can of soda!). Slowly reduce your calories over time. Talk to your health care team about your goals.

- **Record Your Progress.** Write down all the things you eat and drink and the number of minutes you are active. Keeping a diary is one of the best ways to stay focused and reach your goals.

Role of the Individual in Helping Prevent Diabetes

- **Seek Help**. You don't have to prevent diabetes alone. Ask your family and friends to help you out. Involve them in your activities. You can help each other move more, eat less, and live a healthy life. Go for a walk together or play a pick-up game of basketball. Join a support group in your area to help you stay on track.
- **Keep at It**. Making even small changes is hard in the beginning. Try to add one new change a week. If you get off track, start again and keep at it.

Get Moving

Did you know that as you get older, you have a greater chance of getting type 2 diabetes? It's true. You have a greater chance of getting diabetes if you are age 45 or older, are overweight or obese, or have a family history of diabetes.

You can take steps to prevent or delay getting type 2 diabetes. If you are overweight, losing a modest amount of weight can help. A modest weight loss for a 200-pound person who wants to prevent or delay type 2 diabetes is about 10 to 14 pounds. Read this section to find out how.

Step 1: Eat well to help prevent or delay type 2 diabetes.

Taking steps to lose weight can include eating smaller meal portions and choosing healthy foods. Here are a few tips to help you get started with both.

Choose healthy foods

Eat more fruits and vegetables and fewer high-fat foods to help with weight loss.

- Choose whole grain foods such as whole wheat bread, crackers, cereals, brown rice, oatmeal, and barley.
- Eat a mix of colorful fruits and vegetables.
- Choose fish, lean meat, and chicken and turkey without the skin.
- Eat foods that have been baked, broiled, or grilled instead of fried.
- Drink water instead of juice and regular soda.

- Choose low-fat or skim milk, yogurt, and cheese.

Reduce portion sizes

Eat smaller amounts of food to help with weight loss.

- Fill half of your plate with fruits and vegetables. Fill one quarter with a lean protein, such as chicken or turkey without the skin or beans. Fill one quarter with a whole grain, such as brown rice or whole wheat pasta.
- Share your main dish when eating out or wrap half of it to go.
- Eat a small serving of dessert at the end of a healthy meal, but not every day. Sweets and desserts have a lot of fat and sugar.
- Eat small amounts of heart-healthy fats. Examples include nuts, seeds, and vegetable oils. For most nuts and seeds without the shell, a small amount would be 1 ounce or a small handful.

Step 2: Start now to get moving—and have fun.

Moving more and sitting less can help you lose weight or stay at a healthy weight. It also can also help you improve your strength and become more flexible. Ask your doctor how you can safely start to be more active.

Find ways to move more every day

Add more activity each day until you reach at least 30 minutes a day, 5 days a week.

- Get off the couch, turn on the music, and dance!
- Do not sit for long periods of time.
- Stretch and move around during commercial breaks.
- Walk around the house while you talk on the phone.
- Park your car farther away and walk if it is safe.

Brisk walking is a great way to be active

During a brisk walk, you walk faster than your normal pace. Here are some tips to get you started:

- Start with 10 minutes a day if you are not active.

Role of the Individual in Helping Prevent Diabetes

- Walk slowly for a few minutes to warm up then increase your speed over time.
- Wear walking shoes that fit your feet and provide comfort and support.
- Walk in safe places. Some good places for brisk walking include indoor or outdoor walking paths, a shopping mall, and community centers.

Remember to warm up and stretch. Before you start any activity, warm up slowly. Shrug your shoulders, swing your arms or march in place for 3 to 5 minutes before. Stretch after you have been active when your muscles are warm. Do not bounce or stretch so far that it hurts.

Step 3: Get your friends and family involved.

Making lifestyle changes can be easier with help from your loved ones.

- Offer fruit instead of cookies and chips when your grandkids, friends, and family visit.
- Show the younger people in your life the dances you enjoy.
- Enjoy a walk with friends or family around a park, museum, or zoo.
- Go for a swim with a friend. Moving around in water is gentle on your joints.
- Teach your kids or grandkids how to plant and take care of a garden.

Step 4: Make a plan

Use this section to plan how you will eat healthy foods and move more. Think about what is important to your health and what changes you are willing and able to make. To get started, choose one goal to work on and decide what steps will help you reach your goal.

Take Your First Steps

What's my goal?

(Example: I want to see if I can walk for 30 minutes, 5 days of the week.)

How will I get started?

(Example: I will walk for 10 minutes after lunch.)

What do I need to get ready?

(Example: I will put my walking shoes where I can see them every day.)

What might get in the way of making this change?

(Example: If it is bad weather, I will walk at the mall.)

How will I reward myself for sticking with my plan?

(Example: If I stick with my plan this week, I will watch a movie.)

Step 5: Find out how insurance coverage can help you prevent type 2 diabetes.

Medicare. Medicare covers all or some of the costs of certain exams, tests, and check-ups for people who have a greater chance of getting diabetes. Medicare will also cover certain weight loss services and programs.

Other health insurance. Other plans may also cover the costs of certain exams, tests, check-ups, and diabetes prevention programs approved by the Centers for Disease Control and Prevention (CDC) for people who have a greater chance of getting diabetes. Ask your doctor or insurance company what your plan covers.

Role of the Individual in Helping Prevent Diabetes

Section 14.2

Keep Your Diabetes under Control

Text in this section is excerpted from "Prevent Diabetes Problems: Keep Your diabetes under Control," National Institute of Diabetes and Digestive and Kidney Diseases (NIDDK), National Institutes of Health (NIH), February 2014.

What are diabetes problems?

Diabetes problems are health problems that can happen when you have diabetes. If your diabetes is not under control, you will have too much glucose, also called sugar, in your blood. Having too much glucose in your blood for a long time can affect many important parts of your body, such as your:

- blood vessels and heart
- nerves
- kidneys
- mouth
- eyes
- feet

You can do a lot to prevent or slow down these health problems if you keep your diabetes under control.

This table shows the body parts that can be affected by diabetes and the resulting health problems you may have.

Table 14.1. The body parts that can be affected by diabetes and the resulting health problems

Affected Body Part	Resulting Health Problems You May Have
Blood vessels and heart	• Heart disease
	• Heart attack
	• Stroke

Table 14.1. Continued

Affected Body Part	Resulting Health Problems You May Have
	• High blood pressure
	• Poor blood circulation, or flow, throughout your body
Nerves	• Pain, tingling, weakness, or numbness in your hands, arms, feet, or legs
	• Problems with your bladder, digestion, having sex, and keeping your heartbeats and blood pressure steady
Kidneys	• Protein loss through your urine
	• Buildup of wastes and fluid in your blood
Mouth	• Gum disease and loss of teeth
	• Dry mouth
	• Thrush, or the growth of too much fungus in the mouth
Eyes	• Loss of vision and blindness
Feet	• Sores
	• Infections
	• Amputation

What should my blood glucose numbers be?

Your blood glucose numbers should meet the targets in this chart unless your doctor helps you set different targets. Targets are numbers you aim for. The table shows the target blood glucose numbers—measured in milligrams per deciliter (mg/dL)—for most people with diabetes.

Table 14.2. Target Blood Glucose Numbers (mg/dl) for Most People with Diabetes

Target Blood Glucose Numbers (mg/dl) for Most People with Diabetes	
Time of the Day	Targets
Before meals and when you wake up	70 to 130
1 to 2 hours after eating	180 or below

Role of the Individual in Helping Prevent Diabetes

This table shows target blood glucose numbers for women with diabetes who become pregnant.

Table 14.3. Target Blood Glucose Numbers (mg/dl) for Women with Diabetes Who Become Pregnant

Target Blood Glucose Numbers (mg/dl) for Women with Diabetes Who Become Pregnant	
Time of the Day	Targets
Before meals and when you wake up	60 to 99
1 to 2 hours after eating	129 or below

This chart shows target blood glucose numbers for women who develop diabetes during pregnancy, called gestational diabetes.

Table 14.4. Target Blood Glucose Numbers (mg/dl) for Women with Gestational Diabetes

Target Blood Glucose Numbers (mg/dl) for Women with Gestational Diabetes	
Time of the Day	Targets
Before meals and when you wake up	95 or below
1 hour after eating	140 or below
2 hours after eating	120 or below

Keep track of your blood glucose test results

Keep track of your blood glucose test results by using a record page.
- Make copies of the record page at the end of this booklet or ask your health care team for a blood glucose record book.
- Always bring your record book to your checkups so you can talk with your health care team about reaching your target blood glucose levels. Or you may be able to use an electronic blood glucose tracking system on the Internet or on your cell phone.

How can I check my blood glucose numbers?

You can check your blood glucose numbers at home using a blood glucose meter. Your health care team can teach you how to:

- prick your finger to get a drop of blood for testing
- use your meter to find out the glucose level in the drop of blood

The results of your blood glucose checks can help you make decisions about your diabetes medicines, daily meals and snacks, and physical activity.

Ask your health care team when and how often you need to check your blood glucose. Self-tests are usually done before meals, after meals, and at bedtime.

Your blood glucose test results will help you and your health care team make a plan for keeping your blood glucose under control.

What should I do if my blood glucose numbers are too high or too low?

If your blood glucose numbers are often higher or lower than your targets, tell your health care team. You may need to make changes in how you take care of your diabetes.

High blood glucose, called hyperglycemia, can make you:

- thirsty
- weak or tired
- have headaches
- urinate more often
- have trouble paying attention
- have blurred vision
- have yeast infections

Talk with your health care team if you notice any of these symptoms. Ask what you should do when your blood glucose is too high.

Low blood glucose, called hypoglycemia, can make you:

- hungry
- dizzy or shaky

Role of the Individual in Helping Prevent Diabetes

- confused
- pale
- sweat more
- weak
- anxious or cranky
- have headaches
- have a fast heartbeat

> **Note**
>
> Severe hypoglycemia can cause you to pass out. If that happens, you'll need help bringing your blood glucose level back to normal. Your health care team can teach your family members and friends how to give you an injection of glucagon, a medicine that raises blood glucose levels quickly. If glucagon is not available, someone should call 911 to get you to the nearest emergency room for treatment.

If you have any of these symptoms, check your blood glucose. If your number is too low, have one of these quick sources of glucose:

- three or four glucose tablets
- one serving of glucose gel—the amount equal to 15 grams of carbohydrates
- 1/2 cup, or 4 ounces, of any fruit juice
- 1/2 cup, or 4 ounces, of a regular—not diet—soft drink
- 1 cup, or 8 ounces, of milk
- five or six pieces of hard candy
- 1 tablespoon of sugar or honey

Check your blood glucose again in 15 minutes to make sure it is at your pre-meal target number. If your number is still too low, have another serving of a quick glucose food or drink. Repeat these steps until your blood glucose is at your pre-meal target number or higher.

After you feel better and your blood glucose returns to your target number, eat your regular meals and snacks as planned.

What should my blood pressure be?

Your blood pressure should be below 140/80 unless your doctor helps you set a different goal.

Blood pressure is the force of blood flow inside your blood vessels. Blood pressure is written with two numbers separated by a slash and is said as "140 over 80." The top number is the pressure as your heart beats and pushes blood through your blood vessels. The bottom number is the pressure as your blood vessels relax between heartbeats.

High blood pressure forces your heart to work harder to pump blood. High blood pressure can strain your heart, damage blood vessels, and increase your risk of heart attack, stroke, eye problems, and kidney problems.

Many people with diabetes also have high blood pressure. But keeping your blood pressure at your goal will help prevent damage to your heart, blood vessels, and other parts of your body. Healthy meal planning, medicines, and physical activity can help you reach your blood pressure goal.

> Have your blood pressure checked at every medical visit. Ask your doctor whether you need medicine to control your blood pressure.

What should my cholesterol and triglycerides be?

Your cholesterol and triglyceride numbers should meet the targets in this chart unless your doctor helps you set different targets.

Table 14.5. Target Blood Cholesterol Numbers for Most People with Diabetes

Target Blood Cholesterol Numbers for Most People with Diabetes	
Total Cholesterol	Below 200
LDL, or bad, cholesterol	below 100 or below 70 if you have cardiovascular disease or other health problems
HDL, or good, cholesterol	above 40 in men and above 50 in women
Triglycerides	below 150

Role of the Individual in Helping Prevent Diabetes

Cholesterol is a type of fat found in your body's cells, in blood, and in many foods. High cholesterol can lead to heart and blood vessel disease, also called cardiovascular disease. Cardiovascular disease is the biggest health problem for people with diabetes.

LDL cholesterol

LDL cholesterol is known as the bad cholesterol because it builds up in the artery walls that supply blood to your heart. Extra cholesterol in your blood can build up in artery walls if:

- you often eat foods that are high in LDL cholesterol
- high cholesterol runs in your family

HDL cholesterol

HDL cholesterol, or good cholesterol, carries cholesterol from other parts of your body back to your liver, which removes the cholesterol from your body.

Triglycerides

Triglycerides are another form of fat found in your blood and in food. Although triglycerides do not build up in artery walls, they can be a sign that your risk for cardiovascular disease is high.

Total cholesterol

Your total cholesterol number reflects all the cholesterol in the blood, but is mostly due to the amount of your LDL cholesterol.

Meeting your target numbers for cholesterol levels will help prevent heart disease, stroke, and damage to your blood vessels. Keeping cholesterol levels under control can also help with blood flow. Healthy meal planning, medicines, and physical activity can help you reach your target blood cholesterol numbers.

> Have your cholesterol checked at least once a year. Your doctor will send you to a lab to have a small sample of your blood drawn for the cholesterol test. Ask your doctor whether you need medicine called a statin to control your cholesterol.

Eating, diet, and nutrition

Following a healthy eating plan is a key step in living with diabetes and preventing diabetes problems. Your health care team will help you make a healthy eating plan.

Will I need to take diabetes medicines?

If you cannot reach your target blood glucose levels with a healthy eating plan and physical activity, you may need diabetes medicines. The kind of medicines you'll take will depend on your type of diabetes, your schedule, and your other health problems. Diabetes medicines help keep your blood glucose in the target range.

Your doctor will prescribe any medicines you need, including insulin. Insulin helps your blood glucose levels stay on target by moving glucose from your blood to your body's cells. You will need to take insulin if your body no longer makes enough.

Be sure to take your medicines as directed by your doctor.

What steps can I take to prevent diabetes problems?

You can take steps each day to prevent diabetes problems.

Table 14.6. Steps to Prevent Diabetes

Steps
Healthy Eating
• Follow the healthy eating plan that you and your doctor or dietitian have made.
• Learn what to eat to keep your blood glucose levels under control.
• Make wise food choices to help you feel good every day and to lose weight if needed.
Blood Glucose
• Check your blood glucose every day.
• Each time you check your blood glucose, write the number in a record book to share with your health care team.
• Treat low blood glucose quickly.
Physical Activity
• Even small amounts of physical activity help manage diabetes. Aim for 30 to 60 minutes of physical activity most days of the week. Children and adolescents with type 2 diabetes who are 10 to 17 years old should aim for 60 minutes of activity every day.

Role of the Individual in Helping Prevent Diabetes

Table 14.6. Continued

• Not all physical activity has to take place at the same time.
• Do aerobic activities, such as brisk walking, which use your large muscles to make your heart beat faster. The large muscles are those of the upper and lower arms and legs and those that control head, shoulder, and hip movements.
• Do activities to strengthen muscles and bone, such as lifting weights or sit-ups. Aim for two times a week.
• Stretch to increase your flexibility, lower stress, and help prevent muscle soreness after physical activity.
Steps
• Increase daily activity by decreasing time spent watching TV or at the computer. Children and adolescents should limit screen time not related to school to less than 2 hours per day. Limiting screen time can help you meet your physical activity goal.
• Always talk with your doctor before you start a new physical activity program.
Medicines
• Take your medicines as directed, including insulin if ordered by your doctor.
Feet
• Check your feet every day for cuts, blisters, sores, swelling, redness, or sore toe nails.
Mouth
• Brush and floss your teeth every day
Blood Pressure
• Control your blood pressure and cholesterol.
Smoking
• Don't smoke.

What should I discuss with my health care team at each checkup?

This table lists important things that you should discuss with your health care team at each checkup.

Table 14.7. Things to Discuss with Health Care Team

Things to Discuss with Your Health Care Team at Each Checkup	Make Sure to...
Blood glucose records and how you check your blood glucose	• Share your blood glucose records. Your health care team will ask to see how you are checking your blood glucose to make sure you are doing it right.
	• Mention if you often have low or high blood glucose.
Things to Discuss with Your Health Care Team at Each Checkup	**Make Sure to...**
Weight	• Talk about how much you should weigh.
	• Talk about ways to reach your weight goal that will work for you.
Blood pressure	• Talk about your blood pressure numbers.
Cholesterol	• Talk about your cholesterol numbers.
Medicines	• Talk about the medicines you are taking. Mention if you are having any problems.
	• Ask if you should take a low-dose aspirin every day to lower your risk for heart disease.
Feet	• Ask to have your feet checked for problems.
Physical activity plan	• Talk about what you do to stay active.
Meal plan	• Talk about what you eat, how much you eat, and when you eat.
Feelings	• Ask about ways to handle stress.
	• If you are feeling sad or unable to cope with problems, ask for help.
Smoking	• If you smoke, ask for help with quitting.
Mouth	• If you see signs of problems from diabetes in your mouth, tell your doctor and see your dentist.

Role of the Individual in Helping Prevent Diabetes

Prepare a blank record where you can keep track of your blood glucose test results, medicines, and notes about things that affect your blood glucose. Make one copy of the record for each week. This record will help you see whether your diabetes plan is working. Review your record with your health care team at each checkup.

How to use the Daily Diabetes Record

Follow this checklist when completing the daily diabetes record.

Blood Glucose Checks

- Talk with your health care team about the best times to check your blood glucose—before meals, after meals, or at bedtime. Write when to check your blood glucose at the top of the chart.
- Write down your target blood glucose numbers. If needed, record test results taken before and after a meal on either side of the line in the meal boxes. For instance, 180 / 150.
- Circle the blood glucose result each time you're above or below your target.

Medicines

- Under the heading marked "Medicines," write the names of your diabetes medicines and the amounts taken.

Notes

- Write down things that may affect your blood glucose numbers. Some examples are:
    - eating more or less than usual
    - forgetting to take your diabetes medicines
- physical activity—write down what kind and for how long
- being sick
- feeling upset about something—being under stress

Chapter 15

How Staying Healthy Can Help in the Prevention of Diabetes

Chapter Contents

Section 15.1—Keep Your Mouth Healthy 98
Section 15.2—Keep Your Teeth Healthy 102
Section 15.3—Keep Your Kidneys Healthy 104
Section 15.4—Keep Your Heart and Blood
               Vessels Healthy 111
Section 15.5—Keep Your Feet Healthy 115
Section 15.6—Keep Your Eyes Healthy 117

Section 15.1

Keep Your Mouth Healthy

Text in this section is excerpted from "Prevent Diabetes Problems: Keep Your Mouth Healthy," National Institute of Diabetes and Digestive and Kidney Diseases (NIDDK), National Institutes of Health (NIH), July 2014.

How can diabetes affect my mouth?

Too much glucose, also called sugar, in your blood from diabetes can cause pain, infection, and other problems in your mouth. Your mouth includes:

- your teeth
- your gums
- your jaw

tissues such as your tongue, the roof and bottom of your mouth, and the inside of your cheeks

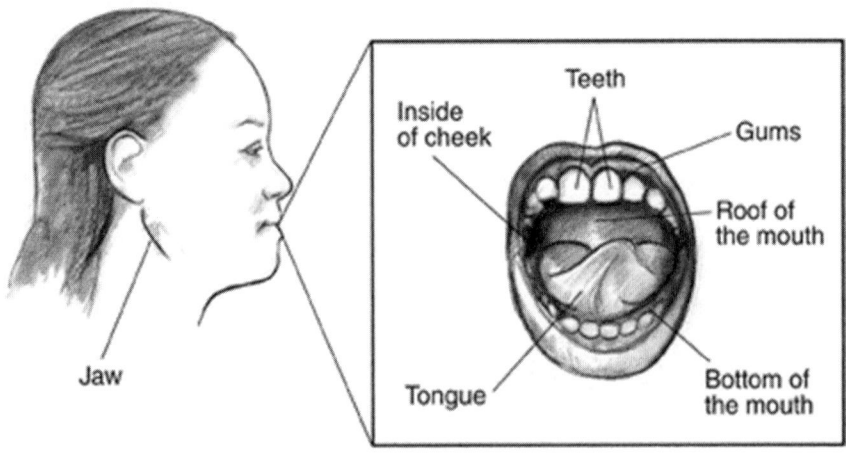

Figure 15.1. *Parts of Mouth*

How Staying Healthy Can Help in the Prevention of Diabetes

Glucose is present in your saliva—the fluid in your mouth that makes it wet. When diabetes is not controlled, high glucose levels in your saliva help harmful bacteria grow. These bacteria combine with food to form a soft, sticky film called plaque. Plaque also comes from eating foods that contain sugars or starches. Some types of plaque cause tooth decay or cavities. Other types of plaque cause gum disease and bad breath.

> high glucose levels = ◐ plaque

Gum disease can be more severe and take longer to heal if you have diabetes. In turn, having gum disease can make your blood glucose hard to control.

How will I know if I have mouth problems from diabetes?

Check your mouth for signs of problems from diabetes. If you notice any problems, see your dentist right away. Some of the first signs of gum disease are swollen, tender, or bleeding gums. Sometimes you won't have any signs of gum disease. You may not know you have it until you have serious damage. Your best defense is to see your dentist twice a year for a cleaning and checkup.

How can I prepare for a visit to my dentist?

Plan ahead. Talk with your doctor and dentist before the visit about the best way to take care of your blood glucose during dental work.

You may be taking a diabetes medicine that can cause low blood glucose, also called hypoglycemia. If you take insulin or other diabetes medicines, take them and eat as usual before visiting the dentist. You may need to bring your diabetes medicines and your snacks or meal with you to the dentist's office.

You may need to postpone any nonemergency dental work if your blood glucose is not under control.

If you feel nervous about visiting the dentist, tell your dentist and the staff about your feelings. Your dentist can adapt the treatment to your needs. Don't let your nerves stop you from having regular checkups. Waiting too long to take care of your mouth may make things worse.

What if my mouth is sore after my dental work?

A sore mouth is common after dental work. If this happens, you might not be able to eat or chew the foods you normally eat for several hours or days. For guidance on how to adjust your usual routine while your mouth is healing, ask your doctor:

- what foods and drinks you should have
- if you should change the time when you take your diabetes medicines
- if you should change the dose of your diabetes medicines
- how often you should check your blood glucose

How does smoking affect my mouth?

Smoking makes problems with your mouth worse. Smoking raises your chances of getting gum disease, oral and throat cancers, and oral fungal infections. Smoking also discolors your teeth and makes your breath smell bad.

Smoking and diabetes are a dangerous mix. Smoking raises your risk for many diabetes problems. If you quit smoking,

- you will lower your risk for heart attack, stroke, nerve disease, kidney disease, and amputation
- your cholesterol and blood pressure levels might improve
- your blood circulation will improve

If you smoke, stop smoking. Ask for help so that you don't have to do it alone. You can start by calling 1–800–QUITNOW or 1–800–784–8669.

How can I keep my mouth healthy?

You can keep your mouth healthy by taking these steps:

- Keep your blood glucose numbers as close to your target as possible. Your doctor will help you set your target blood glucose numbers and teach you what to do if your numbers are too high or too low.
- Eat healthy meals and follow the meal plan that you and your doctor or dietitian have worked out.

How Staying Healthy Can Help in the Prevention of Diabetes

- Brush your teeth at least twice a day with fluoride toothpaste. Fluoride protects against tooth decay.
- Aim for brushing first thing in the morning, before going to bed, and after each meal and sugary or starchy snack.
- Use a soft toothbrush.
- Gently brush your teeth with the toothbrush angled towards the gum line.
- Use small, circular motions.
- Brush the front, back, and top of each tooth. Brush your tongue, too.
- Change your toothbrush every 3 months or sooner if the toothbrush looks worn or the bristles spread out. A new toothbrush removes more plaque.
- Drink water that contains added fluoride or ask your dentist about using a fluoride mouth rinse to prevent tooth decay.
- Ask your dentist about using an anti-plaque or anti-gingivitis mouth rinse to control plaque or prevent gum disease.
- Use dental floss to clean between your teeth at least once a day. Flossing helps prevent plaque from building up on your teeth. When flossing,
  - slide the floss up and down and then curve it around the base of each tooth under the gums
  - use clean sections of floss as you move from tooth to tooth
- Another way of removing plaque between teeth is to use a dental pick or brush—thin tools designed to clean between the teeth. You can buy these picks at drug stores or grocery stores.
- If you wear dentures, keep them clean and take them out at night. Have them adjusted if they become loose or uncomfortable.
- Call your dentist right away if you have any symptoms of mouth problems.
- See your dentist twice a year for a cleaning and checkup. Your dentist may suggest more visits if you need them.
- Follow your dentist's advice.

- If your dentist tells you about a problem, take care of it right away.
- Follow any steps or treatments from your dentist to keep your mouth healthy.
- Tell your dentist that you have diabetes.
- Tell your dentist about any changes in your health or medicines.
- Share the results of some of your diabetes blood tests, such as the A1C test or the fasting blood glucose test.
- Ask if you need antibiotics before and after dental treatment if your diabetes is uncontrolled.
- If you smoke, stop smoking.

Section 15.2

Keep Your Teeth Healthy

Text in this section is excerpted from "Diabetes and You: Healthy Teeth Matter!" National Diabetes Education Program (NDEP), January 2014.

Tips to Keep Your Teeth Healthy

1. Get a dental exam at least once a year, and more often if your dentist says you need one. At your exam, your dentist or dental hygienist will:

- Explain how diabetes affects your teeth and gums.
- Check for problems, such as cavities or gum disease (see next page to learn the signs of gum disease).
- Treat any problems you have with your teeth or gums.
- Teach you how to check for signs of gum disease at home.
- Provide care, such as a fluoride treatment, to keep your mouth healthy.
- Tell you how to treat problems, such as dry mouth.

How Staying Healthy Can Help in the Prevention of Diabetes

2. Work with your dentist to create a health plan for your teeth.

- Ask the best way to take care of your teeth at home.
- Ask how often to come in for a dental visit.
- Ask what to do if you start to have problems with your teeth or gums.
- Ask your dentist to send your exam results to your other doctors after every visit.

3. Take care of your teeth at home.

- Brush with a soft-bristled toothbrush at least two times a day, using toothpaste with fluoride.
- Floss once a day.
- Visit a dentist if you think you have gum disease.
- Limit food and drinks that are high in sugar.

What Are the Signs of Gum Disease?

- Red, swollen, or bleeding gums
- Gums pulling away from teeth
- Sores on the gums
- Loose teeth or change in bite or tooth position
- Bad breath.

How Can Diabetes Harm Your Teeth?

- Diabetes is associated with gum disease, also known as periodontal disease.
- Gum disease can lead to tooth loss.
- Treatment of gum disease in people with type 2 diabetes can lower blood sugar over time.
- Gum disease treatment can lower your chance of having other problems from diabetes, such as heart and kidney disease.
- Gum disease may increase the risk of type 2 diabetes.

> **To-do List for Healthy Teeth**
>
> - Get a dental exam at least once a year.
> - Keep your next dental appointment.
> - Check your mouth for red and swollen gums, bleeding gums, loose teeth, a change in how your bite feels, or bad breath.
> - Ask your dental provider if you are doing a good job of taking care of your teeth and gums at home.
> - Ask your dentist to send your test results to your other doctors after every visit.
> - Keep your blood sugar at a healthy level.

Section 15.3

Keep Your Kidneys Healthy

> Text in this section is excerpted from "Prevent Diabetes Problems: Keep Your Kidneys Healthy," National Institute of Diabetes and Digestive and Kidney Diseases (NIDDK), National Institutes of Health (NIH), February 2014.

What are my kidneys and what do they do?

Your kidneys are two bean-shaped organs, each about the size of a fist. They are located just below your rib cage, one on each side of your spine. Every day, your two kidneys filter about 120 to 150 quarts of blood to produce about 1 to 2 quarts of urine. Urine flows from your kidneys to your bladder through tubes called ureters. Your bladder stores urine until releasing it through urination.

How can diabetes affect my kidneys?

Too much glucose, also called sugar, in your blood from diabetes damages your kidneys' filters. If the filters are damaged, a protein

How Staying Healthy Can Help in the Prevention of Diabetes

called albumin, which you need to stay healthy, leaks out of your blood and into your urine. Damaged kidneys do not do a good job of filtering wastes and extra fluid from your blood. The wastes and extra fluid build up in your blood and make you sick.

Diabetes is a leading cause of kidney disease. Diabetic kidney disease is the medical term for kidney disease caused by diabetes. Diabetic kidney disease affects both kidneys at the same time.

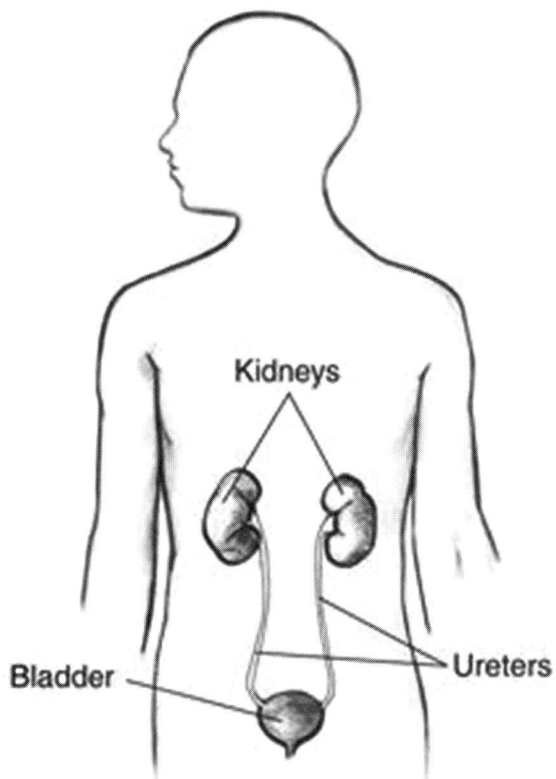

Figure 15.2. *Kidneys*

If kidney disease runs in your family, you are also at risk for kidney disease. Talk with your family members about their medical history and your doctor about having your kidney function tested.

What are blood pressure and high blood pressure?

Blood pressure is the force of blood flow inside your blood vessels. Blood pressure is written with two numbers separated by a slash. For example, a blood pressure result of 130/80 is said as "130 over 80." The first number is the pressure in your blood vessels as your heart beats and pushes blood through your blood vessels. The second number is the pressure as your blood vessels relax between heartbeats.

High blood pressure forces your heart to work harder to pump blood. High blood pressure can strain your heart, damage your blood vessels, and increase your risk of heart attack, stroke, eye problems, and kidney problems.

How does high blood pressure affect my kidneys if I have diabetes?

High blood pressure is the other leading cause of kidney disease in people with diabetes. High blood pressure also is a result of damage from kidney disease. If you have high blood pressure, your kidneys may already be damaged. Even a small rise in blood pressure can quickly make kidney disease worse.

What should my blood pressure be?

Your blood pressure goal should either be below 140/80 or 140/90 depending on whether you have kidney disease and how severe it is. Discuss your personal goal with your doctor.

Many people with diabetes have high blood pressure. However, keeping your blood pressure at your goal will help prevent damage to your kidneys, heart, brain, blood vessels, and other parts of your body. Meal planning, medicines, and physical activity can help you reach your blood pressure goal.

> **Have your blood pressure checked**
>
> Have your blood pressure checked at every health care visit. Ask your doctor if you need medicine to control your blood pressure. Medicine that helps control your blood pressure can slow progression of kidney disease.

How Staying Healthy Can Help in the Prevention of Diabetes

Two types of blood pressure-lowering medicines, angiotensin-converting enzyme (ACE) inhibitors and angiotensin receptor blockers (ARBs), have been found to slow progression of kidney disease in people with diabetes.

What are the symptoms of diabetic kidney disease?

In the early stages, diabetic kidney disease does not have any symptoms. Kidney disease happens so slowly that you may not feel sick at all for many years. You may not feel sick even when your kidneys do only half the job of healthy kidneys. Only your doctor can tell if you have kidney disease by checking the protein, or albumin, level in your urine at least once a year.

The first symptom of diabetic kidney disease is often swelling in parts of your body, such as your hands, face, feet, or ankles. Also, large amounts of protein in your urine may cause urine to look foamy. Once your kidney function starts to decrease, other symptoms may include:

- increased or decreased urination
- feeling drowsy or tired
- feeling itchy or numb
- dry skin
- headaches
- weight loss
- not feeling hungry
- feeling sick to your stomach
- vomiting
- sleep problems
- trouble staying focused
- darkened skin
- muscle cramps

How can I find out if I have diabetic kidney disease?

The following tests can tell you and your doctor if you have diabetic kidney disease:

Blood pressure test

- Your doctor will use a blood pressure cuff to check your blood pressure. You should have this test done at every health care visit.

Albumin and creatinine measurement

Your doctor will ask you for a sample of your urine to look for albumin. A high level of albumin in your urine may mean you have kidney disease. The urine sample is sent to a lab for a test that looks at the amount of albumin compared with the amount of creatinine, a waste product also in your urine. A urine albumin-to-creatinine ratio test result above 30 is a warning sign of kidney disease. You should have this test at least once a year.

Estimated glomerular filtration rate (eGFR) test.

- Blood drawn at your doctor's office and sent to a lab can be tested to measure how much blood your kidneys filter each minute. If your kidneys are not filtering enough blood, you may have kidney damage or kidney failure. You should have this test at least once a year. The test results show the following:
    - eGFR of 60 or above is in the normal range
    - eGFR below 60 may mean you have kidney disease
    - eGFR of 15 or below may mean you have kidney failure

If your blood and urine test results show evidence of kidney damage or disease, your doctor may suggest more tests to help find out whether you have other health problems causing the damage. Other tests can include blood and urine samples for additional lab tests and imaging tests, or pictures, of your kidneys. Your doctor also may need to perform a biopsy, in which a small piece of tissue is removed from your kidney to look at with a microscope.

What can I do if I have diabetic kidney disease?

Once you have diabetic kidney disease, you can slow it down or stop it from getting worse by watching your blood glucose and blood pressure numbers closely to keep them under control.

If you have high blood pressure or protein in your urine, you can take an ACE inhibitor or ARB to control your blood pressure and reduce kidney damage. If you are pregnant, you should not take an ACE inhibitor or ARB.

See your doctor often. Have your urine and blood tested as your doctor advises to see how well your kidneys are working. You also may need to see a nephrologist—a doctor who specializes in kidney disease.

How does smoking affect my diabetes and kidneys?

If you already have kidney disease, smoking can worsen any blood vessel, heart, and kidney problems. Kidney cancer is also more common in smokers.

How Staying Healthy Can Help in the Prevention of Diabetes

Smoking and diabetes are a dangerous mix. Smoking raises your risk for many diabetes problems. If you quit smoking,

- you will lower your risk for heart attack, stroke, nerve disease, kidney disease, and amputation, which is surgery to cut off a body part
- your cholesterol and blood pressure levels might improve
- your blood circulation will improve

If you smoke, stop smoking. Ask for help so that you don't have to do it alone. You can start by calling 1–800–QUITNOW or 1–800–784–8669.

How can I keep my kidneys healthy?

You can keep your kidneys healthy by taking these steps:

- Keep your blood glucose numbers as close to your target as possible. Your doctor will work with you to set your target blood glucose numbers and teach you what to do if your numbers are too high or too low.
- Keep your blood pressure numbers as close to your personal goal as possible. If you take blood pressure medicine, take it as your doctor advises.
- Eat healthy meals and follow the meal plan that you and your doctor or dietitian have worked out. If you already have kidney disease, you may have to avoid a diet high in protein, fat, sodium, and potassium.
- If you choose hemodialysis, watch how much liquid you drink. Your dietitian will help you figure out how much liquid to drink each day.
- At least once a year, have these tests for kidney disease:
  - blood pressure test
  - albumin and creatinine measurement
  - eGFR
- Have any other kidney tests your doctor thinks you need.
- Avoid taking painkillers often. Daily use of nonsteroidal anti-inflammatory drugs, such as the arthritis-type painkillers ibuprofen and naproxen, can damage your kidneys. If you are dealing

with chronic, or long lasting, pain from a health problem such as arthritis, work with your doctor to find a way to control your pain without putting your kidneys at risk.
- See a doctor right away for bladder or kidney infections.
- You may have an infection if you have these symptoms:
  - pain or burning when you urinate
  - a frequent urge to urinate
  - urine that looks cloudy, reddish, or dark
  - fever or a shaky feeling
  - pain in your back or on your side below your ribs
- If you smoke, stop smoking.

Eating, Diet, and Nutrition

Your dietitian or doctor may suggest a special eating plan for you. You may have to avoid a diet high in protein, fat, sodium, and potassium.

Cut back on protein, especially animal products such as meat.

- Damaged kidneys may fail to remove protein waste products from your blood. Diets high in protein make your kidneys work harder and fail sooner.

Avoid a high-fat diet.

- High-fat diets are high in cholesterol. Cholesterol is a type of fat found in your body's cells, blood, and many foods. Your body needs some cholesterol to work the right way. For example, your body uses cholesterol to make certain essential hormones and maintain nerve function. However, your body makes all the cholesterol it needs. If you often eat foods that are high in cholesterol, or if high cholesterol runs in your family, extra cholesterol in your blood can build up over time in the walls of your blood vessels and arteries. High blood cholesterol can lead to heart disease and stroke, some of the biggest health problems for people with diabetes.

Avoid high-sodium foods.

- Sodium is a mineral found in salt and other foods. High levels of sodium may raise your blood pressure. Some high-sodium foods include canned food, frozen dinners, and hot dogs. The amount of sodium is listed on the food label, so you can see which foods have the highest levels. Try to limit your sodium to less than a teaspoon a day, or about 2,300 milligrams (mg) a day. If you have high blood pressure or are African American, middle-aged, or older, aim for no more than 1,500 mg of sodium per day. Ask your doctor or your dietitian about how much sodium you can have.

Ask your doctor about the amount of potassium you need.
- Potassium is a mineral that helps your heartbeat stay regular and muscles work right. Healthy kidneys keep the right amount of potassium in your body. However, if you have severe kidney damage, high levels of potassium may cause an abnormal heart rhythm or even make your heart stop, called cardiac arrest. Some high-potassium foods include apricots, bananas, oranges, and potatoes.

Section 15.4

Keep Your Heart and Blood Vessels Healthy

Text in this section is excerpted from "Prevent Diabetes Problems: Keep Your Heart and Blood Vessels Healthy," National Institute of Diabetes and Digestive and Kidney Diseases (NIDDK), National Institutes of Health (NIH), August 2013.

What do my heart and blood vessels do?

Your heart and blood vessels make up your circulatory system. Your heart is a muscle that pumps blood through your body. Your heart pumps blood carrying oxygen to large blood vessels, called arteries, and small blood vessels, called capillaries. Other blood vessels, called veins, carry blood back to the heart.

How do my blood vessels get clogged?

Several things, including having diabetes, can make your blood cholesterol level too high. Cholesterol is a substance that is made by the body and used for many important functions. Cholesterol is also found in some food derived from animals. When cholesterol is too high, the insides of large blood vessels become narrowed or clogged. This problem is called atherosclerosis.

Narrowed and clogged blood vessels make it harder for enough blood to get to all parts of your body. This condition can cause problems.

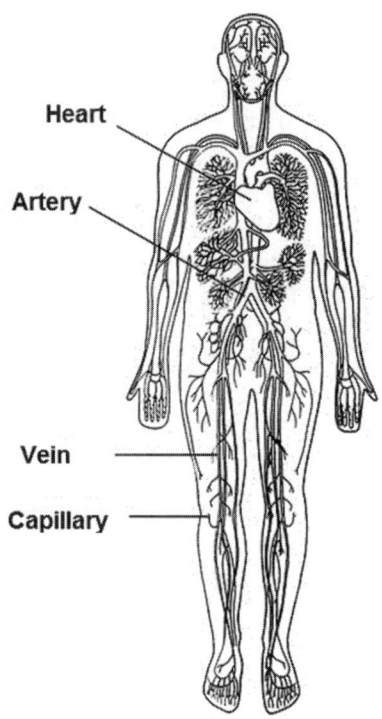

Figure 15.3. *Blood Vessels In Human Body*

What can happen when blood vessels are clogged?

When blood vessels become narrowed and clogged, you can have serious health problems:

Chest pain, also called angina

- When you have angina, you feel pain in your chest, arms, shoulders, or back. You may feel the pain more when your heart beats faster, such as when you exercise. The pain may go away when you rest. You also may sweat a lot and feel very weak. If you do

How Staying Healthy Can Help in the Prevention of Diabetes

not get treatment, chest pain may happen more often. If diabetes has damaged your heart nerves, you may not feel the chest pain. If you have chest pain with activity, contact your doctor.

Heart attack

- A heart attack happens when a blood vessel in or near your heart becomes blocked. Then your heart muscle can't get enough blood. When an area of your heart muscle stops working, your heart becomes weaker. During a heart attack, you may have chest pain along with nausea, indigestion, extreme weakness, and sweating. Or you may have no symptoms at all. If you have chest pain that persists, call 911. Delay in getting treatment may make a heart attack worse.

Stroke

- A stroke can happen when the blood supply to your brain is blocked. Then your brain can be damaged.

Cross section of a healthy blood vessel

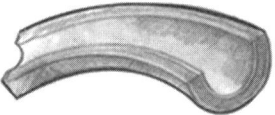

Cross section of a narrowed blood vessel

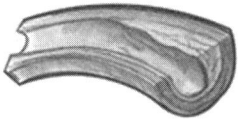

Figure 15.4. *Cross section of healthy and narrowed blood vessel*

How do narrowed blood vessels cause high blood pressure?

Narrowed blood vessels leave a smaller opening for blood to flow through. Having narrowed blood vessels is like turning on a garden hose and holding your thumb over the opening. The smaller opening makes the water shoot out with more pressure. In the same way, narrowed blood vessels lead to high blood pressure. Other factors, such as kidney problems and being overweight, also can lead to high blood pressure.

Many people with diabetes also have high blood pressure. If you have heart, eye, or kidney problems from diabetes, high blood pressure can make them worse.

You will see your blood pressure written with two numbers separated by a slash. For example, your reading might be 120/70, said as "120 over 70." For most people with diabetes, the target is to keep the first number below 140 and the second number below 80, unless their doctor sets a different target.

If you have high blood pressure, ask your doctor how to lower it. Your doctor may ask you to take blood pressure medicine every day. Some types of blood pressure medicine can also help keep your kidneys healthy.

You may also be able to control your blood pressure by:

- eating more fruits and vegetables
- eating less salt and high-sodium foods
- losing weight if you need to
- being physically active
- not smoking
- limiting alcoholic drinks

How can clogged blood vessels hurt my legs and feet?

Peripheral arterial disease, also called PAD, can happen when the openings in your blood vessels become narrow and your legs and feet don't get enough blood. You may feel pain in your legs when you walk or exercise. Some people also have numbness or tingling in their feet or legs or have sores that heal slowly.

What can I do to prevent or control PAD?

- Don't smoke.
- Keep blood glucose and blood pressure under control.
- Keep blood fats close to normal.
- Be physically active.
- Ask your doctor if you should take aspirin every day.

You also may need surgery to treat PAD.

Section 15.5

Keep Your Feet Healthy

Text in this section is excerpted from "Diabetes and You: Healthy Feet Matter!" National Diabetes Education Program (NDEP), January 2014.

How can diabetes harm your feet?

- Diabetes is the main cause for nontraumatic loss of a toe, foot, or leg. Almost half of these cases could be prevented with daily foot care.
- People who have diabetes can lose feeling in their feet. When that happens, it can be hard to tell when you have a problem, like a blister, sore, callus, or cut on your foot.
- Diabetes can reduce the amount of blood flow to your feet.
- Numbness and less blood flow in the feet can slow the time it takes for sores to heal and can lead to foot problems.

What is a podiatrist?

A podiatrist is a medical doctor who specializes in finding and treating foot and ankle problems.

Tips to keep your feet healthy

Have a podiatrist check your feet at least once a year.

Work with your podiatrist to create a foot care plan to help you take care of your feet.

Ask your podiatrist if you qualify for special shoes. These might be covered by Medicare or other insurance plans.

Ask your podiatrist to send your exam results to your other doctors after every visit.

Be sure to keep your next podiatrist appointment!

Check your feet every day.

Set a time every day to look at your bare feet for calluses, cuts, sores, blisters, red spots, and swelling.

Use a mirror to check the bottoms of your feet if you have trouble seeing your feet. You can also ask a family member to help you.

Wash your feet every day.

Use warm water, not hot, to wash your feet. Do not soak your feet.

Always check bath water with your hands first to make sure it is not too hot. Sometimes people with diabetes cannot feel how hot the water is with their feet.

Dry your feet well. Be sure to dry between the toes.

Keep the skin soft and smooth.

Rub a thin coat of lotion over the tops and bottoms of your feet.

Do not put lotion between your toes. Wetness between your toes can cause an infection.

Check with a podiatrist about the best way to trim your toenails and to care for corns and calluses.

Over-the-counter products for corns and calluses or sharp objects may harm your skin. Do not use them.

Wear shoes and socks at all times.

Do not walk barefoot. It is easy to step on something and hurt your feet.

Wear shoes that fit well and protect your feet.

Check inside your shoes before you put them on to make sure the lining is smooth and there are no objects in them.

Protect your feet from hot and cold.

Wear shoes at the beach and on hot pavement.

Do not use hot water bottles or heating pads on your feet. You may burn your feet.

Keep the blood in your feet flowing.

Put your feet up on a chair, couch, or footrest when sitting.

How Staying Healthy Can Help in the Prevention of Diabetes

Wiggle your toes and move your ankles up and down for 5 minutes, two or three times a day.

Do not cross your legs for long periods of time.

To-do List for Healthy Feet

- Have a podiatrist examine your feet at least once a year.
- Keep your next podiatrist appointment.
- Ask your podiatrist to send your test results to your other doctors after every visit.
- Ask your primary care provider to check your feet at every visit.
- Check your feet every day.
- Keep your blood sugar at a healthy level.

Section 15.6

Keep Your Eyes Healthy

Text in this section is excerpted from "Prevent Diabetes Problems: Keep Your Eyes Healthy," National Institute of Diabetes and Digestive and Kidney Diseases, (NIDDK), National Institutes of Health (NIH), July 2014.

How can diabetes affect my eyes?

Too much glucose, also called sugar, in your blood from diabetes can damage four parts of your eye:

Retina.

- The retina is the tissue that lines the back of your eye. The retina converts light coming into your eye into visual messages through the optic nerve to your brain. The macula is the small, sensitive, center part of the retina that gives sharp, detailed vision.

Lens

- The lens of your eye is clear and is located behind the iris, the colored part of your eye. The lens helps to focus light, or an image, on the retina.

Vitreous gel

- The vitreous gel is a clear, colorless mass that fills the rear of your eye, between the retina and lens.

Optic nerve.

- The optic nerve, at the back of your eye, is your eye's largest sensory nerve. The optic nerve connects your eye to your brain, carries visual messages from the retina to your brain, and sends messages between your brain and your eye muscles.

Diabetes damage to your eyes—called diabetic eye disease—can cause permanent vision loss, including low vision and blindness. Low vision means that even with regular glasses, contact lenses, medicine, or surgery, you can't see well enough to easily complete everyday tasks.

How does diabetes affect the retina?

Over time, having high blood glucose levels from diabetes can damage the tiny blood vessels on the retina. Diabetic retinopathy is the medical term for damage to the retina from diabetes.

Retina damage happens slowly. First, the retina's blood vessels swell. As retina damage worsens, the blood vessels become blocked and cut off the retina's oxygen supply. In response, new, weak blood vessels grow on the retina and the surface of the vitreous gel. These blood vessels break easily and leak blood into the vitreous gel. The leaking blood keeps light from reaching the retina.

When that happens, you may see floating spots or almost total darkness. One of your eyes may be damaged more than the other, or both eyes may have the same amount of damage. Sometimes the blood clears out by itself. However, you might need surgery to remove the blood.

Over the years, the swollen and weak blood vessels can form scar tissue and pull the retina away from the back of your eye. If the retina pulls away, a condition called detached retina, you may see floating spots or flashing lights. You may feel as if a curtain has been pulled

How Staying Healthy Can Help in the Prevention of Diabetes

over part of what you are looking at. A detached retina can cause vision loss or blindness if you don't take care of it quickly. See an ophthalmologist—a doctor who diagnoses and treats all eye diseases—right away if you have these symptoms.

Some people with diabetic retinopathy also have a problem called macular edema. Macular edema, or swelling, can happen in any stage of retinopathy. Swelling in the macula is caused by leaking fluid from the retina's damaged blood vessels.

Macular edema is the most common cause of vision loss for people with diabetes. Your vision loss can be mild to severe if the edema is not treated, so it is important to have an eye exam at least once a year. You can have an eye exam with an ophthalmologist or an optometrist—a primary eye care provider who prescribes glasses and contact lenses and diagnoses and treats certain conditions and diseases of the eye.

What are the symptoms of diabetes retina problems?

Often, no symptoms appear during the early stages of diabetes retina problems. As retina problems worsen, your symptoms might include:

- blurry or double vision
- rings, flashing lights, or blank spots in your vision
- dark or floating spots in your vision
- pain or pressure in one or both of your eyes
- trouble seeing things out of the corners of your eyes

How can my eye doctor tell whether I have diabetes retina problems?

Your eye doctor can tell whether you have diabetes retina problems during a dilated eye exam. In a dilated eye exam, your eye doctor will use eye drops to enlarge your pupils. Your pupil is the opening at the center of the iris.

Enlarging your pupils allows your eye doctor to see more of the inside of your eyes to check for signs of disease. Your eye doctor will use a special magnifying lens to look at your retina and optic nerve for signs of damage and other eye problems.

At the time of your dilated eye exam, your eye doctor also will conduct other tests to measure:

- pressure in your eyes
- your side, or peripheral, vision
- how well you see at various distances

Have a dilated eye exam at least once a year, even if your vision seems fine. Regular exams can prevent most instances of severe vision loss or blindness from diabetes eye problems. These exams can also help you protect your vision and make sure you are seeing at your best.

You may need to see an ophthalmologist to have a test called an eye angiogram.

For this test, you will be given eye drops to dilate your pupils. You will be asked to place your chin on a camera's chin rest and your forehead against a support bar to keep your head still during the test. Your ophthalmologist will take pictures of the insides of your eyes. A dye is injected into a vein in your arm. As the dye reaches your eyes and moves through your eyes' blood vessels, the camera takes more pictures.

This test will show whether you have abnormal or leaking blood vessels on your retina and help your ophthalmologist decide the best treatment.

Will I have diabetes retina problems?

The longer you've had diabetes, the more likely you are to have diabetes retina problems. You are less likely to have diabetes retina problems, or will have milder problems if you have them, if you keep your blood glucose numbers close to your targets. Targets are numbers you aim for.

Does pregnancy affect diabetes retina problems?

Changes in your body during pregnancy might cause diabetes retina problems to occur or worsen.

If you have diabetes and are planning to get pregnant soon, you should have a dilated eye exam and talk with your eye doctor about diabetes retina problems. If you need surgery for your eyes, you may want to have it before you get pregnant.

How Staying Healthy Can Help in the Prevention of Diabetes

If you have diabetes and are already pregnant, you should have a dilated eye exam during your first 3 months of pregnancy or as soon as possible. Talk with your eye doctor about how often you should have dilated eye exams throughout your pregnancy to keep your eyes healthy.

If you have gestational diabetes, a type of diabetes that develops only during pregnancy, you do not have an increased risk of getting diabetic retinopathy unless the diabetes continues after your pregnancy.

What other eye problems can occur in people with diabetes?

People with diabetes can have the following eye problems more often and at a younger age than people who do not have diabetes:

Cataract

- A cataract is a clouding of the normally clear lens that causes blurry vision. You need surgery to remove a cataract. During surgery, the ophthalmologist takes the lens out and puts in a plastic lens that is similar to a contact lens. The plastic lens stays in your eye permanently.

Glaucoma

- Glaucoma is a group of diseases that may be caused by an increase in eye pressure. Glaucoma can damage the optic nerve and result in vision loss and blindness. People with diabetes are more likely to get a severe type of glaucoma in which abnormal blood vessels grow in the front part of your eye. Your ophthalmologist will treat glaucoma with eye drops, pills, or surgery to control your eye pressure.

Neuropathy

- Neuropathy is nerve damage. Damage to the nerves in the feet or legs is the most common nerve damage from diabetes. However, diabetes can also affect the nerves to the eye. Having high blood glucose from diabetes causes decreased blood supply to the optic nerve. You may suddenly have double vision, drooping of your eyelid, or pain over your eye. Some people have full or partial paralysis of their eye muscles. This type of neuropathy tends to improve by itself over a period of weeks to months. If it doesn't, you may need to wear a patch over one eye or use a special lens to try to align your eyes.

What can I do if I already have some vision loss from diabetes retina problems?

If you already have some vision loss from diabetes retina problems that cannot be corrected by treatment, ask your eye doctor about low vision services and devices that can help you make the most of your remaining vision. Ask for a referral to a specialist in low vision. Many community organizations and agencies offer information about low vision counseling and training, and other special services for people with vision problems.

How can I keep my eyes healthy?

You can keep your eyes healthy by taking these steps:

- Keep your blood glucose numbers as close to your targets as you can. Improving your blood glucose numbers can greatly lower your risk for retinopathy. Your doctor will work with you to set your target blood glucose numbers and teach you what to do if your numbers are too high or too low.

- Keep your blood pressure as close to your target as you can. High blood pressure can damage the tiny blood vessels on the retina. Have your blood pressure checked at every medical visit. Ask your doctor whether you need medicine or a combination of medicines to control your blood pressure. If your doctor prescribes blood pressure medicine, take it regularly.

- Have a healthy diet and be physically active to reduce your need for medicines to control your blood glucose, blood pressure, cholesterol, and triglycerides.

- If you smoke, stop smoking.

- Call your eye doctor right away if you have any signs of eye problems, especially sudden vision loss.

- Have a dilated eye exam at least once a year, even if your vision seems fine.

Chapter 16

Diabetes Prevention – Questions for Your Doctor

Talk with your doctor or nurse about steps you can take to prevent type 2 diabetes.

Type 2 Diabetes – What do I ask the doctor?

Visiting the doctor can be stressful. It helps to have questions written down before your appointment. Print out this list of questions, and take it with you the next time you visit the doctor. Take notes to help you remember your doctor's answers.

- Am I at risk for prediabetes or type 2 diabetes?
- How can I find out if I have diabetes?
- Are there any warning signs of diabetes I should watch for?
- Does my weight put me at risk for diabetes?
- If I'm overweight, how many pounds do I need to lose to prevent or delay diabetes?
- How much physical activity should I get to prevent or delay diabetes?

This chapter includes excerpts from "Preventing Diabetes: Questions for the doctor," Office of Disease Prevention and Health Promotion (ODPHP), July 30, 2015; and text from "Gestational Diabetes Screening: Questions for the doctor," Office of Disease Prevention and Health Promotion (ODPHP), March 30, 2015.

- What changes can I make to my diet to prevent or delay diabetes?
- What are some healthy ways to lose weight and keep it off?
- What are my blood pressure numbers and cholesterol levels, and what should they be?
- Do my blood pressure numbers and cholesterol levels put me at risk for diabetes?
- Is there any information about preventing diabetes that I could take home?
- Are there any local diabetes prevention programs that you could recommend?

Getting tested for gestational diabetes is part of regular prenatal care (care during pregnancy). The test is usually done between 24 and 28 weeks of pregnancy.

Under the Affordable Care Act, health insurance plans must cover testing for gestational diabetes. Depending on your plan, you may be able to get screened at no cost to you.

Gestational Diabetes – What do I ask the doctor?

Visiting the doctor can be stressful. It helps to have questions written down before your appointment. Print this list of questions, and take it with you the next time you visit your doctor or midwife.

- What puts me at risk for gestational diabetes?
- What can I do to lower my risk?
- How will you test me for gestational diabetes?
- How could gestational diabetes affect my baby's health?
- How could gestational diabetes affect my health?
- If I have gestational diabetes, what happens next?

Chapter 17

Team Care Approach for Diabetes Management

A team approach to diabetes care can effectively help people cope with the vast array of complications that can arise from diabetes. People with diabetes can lower their risk for microvascular complications, such as eye disease and kidney disease; macrovascular complications, such as heart disease and stroke; and other diabetes complications, such as nerve damage, by:

- Controlling their ABCs (A1C, blood pressure, cholesterol, and smoking cessation).
- Following an individualized meal plan.
- Engaging in regular physical activity.
- Avoiding tobacco use.
- Taking medicines as prescribed.
- Coping effectively with the demands of a complex chronic disease.

Text in this chapter is excerpted from "Working Together to Manage Diabetes: A Guide for Pharmacy, Podiatry, Optometry, and Dentistry," Centers for Disease Control and Prevention (CDC), January 2014.

Patients who increase their use of effective behavioral interventions to lower the risk of diabetes—and treatments to improve glycemic control and cardiovascular risk profiles—can prevent or delay progression to kidney failure, vision loss, nerve damage, lower-extremity amputation, and cardiovascular disease. This in turn can lead to increased patient satisfaction with care, better quality of life, improved health outcomes, and ultimately, lower health care costs.

PPOD and the Team Approach

PPOD providers (Pharmacy, Podiatry, Optometry, and Dentistry) are well positioned to advise and educate patients about diabetes and play an integral role in the team care approach to diabetes care. A multidisciplinary team approach is critical to success in diabetes care and complications prevention. Evidence indicates that a team approach:

- Can facilitate diabetes management.
- Can lower the risk for chronic disease complications.
- Help educate about ways to reduce risk factors for type 2 diabetes.

There are many other possible members of the health care team in addition to physicians (e.g., primary care, endocrinologist, obstetrician-gynecologist, and ophthalmologist). This team could include (but is not limited to):

- Pharmacists
- Podiatrists
- Optometrists
- Dental care professionals
- Primary care physicians
- Physician assistants
- Nurse practitioners
- Dietitians
- Certified diabetes educators
- Community health workers
- Mental health professionals

Team Care Approach for Diabetes Management

Clinical care teams can be augmented by including the resources and support of community partners such as:

- School nurses
- Trained peer leaders

All of these team members play important roles in the delivery of care for people with diabetes.

Chapter 18

Tips to Prevent Type 2 Diabetes

Reduce Portion Sizes

Portion size is the amount of food you eat, such as 1 cup of fruit or 6 ounces of meat. If you are trying to eat smaller portions, eat a half of a bagel instead of a whole bagel or have a 3-ounce hamburger instead of a 6-ounce hamburger. Three ounces is about the size of your fist or a deck of cards.

1. Drink a large glass of water 10 minutes before your meal so you feel less hungry.
2. Keep meat, chicken, turkey, and fish portions to about 3 ounces.
3. Share one dessert.
4. Use teaspoons, salad forks, or child-size forks, spoons, and knives to help you take smaller bites and eat less.
5. Make less food look like more by serving your meal on a salad or breakfast plate.

Text in this chapter is excerpted from "Choose More than 50 Ways to Prevent Type 2 Diabetes," National Diabetes Education Program (NDEP), September 1, 2014.

6. Eat slowly. It takes 20 minutes for your stomach to send a signal to your brain that you are full.

7. Listen to music while you eat instead of watching TV (people tend to eat more while watching TV).

Move More Each Day

Find ways to be more active each day. Try to be active for at least 30 minutes, 5 days a week. Walking is a great way to get started and you can do it almost anywhere at any time. Bike riding, swimming, and dancing are also good ways to move more.

If you are looking for a safe place to be active, contact your local parks department or health department to ask about walking maps, community centers, and nearby parks.

8. Show your kids the dances you used to do when you were their age.

9. Turn up the music and jam while doing household chores.

10. Work out with a video that shows you how to get active.

11. Deliver a message in person to a co-worker instead of sending an e-mail.

12. Take the stairs to your office. Or take the stairs as far as you can, and then take the elevator the rest of the way.

13. Catch up with friends during a walk instead of by phone.

14. March in place while you watch TV.

15. Choose a place to walk that is safe, such as your local mall.

16. Get off of the bus one stop early and walk the rest of the way home or to work if it is safe.

17. Buy a mix of vegetables when you go food shopping.

18. Choose veggie toppings like spinach, broccoli, and peppers for your pizza.

19. Try eating foods from other countries. Many of these dishes have more vegetables, whole grains, and beans.

20. Buy frozen and low-salt (sodium) canned vegetables. They may cost less and keep longer than fresh ones.

Tips to Prevent Type 2 Diabetes

21. Serve your favorite vegetable and a salad with low-fat macaroni and cheese.
22. Stir fry, broil, or bake with non-stick spray or low-salt broth. Cook with less oil and butter.
23. Try not to snack while cooking or cleaning the kitchen.
24. Cook with smaller amounts of cured meats (smoked turkey and turkey bacon). They are high in salt.
25. Cook with a mix of spices instead of salt.
26. Try different recipes for baking or broiling meat, chicken, and fish.
27. Choose foods with little or no added sugar to reduce calories.
28. Choose brown rice instead of white rice.
29. Have a big vegetable salad with low-calorie salad dressing when eating out. Share your main dish with a friend or have the other half wrapped to go.
30. Make healthy choices at fast food restaurants. Try grilled chicken (with skin removed) instead of a cheeseburger.
31. Skip the fries and chips and choose a salad.
32. Order a fruit salad instead of ice cream or cake.
33. Find a water bottle you really like (from a church or club event, favorite sports team, etc.) and drink water from it every day.
34. Peel and eat an orange instead of drinking orange juice.
35. If you drink whole milk, try changing to 2% milk. It has less fat than whole milk. Once you get used to 2% milk, try 1% or fat-free (skim) milk. This will help you reduce the amount of fat and calories you take in each day.
36. Drink water instead of juice and regular soda.
37. Make at least half of your grains whole grains, such as whole grain breads and cereals, brown rice, and quinoa.
38. Use whole grain bread for toast and sandwiches.
39. Keep a healthy snack with you, such as fresh fruit, a handful of nuts, and whole grain crackers.

40. Slow down at snack time. Eating a bag of low-fat popcorn takes longer than eating a candy bar.
41. Share a bowl of fruit with family and friends.
42. Eat a healthy snack or meal before shopping for food. Do not shop on an empty stomach.
43. Shop at your local farmers market for fresh, local food.
44. Make a list of food you need to buy before you go to the store.
45. Keep a written record of what you eat for a week. It can help you see when you tend to overeat or eat foods high in fat or calories.
46. Compare food labels on packages.
47. Choose foods lower in saturated fats, trans fats, cholesterol (ko-LESS-tuh-ruhl), calories, salt, and added sugars.

Take Care of Your Mind, Body, and Soul

48. Take time to change the way you eat and get active. Try one new food or activity a week.
49. Find ways to relax. Try deep breathing, taking a walk, or listening to your favorite music.
50. Pamper yourself. Read a book, take a long bath, or meditate.
51. Think before you eat. Try not to eat when you are bored, upset, or unhappy.

Be Creative

Honor your health as your most precious gift. There are many more ways to prevent or delay type 2 diabetes by making healthy food choices and moving more. Discover your own and share them with your family, friends, and neighbors.

Chapter 19

Diagnosis of Diabetes

How are diabetes and prediabetes diagnosed?

Blood tests are used to diagnosis diabetes and prediabetes because early in the disease type 2 diabetes may have no symptoms. All diabetes blood tests involve drawing blood at a health care provider's office or commercial facility and sending the sample to a lab for analysis. Lab analysis of blood is needed to ensure test results are accurate. Glucose measuring devices used in a health care provider's office, such as finger-stick devices, are not accurate enough for diagnosis but may be used as a quick indicator of high blood glucose.

Testing enables health care providers to find and treat diabetes before complications occur and to find and treat prediabetes, which can delay or prevent type 2 diabetes from developing.

Any one of the following tests can be used for diagnosis:*

- An A1C test, also called the hemoglobin A1C, HbA1C, or glycohemoglobin test
- A fasting plasma glucose (FPG) test
- An oral glucose tolerance test (OGTT)

*Not all tests are recommended for diagnosing all types of diabetes. See the individual test descriptions for details.

Text in this chapter is excerpted from "Diagnosis of Diabetes and Prediabetes," National Institute of Diabetes and Digestive and Kidney Diseases (NIDDK), National Institutes of Health (NIH), June 2014.

Another blood test, the random plasma glucose (RPG) test, is sometimes used to diagnose diabetes during a regular health checkup. If the RPG measures 200 micrograms per deciliter or above, and the individual also shows symptoms of diabetes, then a health care provider may diagnose diabetes.

Symptoms of diabetes include:

- Increased urination
- Increased thirst
- Unexplained weight loss

Other symptoms can include fatigue, blurred vision, increased hunger, and sores that do not heal.

Any test used to diagnose diabetes requires confirmation with a second measurement unless clear symptoms of diabetes exist.

Changes in Diagnostic Testing

In the past, the A1C test was used to monitor blood glucose levels but not for diagnosis. The A1C test has now been standardized, and in 2009, an international expert committee recommended it be used for diagnosis of type 2 diabetes and prediabetes.

Fasting Plasma Glucose Test

The FPG test is used to detect diabetes and prediabetes. The FPG test has been the most common test used for diagnosing diabetes because it is more convenient than the OGTT and less expensive. The FPG test measures blood glucose in a person who has fasted for at least 8 hours and is most reliable when given in the morning.

People with a fasting glucose level of 100 to 125 mg/dL have impaired fasting glucose (IFG), or prediabetes. A level of 126 mg/dL or above, confirmed by repeating the test on another day, means a person has diabetes.

Oral Glucose Tolerance Test

The OGTT can be used to diagnose diabetes, prediabetes, and gestational diabetes. Research has shown that the OGTT is more sensitive than the FPG test, but it is less convenient to administer. When used to test for diabetes or prediabetes, the OGTT measures blood glucose

Diagnosis of Diabetes

after a person fasts for at least 8 hours and 2 hours after the person drinks a liquid containing 75 grams of glucose dissolved in water.

If the 2-hour blood glucose level is between 140 and 199 mg/dL, the person has a type of prediabetes called impaired glucose tolerance (IGT). If confirmed by a second test, a 2-hour glucose level of 200 mg/dL or above means a person has diabetes.

Are diabetes blood test results always accurate?

All laboratory test results can vary from day to day and from test to test. Results can vary:

- within the person being tested. A person's blood glucose levels normally move up and down depending on meals, exercise, sickness, and stress.

- between different tests. Each test measures blood glucose levels in a different way.

- within the same test. Even when the same blood sample is repeatedly measured in the same laboratory, the results may vary due to small changes in temperature, equipment, or sample handling.

- Although all these tests can be used to indicate diabetes, in some people one test will indicate a diagnosis of diabetes when another test does not. People with differing test results may be in an early stage of the disease, where blood glucose levels have not risen high enough to show on every test.

Health care providers take all these variations into account when considering test results and repeat laboratory tests for confirmation. Diabetes develops over time, so even with variations in test results, health care providers can tell when overall blood glucose levels are becoming too high.

Diagnosis of Gestational Diabetes

Health care providers test for gestational diabetes using the OGTT. Women may be tested during their first visit to the health care provider after becoming pregnant or between 24 to 28 weeks of pregnancy depending on their risk factors and symptoms. Women found to have diabetes at the first visit to the health care provider after becoming pregnant may be diagnosed with type 2 diabetes.

Defining Safe Blood Glucose Levels for Pregnancy

Many studies have shown that gestational diabetes can cause complications for the mother and baby. An international, multicenter study, the Hyperglycemia and Adverse Pregnancy Outcome (HAPO) study, showed that the higher a pregnant woman's blood glucose is, the higher her risk of pregnancy complications. The HAPO researchers found that pregnancy complications can occur at blood glucose levels that were once considered to be normal.

Based on the results of the HAPO study, new guidelines for diagnosis of gestational diabetes were recommended by the International Association of the Diabetes and Pregnancy Study Groups in 2011. So far, the new guidelines have been adopted by the American Diabetes Association (ADA), but not by the American College of Obstetricians and Gynecologists (ACOG), or other medical organizations. Researchers estimate these new guidelines, if widely adopted, will increase the proportion of pregnant women diagnosed with gestational diabetes to nearly 18 percent.

Both ADA and ACOG guidelines for using the OGTT in diagnosing gestational diabetes are shown in the following tables.

Table 19.1. Recommendations for Testing Pregnant Women for Diabetes

Time of testing	ACOG	ADA
At first visit during pregnancy	No recommendation	Test women with risk factors for diabetes using standard testing for diagnosis of type 2 diabetes. Women found to have diabetes at this time should be diagnosed with type 2 diabetes, not gestational diabetes.
At 24 to 28 weeks of pregnancy	Test women for diabetes based on their history, risk factors, or a 50-gram, 1-hour, nonfasting, glucose challenge test—a modified OGTT. If score is 130–140 mg/dL, test again with fasting, 100-gram, 3-hour OGTT.*	Test all women for diabetes who are not already diagnosed, using a fasting, 75-gram, 2-hour OGTT.*

*See "OGTT Levels for Diagnosis of Gestational Diabetes" for blood glucose levels.

Diagnosis of Diabetes

Table 19.2. OGTT Levels for Diagnosis of Gestational Diabetes

Time of Sample Collection	ACOG Levels** (mg/dL)	ADA Levels (mg/dL)
	100-gram Glucose Drink	75-gram Glucose Drink
Fasting, before drinking glucose	95 or above	92 or above
1 hour after drinking glucose	180 or above	180 or above
2 hours after drinking glucose	155 or above	153 or above
3 hours after drinking glucose	140 or above	Not used
Requirements for Diagnosis	TWO or more of the above levels must be met	ONE or more of the above levels must be met

**Carpenter and Coustan Conversion, some labs use different numbers.

Who should be tested for diabetes and prediabetes?

Adults, pregnant women, children, and teens should be tested for diabetes and prediabetes according to their risk factors.

Adults

Anyone age 45 or older should consider getting tested for diabetes or prediabetes. Testing is strongly recommended for people older than age 45 who are overweight or obese. People younger than 45 should consider testing if they are overweight or obese and have one or more of the following risk factors:

- physical inactivity
- parent, brother, or sister with diabetes
- family background that is African American, Alaska Native, American Indian, Asian American, Hispanic/Latino, or Pacific Islander American
- history of giving birth to at least one baby weighing more than 9 pounds
- history of gestational diabetes
- high blood pressure—140/90 mmHg or higher—or being diagnosed with high blood pressure

- high-density lipoprotein or HDL, cholesterol—"good" cholesterol—level below 35 mg/dL or a triglyceride level above 250 mg/dL
- polycystic ovary syndrome, also called PCOS
- prediabetes—an A1C level of 5.7 to 6.4 percent; an FPG test result of 100–125 mg/dL, indicating IFG; or a 2-hour OGTT result of 140–199 mg/dL, indicating IGT
- acanthosis nigricans, a condition associated with insulin resistance and characterized by a dark, velvety rash around the neck or armpits
- history of cardiovascular disease—disease affecting the heart and blood vessels

In addition to weight, the location of excess fat on the body can be important. A waist measurement of 40 inches or more for men and 35 inches or more for women is linked to insulin resistance and increases a person's risk for type 2 diabetes. This is true even if a person's body mass index (BMI) falls within the normal range.

How to Measure the Waist

To measure the waist, a person should:

- place a tape measure around the bare abdomen just above the hip bone
- make sure the tape is snug but isn't digging into the skin and is parallel to the floor
- relax, exhale, and measure

If results of testing are normal, testing should be repeated at least every 3 years. Health care providers may recommend more frequent testing depending on initial results and risk status. People whose test results indicate they have prediabetes may be tested again in 1 year and should take steps to prevent or delay type 2 diabetes.

Pregnant Women

All pregnant women with risk factors for type 2 diabetes should be tested using standard diabetes blood tests during their first visit to the health care provider during pregnancy to see if they had undiagnosed diabetes before becoming pregnant. After that, pregnant women should be tested for gestational diabetes between 24 and 28 weeks of their pregnancy using the OGTT.

Women who develop gestational diabetes should also have follow-up testing 6 to 12 weeks after the baby is born to find out if they have type 2 diabetes or prediabetes. If results of testing are normal, testing should be repeated at least every 3 years. Blood glucose tests, rather than the A1C test, should be used for testing within 12 weeks of delivery.

Children and Teens

Type 2 diabetes has become increasingly common in children and teens. Children are at high risk for developing type 2 diabetes and should be tested if they are

- overweight or obese and have other risk factors, such as a family history of diabetes
- older than age 10 or have already gone through puberty

Body Mass Index (BMI)

Body mass index is a measurement of body weight relative to height for adults age 20 or older. To use the chart:

- find the person's height in the left-hand column
- move across the row to find the number closest to the person's weight
- find the number at the top of that column

The number at the top of the column is the person's BMI. The words above the BMI number indicate whether the person is normal weight, overweight, or obese. People who are overweight or obese should consider talking with a health care provider about ways to lose weight and reduce the risk of diabetes.

The BMI has certain limitations. The BMI may overestimate body fat in athletes and others who have a muscular build and underestimate body fat in older adults and others who have lost muscle.

The BMI for children and teens must be determined based on age, height, weight, and sex.

What steps can delay or prevent type 2 diabetes?

A major research study, the Diabetes Prevention Program (DPP), proved that people with prediabetes were able to sharply reduce their risk of developing diabetes during the study by losing 5 to 7 percent of their body weight through dietary changes and increased physical activity.

Study participants followed a low-fat, low-calorie diet and engaged in regular physical activity, such as walking briskly five times a week for 30 minutes. These strategies worked well for both men and women in all racial and ethnic groups, but were especially effective for participants age 60 and older. A follow-up study, the Diabetes Prevention Program Outcomes Study (DPPOS), showed losing weight and being physically active provide lasting results. Ten years after the DPP, modest weight loss delayed onset of type 2 diabetes by an average of 4 years.

The diabetes medication metformin also lowers the risk of type 2 diabetes in people with prediabetes, especially those who are younger and heavier and women who have had gestational diabetes. The DPPOS showed that metformin delayed type 2 diabetes by 2 years. People at high risk should ask their health care provider if they should take metformin to prevent type 2 diabetes. Metformin is a medication that makes insulin work better and can reduce the risk of type 2 diabetes.

Chapter 20

Blood Sugar Number

Chapter Contents

Section 20.1—Blood Sugar Test 142
Section 20.2—FAQs on Blood Sugar Test and
 Blood Glucose Monitoring Devices 144

Section 20.1

Blood Sugar Test

Text in this section is excerpted from "Know Your Blood Sugar Numbers," National Diabetes Education Program (NDEP), July 1, 2014.

If you have diabetes, keeping your blood sugar (glucose) numbers in your target range can help you feel good today and stay healthy in the future.

There are two ways to measure blood sugar

1. Self-tests are the blood sugar checks you do yourself. They show what your blood sugar is at the time you test.
2. The A1C is a lab test that measures your average blood sugar level over the last 2 to 3 months. It shows whether your blood sugar stayed close to your target range most of the time, or was too high or too low.

Both ways help you and your health care team to get a picture of how your diabetes care plan is working.

About self-tests for blood sugar

Why should I do self-tests?

Self-tests can help you learn how being active, having stress, taking medicine and eating food can make your blood sugar go up or down. They give you the facts you need to make wise choices as you go through the day.

Keep a record of your results. Look for times when your blood sugar is often too high or too low. Talk about your results with your health care team at each visit. Ask what you can do when your sugar is out of your target range.

How do I check my blood sugar?

Blood sugar meters use a small drop of blood to tell you how much sugar is in your blood at that moment. Ask your health care team how to get the supplies you need. They will also show you how to use them.

What is a good target range for my self-tests?

Many people with diabetes aim to keep their blood sugar between 70 and 130 before meals. About 2 hours after a meal starts, they aim for less than 180. Your target ranges may be different if you are an older adult (over 65), have other health problems like heart disease, or your blood sugar often gets too low. Talk with your health care team about the best target range for you.

Can my blood sugar get too low?

Yes it can. If you feel shaky, sweaty, or hungry, do a check to see if it is below your target range.

Carry something sweet with you at all times, such as 4 hard candies or glucose tablets. If your blood sugar is too low, eat the candy or glucose tablets right away. Let your health care team know if this happens often. Ask how you can prevent it.

How often should I check my blood sugar?

Self-tests are often done before meals, after meals, and at bedtime. People who take insulin need to check more than those who do not take insulin. Discuss your self-test schedule with your health care team.

Are there other numbers I need to know?

Yes, you need tests of your blood pressure and cholesterol (a blood fat). You and your health care team need to decide the best targets for these too. Keeping them in your target range can help lower your chances for having a heart attack or stroke.

How do I pay for these tests?

Medicare and most insurance pay for the A1C, cholesterol, and some self-test supplies. Check with your insurance plan or ask your health care team for help.

What is in it for me?

Finding the time to check your blood sugar can be a struggle. It is also hard when your sugar levels do not seem to match your efforts to manage your diabetes. Keep in mind that your self-test and A1C results are numbers to help you, not to judge you. Many people find that self-testing and using the results to manage their diabetes pays off. They are more able to take charge of their diabetes so that they can feel good today and stay healthy in the future.

Section 20.2

FAQs on Blood Sugar Test and Blood Glucose Monitoring Devices

Text in this section is excerpted from "Blood Glucose Monitoring Devices," U.S. Food and Drug Administration (FDA), January 26, 2015.

What does this test do?

This is a test system for use at home to measure the amount of sugar (glucose) in your blood.

What type of test is this?

This is a quantitative test, which means that you will find out the amount of glucose present in your blood sample.

Why should you take this test?

You should take this test if you have diabetes and you need to monitor your blood sugar (glucose) levels. You and your doctor can use the results to:

- determine your daily adjustments in treatment
- know if you have dangerously high or low levels of glucose
- understand how your diet and exercise change your glucose levels

Blood Sugar Number

The Diabetes Control and Complications Trial (1993) showed that good glucose control using home monitors led to fewer disease complications.

How often should you test your glucose?

Follow your doctor's recommendations about how often you test your glucose. You may need to test yourself several times each day to determine adjustments in your diet or treatment.

What should your glucose levels be?

According to the American Diabetes Association (Standards of Medical Care in Diabetes 2011, Diabetes Care, January 2011, vol.34, Supplement 1, S11-S61) the blood glucose levels for an adult without diabetes are below 100 mg/dL before meals and fasting and are less than 140 mg/dL two hours after meals.

People with diabetes should consult their doctor or health care provider to set appropriate blood glucose goals. You should treat your low or high blood glucose as recommended by your health care provider.

How accurate is this test?

The accuracy of this test depends on many factors including:

- the quality of your meter
- the quality of your test strips
- how well you perform the test. For example, you should wash and dry your hands before testing and closely follow the instructions for operating your meter.
- your hematocrit (the amount of red blood cells in the blood). If you are severely dehydrated or anemic, your test results may be less accurate. Your health care provider can tell you if your hematocrit is low or high, and can discuss with you how it may affect your glucose testing.
- interfering substances (Some substances, such as Vitamin C, Tylenol, and uric acid, may interfere with your glucose testing). Check the instructions for your meter and test strips to find out what substances may affect the testing accuracy.

- altitude, temperature, and humidity (High altitude, low and high temperatures, and humidity can cause unpredictable effects on glucose results). Check the meter manual and test strip package insert for more information. store and handle the meter and strips according to manufacturer's instructions. It is important to store test strip vials closed.

How do you take this test?

Before you test your blood glucose, you must read and understand the instructions for your meter. In general, you prick your finger with a lancet to get a drop of blood. Then you place the blood on a disposable "test strip" that is inserted in your meter. The test strip contains chemicals that react with glucose. Some meters measure the amount of electricity that passes through the test strip. Others measure how much light reflects from it. In the U.S., meters report results in milligrams of glucose per deciliter of blood, or mg/dl.

You can get information about your meter and test strips from several different sources, including the toll-free number in the manual that comes with your meter or on the manufacturer's web site. If you have an urgent problem, always contact your health care provider or a local emergency room for advice.

How do you choose a Glucose Meter?

There are many different types of meters available for purchase that differ in several ways, including:

- accuracy
- amount of blood needed for each test
- how easy it is to use
- pain associated with using the product
- testing speed
- overall size
- ability to store test results in memory
- likelihood of interferences
- ability to transmit data to a computer

Blood Sugar Number

- cost of the meter
- cost of the test strips used
- doctor's recommendation
- technical support provided by the manufacturer
- special features such as automatic timing, error codes, large display screen, or spoken instructions or results

Talk to your health care provider about the right glucose meter for you, and how to use it.

How can you check your meter's performance?

There are three ways to make sure your meter works properly:

1. Use liquid control solutions:

- every time you open a new container of test strips
- occasionally as you use the container of test strips
- if you drop the meter
- whenever you get unusual results
- To test a liquid control solution, you test a drop of these solutions just like you test a drop of your blood. The value you get should match the value written on the test strip vial label.

2. Use electronic checks. Every time you turn on your meter, it does an electronic check. If it detects a problem it will give you an error code. Look in your meter's manual to see what the error codes mean and how to fix the problem. If you are unsure if your meter is working properly, call the toll-free number in your meter's manual, or contact your health care provider.

3. Compare your meter with a blood glucose test performed in a laboratory. Take your meter with you to your next appointment with your health care provider. Ask your provider to watch your testing technique to make sure you are using the meter correctly. Ask your health care provider to have your blood tested with a laboratory method. If the values you obtain on your glucose meter match the laboratory values, then your meter is working well and you are using good technique.

What should you do if your meter malfunctions?

If your meter malfunctions, you should tell your health care provider and contact the company that made your meter and strips.

Can you test blood glucose from sites other than your fingers?

Some meters allow you to test blood from sites other than the fingertip. Examples of such alternative sampling sites are your palm, upper arm, forearm, thigh, or calf. Alternative site testing (AST) should not be performed at times when your blood glucose may be changing rapidly, as these alternative sampling sites may provide inaccurate results at those times. You should use only blood from your fingertip to test if any of the following applies:

- you have just taken insulin
- you think your blood sugar is low
- you are not aware of symptoms when you become hypoglycemic
- the results do not agree with the way you feel
- you have just eaten
- you have just exercised
- you are ill
- you are under stress

Also, you should never use results from an alternative sampling site to calibrate a continuous glucose monitor (CGM), or in insulin dosing calculations.

Chapter 21

The A1C Test and Diabetes

What is the A1C test?

The A1C test is a blood test that provides information about a person's average levels of blood glucose, also called blood sugar, over the past 3 months. The A1C test is sometimes called the hemoglobin A1C, HbA1c, or glycohemoglobin test. The A1C test is the primary test used for diabetes management and diabetes research.

How does the A1C test work?

The A1C test is based on the attachment of glucose to hemoglobin, the protein in red blood cells that carries oxygen. In the body, red blood cells are constantly forming and dying, but typically they live for about 3 months. Thus, the A1C test reflects the average of a person's blood glucose levels over the past 3 months. The A1C test result is reported as a percentage. The higher the percentage, the higher a person's blood glucose levels have been. A normal A1C level is below 5.7 percent.

Text in this chapter is excerpted from "The A1C Test and Diabetes," National Institute of Diabetes and Digestive and Kidney Diseases (NIDDK), National Institutes of Health (NIH), March 2014.

Can the A1C test be used to diagnose type 2 diabetes and prediabetes?

Yes. In 2009, an international expert committee recommended the A1C test as one of the tests available to help diagnose type 2 diabetes and prediabetes. Previously, only the traditional blood glucose tests were used to diagnose diabetes and prediabetes.

Because the A1C test does not require fasting and blood can be drawn for the test at any time of day, experts are hoping its convenience will allow more people to get tested—thus, decreasing the number of people with undiagnosed diabetes. However, some medical organizations continue to recommend using blood glucose tests for diagnosis.

How is the A1C test used to diagnose type 2 diabetes and prediabetes?

The A1C test can be used to diagnose type 2 diabetes and prediabetes alone or in combination with other diabetes tests. When the A1C test is used for diagnosis, the blood sample must be sent to a laboratory that uses an NGSP-certified method for analysis to ensure the results are standardized.

Blood samples analyzed in a health care provider's office, known as point-of-care (POC) tests, are not standardized for diagnosing diabetes. The following table provides the percentages that indicate diagnoses of normal, diabetes, and prediabetes according to A1C levels.

Table 21.1. Diagnosing Diabetes Level

Diagnosis*	A1C Level
Normal	below 5.7 percent
Diabetes	6.5 percent or above
Prediabetes	5.7 to 6.4 percent

*Any test for diagnosis of diabetes requires confirmation with a second measurement unless there are clear symptoms of diabetes.

Having prediabetes is a risk factor for getting type 2 diabetes. People with prediabetes may be retested each year. Within the prediabetes A1C range of 5.7 to 6.4 percent, the higher the A1C, the greater the risk of diabetes. Those with prediabetes are likely to develop type 2 diabetes within 10 years, but they can take steps to prevent or delay diabetes.

The A1C Test and Diabetes

Is the A1C test used during pregnancy?

The A1C test may be used at the first visit to the health care provider during pregnancy to see if women with risk factors had undiagnosed diabetes before becoming pregnant. After that, the oral glucose tolerance test (OGTT) is used to test for diabetes that develops during pregnancy—known as gestational diabetes. After delivery, women who had gestational diabetes should be tested for persistent diabetes. Blood glucose tests, rather than the A1C test, should be used for testing within 12 weeks of delivery.

Can blood glucose tests still be used for diagnosing type 2 diabetes and prediabetes?

Yes. The standard blood glucose tests used for diagnosing type 2 diabetes and prediabetes-the fasting plasma glucose (FPG) test and the OGTT—are still recommended. The random plasma glucose test, also called the casual glucose test, may be used for diagnosing diabetes when symptoms of diabetes are present. In some cases, the A1C test is used to help health care providers confirm the results of a blood glucose test.

Can the A1C test result in a different diagnosis than the blood glucose tests?

Yes. In some people, a blood glucose test may indicate a diagnosis of diabetes while an A1C test does not. The reverse can also occur—an A1C test may indicate a diagnosis of diabetes even though a blood glucose test does not. Because of these variations in test results, health care providers repeat tests before making a diagnosis.

People with differing test results may be in an early stage of the disease, where blood glucose levels have not risen high enough to show on every test. Sometimes, making simple changes in lifestyle—losing a small amount of weight and increasing physical activity—can help people in this early stage reverse diabetes or delay its onset.

How accurate is the A1C test?

The A1C test result can be up to 0.5 percent higher or lower than the actual percentage. This means an A1C measured as 7.0 percent could indicate a true A1C anywhere in the range from 6.5 to 7.5 percent.

To put the A1C test into perspective, an FPG test result of 126 mg/dL obtained from a laboratory test accounting for typical variability within an individual person could indicate a true FPG anywhere in the range from 110 to 142 mg/dL. This variation will be even greater if the blood sample is not processed promptly or is not put on ice, causing blood glucose levels in the sample to decrease.

Are diabetes blood test results always accurate?

All laboratory test results can vary from day to day and from test to test. Results can vary:

- **within the person being tested.** A person's blood glucose levels normally move up and down depending on meals, exercise, sickness, and stress.

- **between different tests.** Each test measures blood glucose levels in a different way. For example, the FPG test measures glucose that is floating free in the blood after fasting and only shows the blood glucose level at the time of the test. Repeated blood glucose tests, such as self-monitoring several times a day with a home meter, can record the natural variations of blood glucose levels during the day. The A1C test represents the amount of glucose attached to hemoglobin, so it reflects an average of all the blood glucose levels a person may experience over 3 months. The A1C test will not show day-to-day changes.

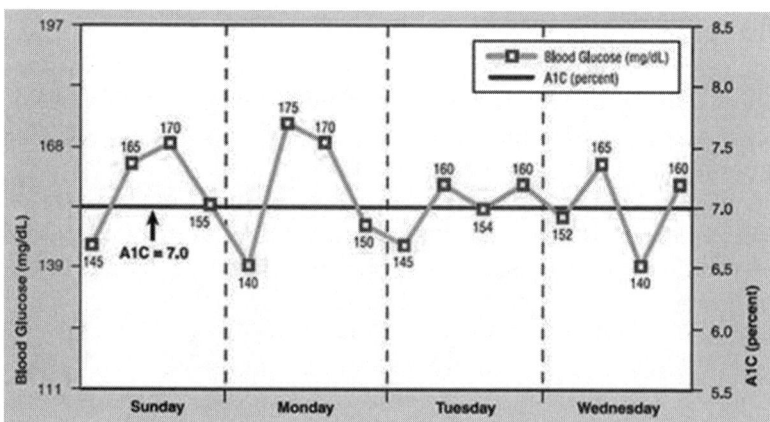

Figure 21.1. *Blood Glucose Measurements Compared with A1C Measurements over 4 Days. The straight black line indicates an A1C measurement of 7.0 percent. The zigzag line shows blood glucose test results from self-monitoring four times a day over a 4-day period.*

- **within the same test.** Even when the same blood sample is repeatedly measured in the same laboratory, the results may vary due to small changes in temperature, equipment, or sample handling.

Health care providers take these variations into account when considering test results and repeat laboratory tests for confirmation. Diabetes develops over time, so even with variations in test results, health care providers can tell when overall blood glucose levels are becoming too high.

Comparing test results from different laboratories can be misleading. People should consider requesting new laboratory tests when they change health care providers, or if their health care provider's office changes the laboratory or clinic it uses for blood testing.

Can the A1C test give false results?

Yes, for some people. The A1C test can be unreliable for diagnosing or monitoring diabetes in people with certain conditions that are known to interfere with the results. Interference should be suspected when A1C results seem very different from the results of a blood glucose test.

People of African, Mediterranean, or Southeast Asian descent, or people with family members with sickle cell anemia or a thalassemia are particularly at risk of interference. People in these groups may have a less common type of hemoglobin, known as a hemoglobin variant, that can interfere with some A1C tests. Most people with a hemoglobin variant have no symptoms and may not know that they carry this type of hemoglobin.

Not all of the A1C tests are unreliable for people with a hemoglobin variant. People with false results from one type of A1C test may need a different type of A1C test for measuring their average blood glucose level.

False A1C results may also occur in people with other problems that affect their blood or hemoglobin. For example, a falsely low A1C result can occur in people with:

- anemia
- heavy bleeding

A falsely elevated A1C result can occur in people who,

- are very low in iron, for example, those with iron deficiency anemia

Other causes of false A1C results include:

- kidney failure
- liver disease

How is the A1C test used after diagnosis of diabetes?

The American Diabetes Association recommends that people with diabetes who are meeting treatment goals and have stable blood glucose levels have the A1C test twice a year. Health care providers may repeat the A1C test as often as four times a year until blood glucose levels reach recommended levels.

The A1C test helps health care providers adjust medication to reduce the risk of long-term diabetes complications. Studies have demonstrated substantial reductions in long-term complications with the lowering of A1C levels.

When the A1C test is used for monitoring blood glucose levels in a person with diabetes, the blood sample can be analyzed in a health care provider's office using a POC test to give immediate results. However, POC tests are less reliable and not as accurate as most laboratory tests.

How does the A1C relate to estimated average glucose?

Estimated average glucose (eAG) is calculated from the A1C. Some laboratories report eAG with the A1C test results. The eAG number helps people with diabetes relate their A1C to daily glucose monitoring levels. The eAG calculation converts the A1C percentage to the same units used by home glucose meters—milligrams per deciliter (mg/dL).

The eAG number will not match daily glucose readings because it is a long-term average rather than the blood glucose level at a single time, as measured with the home glucose meter. The following table shows the relationship between the A1C and the eAG.

What A1C target should people have?

People will have different A1C targets depending on their diabetes history and their general health. People should discuss their A1C target with their health care provider. Studies have shown that people with diabetes can reduce the risk of diabetes complications by keeping A1C levels below 7 percent.

Maintaining good blood glucose control will benefit those with new-onset diabetes for many years to come. However, an A1C level

The A1C Test and Diabetes

that is safe for one person may not be safe for another. For example, keeping an A1C level below 7 percent may not be safe if it leads to problems with hypoglycemia, also called low blood glucose.

Less strict blood glucose control, or an A1C between 7 and 8 percent—or even higher in some circumstances—may be appropriate in people who have:

- limited life-expectancy
- long-standing diabetes and difficulty attaining a lower goal
- severe hypoglycemia
- advanced diabetes complications such as chronic kidney disease, nerve problems, or cardiovascular disease

Will the A1C test show changes in blood glucose levels?

Large changes in a person's blood glucose levels over the past month will show up in their A1C test result, but the A1C does not show sudden, temporary increases or decreases in blood glucose levels. Even though the A1C represents a long-term average, blood glucose levels within the past 30 days have a greater effect on the A1C reading than those in previous months.

Has the A1C test improved?

Yes. A1C laboratory tests are now standardized. In the past, the A1C test was not recommended for diagnosis of type 2 diabetes and prediabetes because the many different types of A1C tests could give varied results. The accuracy has been improved by the National Glycohemoglobin Standardization Program (NGSP), which developed standards for the A1C tests.

The NGSP certifies that manufacturers of A1C tests provide tests that are consistent with those used in a major diabetes study. The study established current A1C goals for blood glucose control that can reduce the occurrence of diabetes complications, such as blindness and blood vessel disease.

Part Three

Medications and Diabetes Care

Chapter 22

Diabetes Treatment

Manage Your Diabetes

Diabetes cannot be cured, but it can be managed. Managing blood glucose (blood sugar) as well as blood pressure and cholesterol is the best defense against the serious complications of diabetes.

Diabetes pills and insulin and diabetes pills are the two kinds of medicines used to lower blood glucose.

People with type 1 diabetes control their blood sugar with insulin — either delivered by injection or a pump. Many people with type 2 diabetes can control blood glucose levels with diet and exercise alone. Others require oral medications or insulin, and some may need both, as well as lifestyle modification.

Taking Diabetes Pills

If your body is still making some insulin, but not enough to keep your blood glucose levels under control, you may need diabetes pills. Some medications are taken once a day; others must be taken more often. Ask your health care team when you should take your pills. Remember to take your medicines every day, even when you feel well.

Text in this chapter is excerpted from "Diabetes," National Institute on Aging (NIA), National Institutes of Health (NIH), August 2014.

Be sure to tell your doctor if your pills make you feel sick or if you have any other problems. Remember, diabetes pills don't lower blood glucose all by themselves. You will still want to follow a meal plan and exercise to help lower your blood glucose.

Taking Insulin

You need insulin if your body has stopped making insulin or if your body doesn't make enough. Everyone with type 1 diabetes needs insulin, and many people with type 2 diabetes do, too.

Insulin can't be taken as a pill. It is usually taken by shots or with an insulin pump or insulin pen. Insulin pumps are small machines, usually worn on the hip, that contain insulin and deliver small steady doses of insulin throughout the day. Some pumps are attached directly to the skin. Other people use an insulin pen, which holds a cartridge of insulin that is dialed to the prescribed dose of insulin and then injected.

Sometimes, people who take diabetes pills may need insulin shots for a while. If you get sick or have surgery, the diabetes pills may no longer work to lower your blood glucose.

Chapter 23

Diabetes Medications

Chapter Contents

Section 23.1—Diabetes Medications – An Overview 162
Section 23.2—Managing Diabetes Medications 166
Section 23.3—Women and Diabetes Medications 169

Section 23.1

Diabetes Medications – An Overview

Text in this section is excerpted from "What I Need to Know about Diabetes Medicines," National Institute of Diabetes and Digestive and Kidney Diseases (NIDDK), National Institutes of Health (NIH), December 2013.

What do diabetes medicines do?

Over time, high levels of blood glucose, also called blood sugar, can cause health problems. These problems include heart disease, heart attacks, strokes, kidney disease, nerve damage, digestive problems, eye disease, and tooth and gum problems. You can help prevent health problems by keeping your blood glucose levels on target.

Everyone with diabetes needs to choose foods wisely and be physically active. If you can't reach your target blood glucose levels with wise food choices and physical activity, you may need diabetes medicines. The kind of medicine you take depends on your type of diabetes, your schedule, and your other health conditions. Diabetes medicines help keep your blood glucose in your target range.

Medicines for Type 1 Diabetes

Type 1 diabetes, once called juvenile diabetes or insulin-dependent diabetes, is usually first found in children, teenagers, or young adults. If you have type 1 diabetes, you must take insulin because your body no longer makes it. You also might need to take other types of diabetes medicines that work with insulin.

Medicines for Type 2 Diabetes

Type 2 diabetes, once called adult-onset diabetes or noninsulin-dependent diabetes, is the most common form of diabetes. It can start when the body doesn't use insulin as it should, a condition called insulin resistance. If the body can't keep up with the need for insulin, you may need diabetes medicines. Many choices are available. Your doctor might prescribe two or more medicines. The ADA recommends that most people start with metformin, a kind of diabetes pill.

Medicines for Gestational Diabetes

Gestational diabetes is diabetes that occurs for the first time during pregnancy. The hormones of pregnancy or a shortage of insulin can cause gestational diabetes. Most women with gestational diabetes control it with meal planning and physical activity. But some women need insulin to reach their target blood glucose levels.

Medicines for Other Types of Diabetes

If you have one of the rare forms of diabetes, such as diabetes caused by other medicines or monogenic diabetes, talk with your doctor about what kind of diabetes medicine would be best for you.

Types of diabetes medicines

Diabetes medicines come in several forms.

Insulin

If your body no longer makes enough insulin, you'll need to take it. Insulin is used for all types of diabetes. Your doctor can help you decide which way of taking insulin is best for you.

- **Taking injections.** You'll give yourself shots using a needle and syringe. The syringe is a hollow tube with a plunger. You will put your dose of insulin into the tube. Some people use an insulin pen, which looks like a pen but has a needle for its point.

- **Using an insulin pump.** An insulin pump is a small machine about the size of a cell phone, worn outside of your body on a belt or in a pocket or pouch. The pump connects to a small plastic tube and a very small needle. The needle is inserted under the skin and stays in for several days. Insulin is pumped from the machine through the tube into your body.

- **Using an insulin jet injector.** The jet injector, which looks like a large pen, sends a fine spray of insulin through the skin with high-pressure air instead of a needle.

- **Using an insulin infuser**. A small tube is inserted just beneath the skin and remains in place for several days. Insulin is injected into the end of the tube instead of through the skin.

What does insulin do?

Insulin helps keep blood glucose levels on target by moving glucose from the blood into your body's cells. Your cells then use glucose for energy. In people who don't have diabetes, the body makes the right amount of insulin on its own. But when you have diabetes, you and your doctor must decide how much insulin you need throughout the day and night.

What are the possible side effects of insulin?

Possible side effects include:

- low blood glucose
- weight gain

How and when should I take my insulin?

Your plan for taking insulin will depend on your daily routine and your type of insulin. Some people with diabetes who use insulin need to take it two, three, or four times a day to reach their blood glucose targets. Others can take a single shot. Your doctor or diabetes educator will help you learn how and when to give yourself insulin.

Diabetes Pills

Along with meal planning and physical activity, diabetes pills help people with type 2 diabetes or gestational diabetes keep their blood glucose levels on target. Several kinds of pills are available. Each works in a different way. Many people take two or three kinds of pills. Some people take combination pills. Combination pills contain two kinds of diabetes medicine in one tablet. Some people take pills and insulin.

Your doctor may ask you to try one kind of pill. If it doesn't help you reach your blood glucose targets, your doctor may ask you to:

- take more of the same pill
- add another kind of pill
- change to another type of pill

Diabetes Medications

- start taking insulin
- start taking another injected medicine

If your doctor suggests that you take insulin or another injected medicine, it doesn't mean your diabetes is getting worse. Instead, it means you need insulin or another type of medicine to reach your blood glucose targets. Everyone is different. What works best for you depends on your usual daily routine, eating habits, and activities, and your other health conditions.

For information about the different kinds of pills and what they do, see the inserts. You'll see the brand name and the generic name—the scientific name—for each medicine. Find your diabetes pills and check off the names.

Injections Other than Insulin

In addition to insulin, two other types of injected medicines are now available. Both work with insulin—either the body's own or injected—to help keep your blood glucose from going too high after you eat. Neither is a substitute for insulin.

What do I need to know about side effects of medicines?

A side effect is an unwanted problem caused by a medicine. For example, some diabetes medicines can cause nausea or an upset stomach when you first start taking them. Before you start a new medicine, ask your doctor about possible side effects and how you can avoid them. If the side effects of your medicine bother you, tell your doctor.

Section 23.2

Managing Diabetes Medications

Text in this section is excerpted from "Diabetes and You: All Medicines Matter!" National Diabetes Education Program (NDEP), January 2014.

Tips to manage your diabetes medicines

Take your medicines as directed. Talk with your pharmacist and your regular doctor if:

- You have any allergic reactions to your medicines.
- You have any problems with your medicines, like forgetting to take them or having a hard time swallowing them, reading the labels, or affording them.
- You have any changes in your diet or health.
- You are pregnant or breastfeeding.

Keep a list of all the medicines you take, and give your pharmacist and all of your health care providers a copy. Be sure the list includes:

- Medicines your doctor has prescribed for you.
- Vitamins and herbal supplements.
- Over-the-counter items, like aspirin, other pain medicine, or cold medicines. Over-the-counter medicines are ones you can buy off the shelf without a doctor's prescription.

Tell your pharmacist about information you learn after visiting your dentist, eye doctor, foot doctor, or other member of your health care team.

- Tell your pharmacist about any new health problems.
- Share new test results with your pharmacist.

Diabetes Medications

How Can Medicine Help Your Diabetes?

- Medicine can help you control your diabetes and blood sugar. Blood sugar that is too high or too low can cause problems with teeth, eyes, and feet, as well as other serious health problems.
- Many people with chronic (lifelong) diseases like diabetes do not take their medicines correctly. This puts them at risk of more serious health problems.
- There are more than 30 different medicines for diabetes. They can be taken by mouth, needle, or pump.
- People with diabetes may need many medicines at once to help them. Doctors choose medicines to best meet people's diabetes needs.

How Can Pharmacists Help?

- Did you know that patients see their pharmacists up to seven times more often than their doctors?
- Pharmacists are often available all day, in the evening, and on weekends.

Questions to ask your pharmacist

- What are the brand and generic (nonbrand) names of my medicines?
- What are each of my medicines for?
- When should I take each medicine?
- How much should I take of each medicine?
- How long should I use this medicine, and can I stop using it if I feel better?
- What should I do if I miss a dose or take too much?
- When will the medicine start to work?
- What are the possible side effects?
- Will my over-the-counter medicines react with my prescription medicines and could they affect my blood sugar levels?
- Will this medicine take the place of anything I already take?
- Are there any other medicines, foods, drinks, or activities that I should avoid?

- Are there programs that can help me if I can't afford my medicines?
- Does the pharmacy have any other special programs that can help me manage my diabetes?
- What is the best way to use my blood glucose meter and other supplies?

Include to-do list for managing your medicines

- Make a list of all the medicines (prescription and over-the-counter), supplements, and vitamins you take, and give a copy to your pharmacist and regular doctor.
- Work with your pharmacist to make a plan to manage your medicine.
- Ask your insurance company or pharmacy if you can save money by filling your prescriptions online or by mail. If you have questions, call the phone number provided and ask to speak with a licensed pharmacist.

Section 23.3

Women and Diabetes Medications

Text in this section is excerpted from "Women and Diabetes – Diabetes Medicines," U.S. Food and Drug Administration (FDA), October 26, 2015.

General tips

There are few kinds of medicines used to treat diabetes. Each kind affects your body in a different way. Some diabetes medicines are taken as pills that you swallow. There are other medicines that you inject. Some people with diabetes need to use medicines every day. What you need depends on your health and the type of diabetes you have.

Your healthcare provider can tell you if you need to use medicine to treat your diabetes.

- Talk to your doctor before you change or stop taking your diabetes medicines.
- People with type 1 diabetes must use insulin.
- Ask your doctor about your target blood sugar level.
- Talk to your doctor or nurse about what you should do if your blood sugar gets too low or too high.
- Ask your doctor if your diabetes medicines will affect your other medicines including your birth control.

Diabetes medicines

The different kinds of diabetes medicines are listed below. These medicines are most often used to treat type 2 diabetes. The brand names and other names are given for each drug. There are also some general tips about each kind of diabetes medicine. Ask your doctor, nurse, or pharmacist to tell you the side effects and warnings for the medicines you are taking. This page does not give all of the side effects or warnings for each medicine.

Meglitinides

How do they work? These pills help your body make more insulin around mealtime.

Table 23.1. List of Meglitindes

Brand Name	Other Name
Prandin	Repaglinide
Starlix	Nateglinide

Some Things to Think About

Before you start taking these medicines, tell your health provider if:
- you have liver or kidney problems
- you are pregnant or breastfeeding

Common Side Effects
- Hypoglycemia (blood sugar that is too low)

Alpha-glucosidase Inhibitors

How do they work?

These pills help your body digest sugar more slowly.

Table 23.2. List of Alpha-glucosidase Inhibitors

Brand Name	Other Name
Glyset	Miglitol
Precose	Acarbose

Some Things to Think About

- These medicines are not likely to cause weight gain or blood sugar that is too low
- Before you start taking this drug, tell your doctor if:
    - you have heart, liver, or kidney problems
    - you are pregnant or breastfeeding

Diabetes Medications

Common Side Effects

- Stomach Pain
- Diarrhea
- Gas
- Abnormal Liver Tests

Sulfonylureas

How do they work?

These pills help your body make more insulin.

Table 23.3. List of Sulfonyureas

Brand Name	Other Name
Amaryl	Glimepiride
Diabeta	Glyburide
Glynase	Chlorpropamide
Diabinese	Glipizide
Glucotrol	Tolbutamide
Glucotrol XL	Tolazamide

Some Things to Think About

- Before you start taking this drug, tell your health care provider if you have heart, liver, or kidney problems.
- Older adults and people with kidney or liver problems may be more likely to have low blood sugar when taking these medicines.

Common Side Effects

- Hypoglycemia (blood sugar that is too low)
- Weight Gain
- Headache
- Dizziness

Biguanides

How do they work?

These pills stop your liver from making too much sugar (glucose). They also help the sugar get into your cells.

Table 23.4. List of Biguanides

Brand Name	Other Name
Fortamet	Metformin
Glucophage	Metformin
Glucophage XR (extended release)	Metformin
Glumetza	Metformin
Riomet	Metformin

Some Things to Think About

- Talk to your doctor about your kidney health before you start and while you are taking this type of medicine.
- These medicines are not likely to cause weight gain or blood sugar that is too low.
- People who drink a lot of alcohol and people with kidney problems may have a rare side effect called lactic acidosis (acid to build up in the blood).

Common Side Effects

- Diarrhea
- Indigestion
- Nausea and Vomiting
- Gas
- Feeling Weak
- Headache

Dopamine Receptor Agonists

How do they work?

This pill affects a chemical called dopamine in your cells. It is not clear how this pill works for diabetes.

Diabetes Medications

Table 23.5. List of Dopamine Receptor Agonists

Brand Name	Other Name
Cycloset	Bromocriptine

One Thing to Think About

- Do not take this medicine if you are breastfeeding.

Common Side Effects

- Nausea
- Headache
- Feel Very Tired
- Feel Dizzy
- Vomiting

SGLT2 Inhibitors

How do they work?

These pills affect the kidney to increase the amount of sugar that goes out in the urine.

Table 23.6. List of SGLT2 Inhibitors

Brand Name	Other Name
Farxiga	Dapagliflozin
Invokana	Canagliflozin
Jardiance	Empagliflozin

Some Things to Think About

- Do not take these drugs if you have severe kidney problems or are on dialysis.
- Before you take these drugs, tell your doctor if you have kidney or liver problems.

Common Side Effects

- Vaginal Yeast Infections

- Urinary Tract Infections
- Changes in Urination

Combination Medicines

Table 23.7. List of Combination Medicines

Brand Name	Other Name
ActoPlus Met	Pioglitazone and Metformin
ActoPlus Met XR (extended release)	Pioglitazone and Metformin
Avandamet	Rosiglitazone and Metformin
Avandaryl	Rosiglitazone and Glimepiride
Duetact	Pioglitazone and Glimepiride
Glucovance	Glyburide and Metformin
Invokamet	Canagliflozin and Metformin
Janumet	Sitagliptin and Metformin
Janumet XR (extended release)	Sitagliptin and Metformin
Kazano	Alogliptin and Metformin
Kombiglyze	Saxagliptin and Metformin
Kombiglyze XR (extended release)	Saxagliptin and Metformin
Metaglip	Glipizide and Metformin
Oseni	Alogliptin and Metformin
PrandiMet	Repaglinide and Metformin
Xigduo XR	Dapagliflozin and Metformin

Some Things to Think About

- These combinations are made up of two kinds of medicines. The side effects depend on which two medicines are in the pill.
- Ask your doctor for the side effects and other facts about the combination drug you are taking.

GLP-1 Receptor Agonists

These are medicines that you inject under your skin. These medicines should not be used instead of insulin.

Diabetes Medications

Table 23.8. List of GLP-1 Receptor Agonists

Brand Name	Other Name
Byetta	Exenatide
Bydureon	Exenatide
Tanzeum	Albiglutide
Trulicity	Dulaglutide
Victoza	Liraglutide

Some Things to Think About

- Some people with diabetes can take these medicines that you inject under your skin.
- These medicines are not the same as insulin.
- Some people feel nauseous when they first start taking these medicines.

Amylin Analog

This is a medicine that you inject under your skin. This medicine should not be used instead of insulin.

Table 23.9. List of Amylin Analog

Brand Name	Other Name
Symlin	Pramlintide Acetate

Some Things to Think About

- People who use insulin can also use Symlin.
- People with type 1 diabetes can also use Symlin.
- Symlin should be taken in a separate injection. Do not mix Symlin and insulin in the same injection.
- This medicine is usually taken before meals.
- Some people feel nauseous when they first start taking this medicine.

What you can do about side effects

Diabetes medicines affect each person differently. These medicines can sometimes cause side effects. The side effects will depend on your body and the type of medicine you are taking. Follow these tips to help you learn how to handle the side effects.

- **Get the facts**. Ask your health care provider for the side effects, warnings, and other facts for the medicines you are taking. This booklet does not give all the facts for each kind of diabetes medicine.

- **Speak up**. Tell someone about any problems you may be having with your medicines. Your doctor may change your medicine or give you tips to help you deal with the side effects.

- **Check the FDA website**. You can find up-to-date safety information about your medicine.

- **Report serious problems with your medicines**. You or your doctor can tell the FDA about serious problems with your medicines. Report online or call FDA at 1-800-332-1088 to request a form.

Questions to ask your doctor

- How will my medicines affect my blood sugar?
- Will it affect my other medicines?
- What are the side effects?
- What do I do if I start having side effects?
- What should I do if I am pregnant, planning to get pregnant, or breastfeeding?
- What else should I know about my diabetes medicines?

Chapter 24

Insulin and Its Role in Diabetes Treatment

Insulin

Insulin helps to take the sugar in your blood to other parts of your body. Diabetes affects how your body makes or uses insulin. Diabetes can make it hard to control how much sugar is in your blood.

There is hope!

There are different kinds of insulin that people with diabetes can use every day to help them stay healthy.

This section gives some basic facts about insulin. Use this section to help you talk to your doctor about the kind of insulin that you are taking.

Do not wait. Diabetes is a serious illness.

Diabetes can cause a heart attack, stroke, blindness, kidney disease, nerve damage and other serious health problems. This is why it is so important for you to get treatment for your diabetes. Treatment can help prevent or slow some of these serious health problems. Exercise, eat a balanced diet, and take your diabetes medicines. You can do it.

Text in this chapter is excerpted from "Insulin," U.S. Food and Drug Administration (FDA), September 28, 2015.

My insulin guide

Ask your health care provider these questions before you start using your insulin.

- How often should I use my insulin?
- Can you show me the right way to inject the insulin?
- Will the insulin affect my other medicines? What about my birth control?
- What are the side effects? What do I do if I start having side effects?
- What is my target blood sugar level?
- How often should I check my blood sugar?
- What should I do if I am pregnant, planning to get pregnant, or breastfeeding?
- How should I store my insulin?

Types of insulin

There are many different types of insulin. The type lets you know how fast the insulin starts working or how long it lasts in your body. Your health care provider will help you find the insulin that is best for you.

- **Rapid-Acting** – This insulin starts working within 15 minutes after you use it. It is mostly gone out of your body after a few hours. It should be taken just before or just after you eat.
- **Short-Acting** – This insulin starts working within 30 minutes to 1 hour after you use it. It is mostly gone out of your body after a few hours. It should be taken 30-45 minutes before you eat.
- **Intermediate-Acting** – This insulin starts working within 2-4 hours after you use it. It reaches its highest level in your blood around 6-8 hours after you use it. It is often used to help control your blood sugar between meals. Some people use this type of insulin in the morning, at bedtime, or both.
- **Long-Acting** – This insulin starts working within 2 to 4 hours after you use it. It can last in the body for up to 24 hours. It is often used in the morning or at bedtime to help control your blood sugar throughout the day.

Insulin and Its Role in Diabetes Treatment

Table 24.1. Types of Insulin

Type of Insulin	Brand Name	Generic Name	Onset	Peak	Duration
Rapid Acting	— NovoLog	— Insulin aspart	15 minutes	30 to 90 minutes	3 to 5 hours
	— Apidra	— Insulin glulisine	15 minutes	30 to 90 minutes	3 to 5 hours
	— Humalog	— Insulin lispro	15 minutes	30 to 90 minutes	3 to 5 hours
Short-acting	— Humulin R — Novolin R	— Regular ®	30 to 60 minutes	2 to 4 hours	5 to 8 hours
Intermediate-acting	— Humulin N — Novolin N	— NPH (N)	1 to 3 hours	8 hours	12 to 16 hours
Long-acting	— Levemir	— Insulin detemir	1 hour	Peakless	20 to 26 hours
	— Lantus	— Insulin glargine			
Pre-mixed NPH (intermediate-acting) and regular (short-acting)	— Humulin 70/30 — Novolin 70/30	— 70% NPH and 30% regular	30 to 60 minutes	Varies	10 to 16 hours
Pre-mixed insulin lispro protamine suspension (intermediate-acting) and insulin lispro (rapid-acting)	— Humalog Mix 75/25	— 75% insulin lispro protamine and 25% insulin lispro	10 to 15 minutes	Varies	10 to 16 hours
Pre-mixed insulin lispro protamine suspension (intermediate-acting) and insulin lispro (rapid-acting)	— Humalog Mix 50/50	— 50% insulin lispro protamine and 50% insulin lispro	10 to 15 minutes	Varies	10 to 16 hours
Pre-mixed insulin aspart protamine suspension (intermediate-acting) and insulin aspart (rapid-acting)	— NovoLog Mix 70/30	— 70% insulin aspart protamine and 30% insulin aspart	5 to 15 minutes	Varies	10 to 16 hours

- **Pre-Mixed** – This is a mix of two different types of insulin. It includes one type that helps to control your blood sugar at meals and another type that helps between meals.

Insulin Tip: Do not store your insulin in a place that is very hot or very cold.

Insulin devices

There are many different ways to inject your insulin. Some people use a needle and syringe to inject their insulin. Others use insulin pens, jet injectors, or pumps. Read the information in this section about the different kinds of insulin devices. Then, talk to your doctor, nurse or pharmacist about the kind that is best for you.

Insulin Needles and Syringes

Needles and syringes are used to inject insulin under the skin. Insulin needles come in different sizes. Most needles have a special coating to help them go through the skin with as little pain as possible.

- Do not share your needles or syringes with others.
- Ask your health care provider which kind of needle is right for you.

Insulin Pens

Insulin pens are devices that look like regular pens with a fine short needle on the tip. The pens have enough insulin in them for a few injections. Some pens have a case filled with insulin that you change when it is empty. Other pens are thrown away when the case is empty.

- Put a new needle on the tip of the pen each time you give yourself an injection (shot).
- Make sure that you use the type of insulin and needle for your kind of pen.
- Do not share your insulin pen or cartridge with others.

Insulin Jet Injectors

Insulin jet injectors use strong air pressure to spray insulin through the skin.

Insulin and Its Role in Diabetes Treatment

- Insulin jet injectors do not use needles.
- Ask your health care provider to show you how to safely use your jet injector.

Insulin Pumps

Insulin pumps are worn on the outside of your body. The pump is connected to your body by a flexible tube that has a tip that sticks under your skin. A cartridge of insulin is put in the pump. The insulin flows through the tube into your body.

- The pump controls how much insulin goes into your body.
- The pump can give you insulin 24 hours a day.

Insulin Tip: There are tools called injection aids that can make it easier for you to inject your insulin. There are tools to help people that have problems seeing and people with physical disabilities. Ask your doctor about tools to help you inject your insulin.

Tips for insulin devices

Each insulin device is different. This section lists some basic tips about insulin devices. Talk to your health care provider to learn everything you should know about your insulin device.

General Tips

- Never share insulin needles (syringes) or devices.
- Ask your doctor or nurse to show you how to inject your insulin.
- Always wash your hands before you inject your insulin.
- Do not inject your insulin in the exact same spot on your body each time.
- The skin may get thick or thin if you use the same spot.
- Inject in the same general area of your body.
- Do not use your insulin if it looks cloudy or looks like something is floating in it. Take it back to the drug store for a new one.
- Do not use insulin needles (syringes), pens, and injectors after the expiration date printed on the label or on the box.

How to Throw Away Used Devices

- Follow the directions on when to throw away the needles, pens or injectors.
- You should throw away your used needles in a hard container like an empty laundry detergent bottle or a metal coffee can.
- Make sure the needles cannot poke through the container.
- Put a label on the container to warn people that it is dangerous.
- Keep the container where children cannot get to it.
- Always put a lid or top on the container.

Insulin side effects

Insulin affects each person differently. Insulin can sometimes cause side effects. The side effects will depend on your body and the type of insulin you are taking. Follow these tips to help you learn how to handle side effects.

- **Get the facts**. Ask your health care provider for the side effects, warnings, and other facts for your insulin. This booklet does not give all facts for each kind of insulin.
- **Speak up**. Tell someone about any problems you may be having with your insulin. Your doctor may change your prescription or give you tips to help you deal with the side effects.
- **Check the FDA website**. You can find up-to-date safety information about your insulin at: www.fda.gov
- **Report serious problems with your insulin or device**. You or your doctor can tell the FDA about serious problems with your medicines.

Call FDA at 1-800-332-1088 to report serious side effects.

Insulin Tip: Talk to your doctor before you change or stop taking your insulin.

Insulin safety tips

- Never drink insulin.
- Do not share insulin needles, pens or cartridges with anyone else.

Insulin and Its Role in Diabetes Treatment

- Talk to your doctor before you change or stop using your insulin.
- Do not inject your insulin in the exact same spot each time.
- Throw away needles in a hard container that can be closed like a laundry detergent bottle.
- Check the expiration date on the insulin before you use it.
- Make a plan about how to handle your insulin when you travel and during an emergency.

Chapter 25

Diabetes and Adult Vaccines

Each year thousands of adults in the United States get sick from diseases that could be prevented by vaccines — some people are hospitalized, and some even die. People with diabetes (both type 1 and type 2) are at higher risk for serious problems from certain vaccine-preventable diseases. **Getting vaccinated is an important step in staying healthy.**

Why Vaccines are Important for You

- Diabetes, even if well managed, can make it harder for your immune system to fight infections, so you may be at risk for more serious complications from an illness compared to people without diabetes.

- Some illnesses, like influenza, can raise your blood glucose to dangerously high levels.

- People with diabetes have higher rates of hepatitis B than the rest of the population. Outbreaks of hepatitis B associated with blood glucose monitoring procedures have happened among people with diabetes.

This chapter includes excerpts from "What You Need to Know about Diabetes and Adult Vaccines," Centers for Disease Control and Prevention (CDC), August 2015; and text from "Diabetes and Hepatitis B Vaccination," Centers for Disease Control and Prevention (CDC), October 2012.

- People with diabetes are at increased risk for death from pneumonia (lung infection), bacteremia (blood infection) and meningitis (infection of the lining of the brain and spinal cord).
- Immunization provides the best protection against vaccine preventable diseases.

Vaccines are one of the safest ways for you to protect your health, even if you are taking prescription medications. Vaccine side effects are usually mild and go away on their own. Severe side effects are very rare.

Getting Vaccinated

You regularly see your provider for diabetes care, and that is a great place to start! If your healthcare professional does not offer the vaccines you need, ask for a referral so you can get the vaccines elsewhere.

Adults can get vaccines at doctors' offices, pharmacies, workplaces, community health clinics, health departments and other locations.

Most health insurance plans cover recommended vaccines. Check with your insurance provider for details and for a list of vaccine providers covered by your plan. If you do not have health insurance, visit www.healthcare.gov to learn more about health insurance options.

What vaccines do you need?

- **Flu vaccine** every year to protect against seasonal flu
- **Pneumococcal vaccines** to protect against serious pneumococcal diseases
- **Hepatitis B vaccine series** to protect against hepatitis B
- **Tdap vaccine** to protect against tetanus, diphtheria, and pertussis (whooping cough)
- **Zoster vaccine** to protect against shingles if you are 60 years or older

There may be other vaccines recommended for you so be sure to talk with your healthcare professional about what is right for you.

What is the recommendation for vaccinating children living with diabetes?

In the United States, the hepatitis B vaccine is now part of the routine childhood vaccination schedule. In 1991, CDC and the ACIP recommended that all children and adolescents be vaccinated for hepatitis B. Estimates of vaccine coverage among infants and children are now over 90%.

What is the recommendation for vaccinating adults younger than 60 years of age?

In 2011, the Centers for Disease Control and Prevention and the Advisory Committee on Immunization Practices (ACIP) released new guidelines that recommend hepatitis B vaccination for all unvaccinated adults with diabetes who are younger than 60 years of age. Vaccination should occur as soon as possible after diagnosis of diabetes; vaccination should also be given to adults diagnosed with diabetes in the past.

What is the recommendation for vaccinating adults 60 years and older?

For unvaccinated adults with diabetes who are 60 years and older, the ACIP recommends hepatitis B vaccination at the discretion of their health care provider. As with other vaccines, the effectiveness of the hepatitis B vaccine decreases with age. Decisions to vaccinate should include the patient's likelihood of acquiring hepatitis B, including the need for assisted blood-glucose monitoring, and overall health status. Hepatitis B vaccination may provide partial, if not full protection for many older adults with diabetes.

Chapter 26

Diabetes Treatment Fraud

As the number of people diagnosed with diabetes continues to grow, illegally sold products promising to prevent, treat, and even cure diabetes are flooding the marketplace.

The U.S. Food and Drug Administration (FDA) is advising consumers not to use such products. They may contain harmful ingredients or may be otherwise unsafe, or may improperly be marketed as over-the-counter (OTC) products when they should be marketed as prescription products. They carry an additional risk if they cause consumers to delay or discontinue effective treatments for diabetes. Without proper disease management, people with diabetes are at a greater risk for developing serious health complications.

"People with chronic or incurable diseases may feel desperate and become easy prey. Bogus products for diabetes are particularly troubling because there are effective options available to help manage this serious disease rather than exposing patients to unproven and risky products," said Gary Coody, R.Ph., national health fraud coordinator for FDA. "Failure to follow well-established treatment plans can lead to, among other things, amputations, kidney disease, blindness and death."

Text in this chapter is excerpted from "Questions and Answers: FDA Alerts Companies to Stop the Illegal Sale of Products Claiming to Treat Diabetes," U.S. Food and Drug Administration (FDA), September 4, 2015.

Warning Letters Issued

Recently, FDA launched an initiative to counter these illegally sold products aimed at consumers who have diabetes. In addition to evaluating numerous consumer complaints, FDA surveyed the marketplace for illegally sold products promising to treat diabetes and its complications.

In July 2013, FDA issued letters warning 15 companies about selling products for diabetes in violation of federal law. These products are sold as dietary supplements; alternative medicines, such as ayurvedics; prescription drugs and over-the-counter drugs, including homeopathic products: Examples of claims observed on these illegally marketed products include:

- "Lower your blood sugar naturally."
- "Lowers A1C levels significantly."
- "You'll lower your chances of having eye disease, kidney disease, nerve damage and heart disease!"
- "It can replace medicine in the treatment of diabetes."
- "For Relief of Diabetic Foot Pain."

Some of the companies also promote unapproved products for other serious diseases, including cancer, sexually transmitted diseases, and macular degeneration.

FDA tested products marketed as "all natural" treatments for diabetes and discovered some of them contained one or more active ingredients found in prescription drugs to treat type 2 diabetes.

Undeclared ingredients can cause serious harm. If consumers and their health care professionals are unaware of the actual ingredients in the products they are taking, these products may interact in dangerous ways with other medications. One possible complication: Patients may end up taking a larger combined dose of the diabetic drugs than they intended, and that may cause a significant unsafe drop in blood sugar levels, a condition known as hypoglycemia.

FDA also looked at sales of prescription drugs from fraudulent online pharmacies. Signs that indicate an online pharmacy is legitimate include: requiring that patients have a valid prescription; providing a physical address in the U.S.; being licensed by a state pharmacy board; and having a state-licensed pharmacist to answer questions. Some fraudulent online pharmacies illegally sell drugs that are not approved in the United States, or sell prescription drug products without meeting necessary requirements.

One website that is subject to a warning letter shipped a prescription diabetes drug without requiring a prescription, and even included an unsolicited free sample of a prescription drug for erectile dysfunction. Moreover, the prescription diabetes drug was dispensed without the medication guide and other precautions required by FDA to ensure the drug is used safely and appropriately.

Although some of these websites may offer for sale what appear to be FDA-approved prescription drugs, FDA cannot confirm that the manufacture or the handling of these drugs follows U.S. regulations or that the drugs are safe and effective for their intended uses. Also, there is a risk the drugs may be counterfeit, contaminated, expired or otherwise unsafe.

Why should consumers be concerned about these products?

Diabetes is a chronic disease requiring diagnosis and management under the supervision of a licensed health care provider. Not only can these illegally sold products be ineffective, they can cause consumers with diabetes to delay seeking proper timely treatment leading to an increased risk for developing serious health complications.

In addition, some of the products may cause harm because they contain undisclosed active pharmaceutical ingredients (also known as APIs), unknown harmful ingredients, may be contaminated, or may be of poor quality.

Products containing undisclosed APIs frequently claim to have similar therapeutic benefit and to be "all natural" or "chemical free" alternatives to available FDA-approved treatments. The FDA is unable to test and identify all products containing potentially harmful hidden ingredients sold to consumers on the Internet and in retail stores. Therefore, consumers should exercise caution before using products claiming to be herbal or all-natural alternatives to FDA-approved prescription drugs. These products should be considered unsafe and should not be used.

More information on how to reduce the risk of encountering a product with an undisclosed ingredient can be found on the FDA's website at Medication Health Fraud.

What should consumers do to protect themselves from these products?

Although the FDA continues to conduct surveillance to minimize the number of violative and potentially dangerous products on the market, we encourage all consumers to exercise caution before using certain products, particularly those targeting chronic diseases such as diabetes. Please talk with your health care provider to discuss treatment options and before using a new product. Consumers can find more information on medication health fraud on the FDA's website.

Consumers using any of the products mentioned in the FDA warning letters are urged to discontinue taking the products and speak with their health care providers. Consumers who suspect they have experienced adverse effects as a result of taking any of these products or other suspicious diabetes products should contact their licensed health care provider immediately.

The FDA encourages consumers and health care providers to report harmful effects experienced from using any product claiming to treat or manage diabetes and diabetes complications to FDA's MedWatch Adverse Event Reporting program by doing one of the following:

- Complete and submit the report online: www.fda.gov/MedWatch/report.htm
- Download form or call 1-800-332-1088 to request a reporting form, then complete and return to the address on the pre-addressed form, or submit by fax to 1-800-FDA-1078

How can I get more information about health fraud scams?

To learn more about identifying and avoiding health fraud scams visit: www.fda.gov/healthfraud.

Chapter 27

New Diabetes Drugs – Tresiba and Ryzodeg 70/30

According to the Centers for Disease Control and Prevention, approximately 21 million people in the United States have been diagnosed with diabetes. Over time, diabetes increases the risk of serious health complications, including heart disease, blindness, nerve, and kidney damage. Improvement in blood sugar control can reduce the risk of some of these long-term complications

Recently the U.S. Food and Drug Administration (FDA) approved Tresiba (insulin degludec injection) and Ryzodeg 70/30 (insulin degludec/insulin aspart injection) to improve blood sugar (glucose) control in adults with diabetes mellitus.

Tresiba

Tresiba is a long-acting insulin analog indicated to improve glycemic control in adults with type 1 and 2 diabetes mellitus. Dosing of Tresiba should be individualized based on the patient's needs. Tresiba is administered subcutaneously once daily at any time of day.

The efficacy and safety of Tresiba used in combination with mealtime insulin for the treatment of patients with type-1 diabetes were evaluated in two 26-week and one 52-week active-controlled clinical trials involving 1,102 participants exposed to Tresiba. The efficacy and safety of Tresiba used in combination with mealtime insulin or used

---

Text in this chapter is excerpted from "New Diabetes Drugs – Tresiba and Ryzodeg 70/30," U.S. Food and Drug Administration (FDA), September 29, 2015.

as add-on to common background oral antidiabetic drugs for the treatment of patients with type-2 diabetes were evaluated in four 26-week and two 52-week active-controlled clinical trials involving 2,702 participants exposed to Tresiba. In participants with type 1 and 2 diabetes who had inadequate blood sugar control at trial entry, treatment with Tresiba provided reductions in HbA1c (hemoglobin A1c or glycosylated hemoglobin, a measure of blood sugar control) in line with reductions achieved with other, previously approved long-acting insulin.

Ryzodeg 70/30

Ryzodeg 70/30 is a mixture of insulin degludec, a long-acting insulin analog, and insulin aspart, a rapid-acting human insulin analog. It is indicated to improve glycemic control in adults with diabetes mellitus.

The efficacy and safety of Ryzodeg 70/30 used in combination with mealtime insulin for the treatment of patients with type 1 diabetes were evaluated in one 26-week active controlled clinical trial involving 362 participants exposed to Ryzodeg 70/30. The efficacy and safety of Ryzodeg 70/30 administered once or twice daily for the treatment of patients with type 2 diabetes were evaluated in four active controlled 26-week clinical trials involving 998 participants exposed to Ryzodeg 70/30. In participants with type 1 and 2 diabetes who had inadequate blood sugar control at trial entry, treatment with Ryzodeg 70/30 provided reductions in HbA1c equivalent to reductions achieved with other, previously approved long-acting or pre-mixed insulin.

Tresiba and Ryzodeg should not be used in those who have increased ketones in their blood or urine (diabetic ketoacidosis). Patients or caregivers should monitor blood glucose in all patients treated with insulin. Insulin regimens should be modified cautiously and only under medical supervision. Tresiba and Ryzodeg may cause low blood sugar (hypoglycemia), which can be life-threatening. Patients should be monitored more closely with changes to insulin dosage, co-administration of other glucose-lowering medications, meal pattern, physical activity, and in patients with renal impairment or hepatic impairment or hypoglycemia unawareness.

Severe, life-threatening, generalized allergy, including anaphylaxis, generalized skin reactions, angioedema, bronchospasm, hypotension, and shock may occur with any insulin.

The most common adverse reactions associated with Tresiba and Ryzodeg in clinical trials were hypoglycemia, allergic reactions, injection site reactions, pitting at the injection site (lipodystrophy), itching, rash, edema, and weight gain.

Part Four

Dietary and Other Lifestyle Issues Important for Diabetes Control

Chapter 28

Eat Right!

Chapter Contents

Section 28.1—Eat Healthy Food 198
Section 28.2—Carbohydrate Counting 204
Section 28.3—Diabetes and Dietary Supplements 210

Section 28.1

Eat Healthy Food

Text in this section is excerpted from "Food Safety for Diabetes Patients," U.S. Department of Health and Human Services (HHS), June 2, 2015; and text from "Tips for Teens with Diabetes: Make Healthy Food Choices," National Diabetes Education Program (NDEP), November 1, 2012.

Food Safety for Diabetes Patients

In addition to cardiovascular disease and kidney problems, diabetes also affects the immune system. These affects leave diabetes patients more prone to infectious disease, such as foodborne illness. A diabetic patient's immune system may not immediately recognize harmful foodborne pathogens increasing a person's risk for infection.

Glucose Levels

High glucose levels suppress the function of white blood cells that fight off infection, increasing one's risk of contracting a foodborne illness. If someone with diabetes contracts a foodborne illness, their blood glucose levels may be affected because the illness impacts what and how much the person can eat.

Gastrointestinal Tract (GI)

Diabetes may cause the stomach to produce low amounts of digestive acid. In addition, nerves may not move food through the GI tract as quickly as in non-diabetic persons. When the stomach holds on to food longer than necessary, bacteria start to multiply. If the amount of unhealthy bacteria in the stomach gets too high, it can lead to foodborne illness.

Kidneys

Kidneys usually work to cleanse the body. For many diabetes patients, their kidneys may not function properly, giving unhealthy bacteria the opportunity to grow out of control.

Eat Right!

Why eat healthy foods?

Healthy foods give you energy to live, learn, and be active.

They help you to:
- Grow at a healthy rate and stay active.
- Keep your blood glucose, also called blood sugar, in balance—not too high and not too low.
- Lose weight slowly, if needed, under your doctor's care.

Do teens with diabetes need to eat special foods?

No, they do not. Meals that are healthy for teens with diabetes are great for everyone—you, your family, and your friends.

How does food affect my body?

Food is the fuel that our bodies use for energy.

The three main sources of fuel are carbohydrates, protein, and fat. The body changes these fuels into glucose for energy or stores them as fat. Eating a balance of foods that contain carbohydrates (carbs for short), protein, and fat every day will help keep your blood glucose close to normal. It may also keep your weight where you and your doctor want it to be.

Fats

Fats are a good source of fuel for the body and help you grow. Fat does not make blood glucose go up but too much fat can make you gain weight. Some fats are better for you than others.

Choose the types of **fats that keep your heart healthy**:
- Small portions of low-fat salad dressing, mayonnaise, and margarine.
- Small amounts of nuts, olives, and olive oil.
- A slice of avocado.

Choose these high fat foods less often. They are **not healthy for your heart**:
- Butter, stick margarine, and regular mayonnaise.

- Fried foods like potato chips and french fries.
- Meats with fat on them, bacon, deli meats, and hot dogs.
- Cakes, cookies, pies, and other desserts.

Protein

Protein helps build strong muscles and bones. Foods with protein do not make blood glucose go up like carbs do. **Having protein in your meal can help you feel less hungry**.

Foods that are a good source of protein include:

- Meat and poultry without skin or extra fat.
- Fish, low-fat cheese, and eggs.
- Natural peanut butter and soy products like tofu.

Carbs

Carbs are a great source of energy for our bodies. Many foods contain carbs. Some are better for you than others. If you eat too many carbs at one time, your blood glucose may get too high. **Learn to eat the right amount at meals and snack times to keep your blood glucose in balance**.

Choose carbs that have lots of fiber:

- Whole grain foods—whole wheat bread and crackers, oatmeal, brown rice, and cereals.
- Lentils and dried peas or beans such as kidney, black, white, split, or black-eyed. These foods are also a good source of protein.
- Fresh fruits and vegetables from every color of the rainbow— red, orange, yellow, white, green, blue, and purple.
- Other good sources of carbs include non or low-fat dairy foods, soy milk, pasta, potatoes, corn, squash, and yams.

Choose these carbs less often:

- white bread
- white rice
- sweetened fruit drinks
- regular soda

Eat Right!

- sweets and desserts

What should I eat?

Find below "Your Healthy Food Guide" which gives ideas about what kinds of foods are good for you. Remember, this is only a guide. Ask your doctor or dietitian about making a meal plan just for you.

Your Healthy Food Guide

Vegetables

Aim for 2 1/2 to 3 cups a day. Here are choices that equal 1 cup:

- 1 cup cut up raw or cooked or vegetables
- 2 cups leafy salad greens
- 1 cup vegetable juice

Fruits

Aim for 1 1/2 to 2 cups a day. Here are choices that equal 1 cup:

- 1 cup cut up raw or cooked fruit
- 1 cup fruit juice
- 1/2 cup dried fruit

    Choose fresh whole fruits as often as you can.

Milk, Yogurt, and Cheese

Aim for 3 cups a day. Here are choices that equal 1 cup:

- 1 cup nonfat or low-fat milk or yogurt
- 1 1/2 ounces cheese

Breads, Cereals, Rice and Pasta

Aim for 6 to 7 ounces a day. Here are choices that equal 1 ounce:

- 1/2 cup of cooked cereal
- 1/2 cup cooked rice or pasta
- 1 cup ready-to-eat cereal

- 1 slice of whole grain bread
- 1/2 small bagel or 1 small muffin

Choose whole grain foods for at least 3 of your 6 choices.

Meat, Poultry, Fish, Dry Beans, Eggs, and Nuts

Aim for 5 to 6 ounces a day. Here are choices that equal 1 ounce:

- 1 ounce lean meat, fish, or chicken
- 1 egg
- 1 tablespoon peanut butter
- 1/2 ounce nuts
- 1/4 cup cooked dry peas or beans such as kidney, white, split, or blackeye
- 1/4 cup tofu

Heart healthy fats

One serving is:

- 1 teaspoon vegetable, olive, or canola oil
- 1 teaspoon tub margarine
- 5 large olives or 1/8 avocado
- 1 tablespoon low-fat mayonnaise
- 2 tablespoons low-fat salad dressing

How much should you eat?

You get most of the fat your body needs from other foods you eat—so choose only a few extra servings of these heart-healthy fats each day.

Regular Soda, Candy, Cookies, and Deserts

If you choose to eat these foods, have a very small amount and not every day.

What about sugar, sweets, and desserts? Am I allowed to eat them again?

Most people like the taste of sweet foods. Small amounts of foods that contain sugar can be part of a healthy meal plan.

Eat Right!

Desserts such as cakes, muffins, pies, cookies, and ice cream contain a lot of fat as well as sugar. If you choose to eat any of these sweet foods, just have a small amount at the end of a healthy meal. Have a piece of fruit if you are still hungry.

Avoid regular soda, sweetened fruit drinks, and sports drinks as they are all high in sugar. Drink water instead.

How much should I eat?

The amount of food you need to eat each day varies with your age, sex, height, and activity level. The amounts in "**Your Healthy Food Guide**" are right for girls age 11 to 17 or boys age 11 to 14 who get 30 to 60 minutes of physical activity each day.

Ask your doctor or dietitian about making a meal plan just for you, especially if you need to lose weight. Being active and eating smaller amounts of food and fewer sweet or fatty foods can help you lose weight in a healthy way. You will keep your heart healthy, too.

It is best to spread your food out over the day. Eat breakfast, lunch, dinner, and a snack—check out your options with your doctor or dietitian. You will have a good supply of energy and you will not get too hungry.

Putting it all together

- Learn about healthy foods and make healthy choices at each meal and snack.
- Ask your health care team to help you make and use a healthy eating plan.
- Choose water to drink.
- Be physically active for at least 60 minutes every day.
- Take the correct amounts of insulin or pills, if you need them to manage your diabetes, and check your blood glucose at the times planned with your health care team.
- Keep screen time to two hours or less a day. This includes time watching TV, playing video or computer games, and using the computer.
- Use this tip sheet to help you reach your goals!

Section 28.2

Carbohydrate Counting

Text in this section is excerpted from "What I need to Know about Carbohydrate Counting and Diabetes," National Institute of Diabetes and Digestive and Kidney Diseases (NIDDK), National Institutes of Health (NIH), December 2013.

What is carbohydrate counting?

Carbohydrate counting, also called carb counting, is a meal planning tool for people with type 1 or type 2 diabetes. Carbohydrate counting involves keeping track of the amount of carbohydrate in the foods you eat each day.

Carbohydrates are one of the main nutrients found in food and drinks. Protein and fat are the other main nutrients. Carbohydrates include sugars, starches, and fiber. Carbohydrate counting can help you control your blood glucose, also called blood sugar, levels because carbohydrates affect your blood glucose more than other nutrients.

Healthy carbohydrates, such as whole grains, fruits, and vegetables, are an important part of a healthy eating plan because they can provide both energy and nutrients, such as vitamins and minerals, and fiber. Fiber can help you prevent constipation, lower your cholesterol levels, and control your weight.

Unhealthy carbohydrates are often food and drinks with added sugars. Although unhealthy carbohydrates can also provide energy, they have little to no nutrients.

The amount of carbohydrate in foods is measured in grams. To count grams of carbohydrate in foods you eat, you'll need to:

- know which foods contain carbohydrates

- learn to estimate the number of grams of carbohydrate in the foods you eat

- add up the number of grams of carbohydrate from each food you eat to get your total for the day

Your doctor can refer you to a dietitian or diabetes educator who can help you develop a healthy eating plan based on carbohydrate counting.

Which foods contain carbohydrates?

Foods that contain carbohydrates include,

- grains, such as bread, noodles, pasta, crackers, cereals, and rice
- fruits, such as apples, bananas, berries, mangoes, melons, and oranges
- dairy products, such as milk and yogurt
- legumes, including dried beans, lentils, and peas
- snack foods and sweets, such as cakes, cookies, candy, and other desserts
- juices, soft drinks, fruit drinks, sports drinks, and energy drinks that contain sugars
- vegetables, especially "starchy" vegetables such as potatoes, corn, and peas

Potatoes, peas, and corn are called starchy vegetables because they are high in starch. These vegetables have more carbohydrates per serving than nonstarchy vegetables.

Examples of nonstarchy vegetables are asparagus, broccoli, carrots, celery, green beans, lettuce and other salad greens, peppers, spinach, tomatoes, and zucchini.

Foods that do not contain carbohydrates include meat, fish, and poultry; most types of cheese; nuts; and oils and other fats.

What happens when I eat foods containing carbohydrates?

When you eat foods containing carbohydrates, your digestive system breaks down the sugars and starches into glucose. Glucose is one of the simplest forms of sugar. Glucose then enters your bloodstream from your digestive tract and raises your blood glucose levels. The hormone insulin, which comes from the pancreas or from insulin shots, helps cells throughout your body absorb glucose and use it for energy. Once glucose moves out of the blood into cells, your blood glucose levels go back down.

How can carbohydrate counting help me?

Carbohydrate counting can help keep your blood glucose levels close to normal. Keeping your blood glucose levels as close to normal as possible may help you,

- stay healthy longer
- prevent or delay diabetes problems such as kidney disease, blindness, nerve damage, and blood vessel disease that can lead to heart attacks, strokes, and amputations—surgery to remove a body part
- feel better and more energetic

You may also need to take diabetes medicines or have insulin shots to control your blood glucose levels. Discuss your blood glucose targets with your doctor. Targets are numbers you aim for. To meet your targets, you will need to balance your carbohydrate intake with physical activity and diabetes medicines or insulin shots.

How much carbohydrate do I need each day?

The daily amount of carbohydrate, protein, and fat for people with diabetes has not been defined—what is best for one person may not be best for another. Everyone needs to get enough carbohydrate to meet the body's needs for energy, vitamins and minerals, and fiber.

Experts suggest that carbohydrate intake for most people should be between 45 and 65 percent of total calories. People on low-calorie diets and people who are physically inactive may want to aim for the lower end of that range.

One gram of carbohydrate provides about 4 calories, so you'll have to divide the number of calories you want to get from carbohydrates by 4 to get the number of grams. For example, if you want to eat 1,800 total calories per day and get 45 percent of your calories from carbohydrates, you would aim for about 200 grams of carbohydrate daily. You would calculate that amount as follows:

- .45 x 1,800 calories = 810 calories
- 810 ÷ 4 = 202.5 grams of carbohydrate

You'll need to spread out your carbohydrate intake throughout the day. A dietitian or diabetes educator can help you learn what foods to eat, how much to eat, and when to eat based on your weight, activity level, medicines, and blood glucose targets.

Eat Right!

How can I find out how much carbohydrate is in the foods I eat?

You will need to learn to estimate the amount of carbohydrate in foods you typically eat. For example, the following amounts of carbohydrate-rich foods each contain about 15 grams of carbohydrate:

- one slice of bread
- one 6-inch tortilla
- 1/3 cup of pasta
- 1/3 cup of rice
- 1/2 cup of canned or fresh fruit or fruit juice or one small piece of fresh fruit, such as a small apple or orange
- 1/2 cup of pinto beans
- 1/2 cup of starchy vegetables such as mashed potatoes, cooked corn, peas, or lima beans
- 3/4 cup of dry cereal or 1/2 cup cooked cereal
- 1 tablespoon of jelly

Some foods are so low in carbohydrates that you may not have to count them unless you eat large amounts. For example, most non-starchy vegetables are low in carbohydrates. A 1/2-cup serving of cooked nonstarchy vegetables or a cup of raw vegetables has only about 5 grams of carbohydrate.

As you become familiar with which foods contain carbohydrates and how many grams of carbohydrate are in food you eat, carbohydrate counting will be easier

Nutrition Labels

You can find out how many grams of carbohydrate are in the foods you eat by checking the nutrition labels on food packages.

Nutrition labels tell you:

- the food's serving size—such as one slice or 1/2 cup
- the total grams of carbohydrate per serving
- other nutrition information, including calories and the amount of protein and fat per serving

If you have two servings instead of one, such as one cup of pinto beans instead of 1/2 cup, you multiply the number of grams of carbohydrate in one serving—for example, 15—by two to get the total number of grams of carbohydrate—30.

15 x 2 = 30

Cooking at Home

To find out the amount of carbohydrate in homemade foods, you'll need to estimate and add up the grams of carbohydrate from the ingredients. You can use books or websites that list the typical carbohydrate content of homemade items to estimate the amount of carbohydrate in a serving.

You can also weigh foods with a scale or measure amounts with measuring cups or spoons to estimate the amount of carbohydrate. For example, if a nutrition label shows that 1 1/2 cups of cereal contain 45 grams of carbohydrate, then 1/2 cup will have 15 grams of carbohydrate and 1 cup will have 30 grams of carbohydrate.

Eating Out

Some restaurants provide nutrition information that lists grams of carbohydrate. You can also use carbohydrate counting food lists to estimate the amount of carbohydrate in restaurant meals.

Can I eat sweets and other foods and drinks with added sugars?

Yes, you can eat sweets and other foods and drinks with added sugars. However, you should limit your intake of these high-carbohydrate foods and drinks because they are often high in calories and low in vitamins, minerals, and fiber. Fiber-rich whole grains, fruits, vegetables, and beans are wiser choices.

Instead of eating sweets every day, try eating them in small amounts once in a while so you don't fill up on foods that are low in nutrition. Ask your dietitian or diabetes educator about including sweets in your eating plan.

What are added sugars?

Added sugars are various forms of sugar added to foods or drinks during processing or preparation. Naturally occurring sugars such as those in milk and fruits are not added sugars but are carbohydrates. The most common sources of added sugars for Americans are:

- sugar-sweetened soft drinks, fruit drinks, sports drinks, and energy drinks
- grain-based desserts, such as cakes, cookies, and doughnuts
- milk-based desserts and products, such as ice cream, sweetened yogurt, and sweetened milk
- candy

> Reading the list of ingredients for foods and drinks can help you find added sugars, such as:
>
> - sugar, raw sugar, brown sugar, and invert sugar—a mixture of fructose and glucose
> - corn syrup and malt syrup
> - high-fructose corn syrup, often used in soft drinks and juices
> - honey, molasses, and agave nectar
> - dextrose, fructose, glucose, lactose, and sucrose
>
> For a healthier eating plan, limit foods and drinks with added sugars.

How can I tell whether carbohydrate counting is working for me?

Checking your blood glucose levels can help you tell whether carbohydrate counting is working for you. You can check your blood glucose levels using a glucose meter.

You should also have an A1C blood test at least twice a year. The A1C test reflects the average amount of glucose in your blood during the past 3 months.

If your blood glucose levels are too high, you may need to make changes in your eating plan or other lifestyle changes. For example, you may need to make wiser food choices, be more physically active, or make changes to your diabetes medicines. Talk with your doctor about what changes you need to make to control your blood glucose levels.

If you use an insulin pump or take more than one daily insulin shot, ask your doctor how to adjust your insulin when you eat something that isn't in your usual eating plan.

Can I use carbohydrate counting if I am pregnant?

You can use carbohydrate counting to help control your blood glucose levels when you are pregnant. Meeting your blood glucose targets during pregnancy is important for your and your baby's health. High blood glucose during pregnancy can harm the baby and increase the baby's chances of having type 2 diabetes later in life.

Women diagnosed with gestational diabetes—a type of diabetes that develops only during pregnancy—can also use carbohydrate counting to help control their blood glucose levels.

Talk with your doctor about using carbohydrate counting to help meet your blood glucose targets during your pregnancy.

Section 28.3

Diabetes and Dietary Supplements

Text in this section is excerpted from "Diabetes and Dietary Supplements," National Center for Complementary and Integrative Health (NCCIH), November 2014.

Diabetes is a group of chronic diseases that affect metabolism—the way the body uses food for energy and growth. Millions of people have diabetes, which can lead to serious health problems if it is not managed well. Conventional medical treatments and following a healthy lifestyle, including watching your weight, can help you prevent, manage, and control many complications of diabetes. Researchers are studying several complementary health approaches, including dietary supplements, to see if they can help people manage type 2 diabetes—the focus of this section—or lower their risk of developing the disease.

Key facts

A healthy diet, physical activity, and blood glucose testing are the basic tools for managing type 2 diabetes. Your health care providers will help you learn to manage your diabetes and track how well you are controlling it. It is very important not to replace proven conventional medical treatment for diabetes with an unproven health product or practice.

Are dietary supplements for diabetes safe?

Some dietary supplements may have side effects, including interacting with your diabetes treatment or increasing your risk of kidney problems.

Are any dietary supplements for diabetes effective?

There is not enough scientific evidence to suggest that any dietary supplements can help prevent or manage type 2 diabetes.

Keep in mind

Tell all your health care providers about any complementary health approaches you use. Give them a full picture of what you do to manage your health. This will help ensure coordinated and safe care.

What the science says

Overall, there is not enough scientific evidence to show that any dietary supplement can help manage or prevent type 2 diabetes. This section addresses some of the many supplements studied for diabetes, with a focus on those that have undergone clinical trials (studies in people).

Alpha-lipoic acid

Alpha-lipoic acid is an antioxidant (a substance that may protect against cell damage). Studies have examined the effects of alpha-lipoic acid supplements on complications of diabetes.

For example:
A 2011 clinical trial of 467 participants with type 2 diabetes found that supplements of 600 milligrams of alpha-lipoic acid daily did not prevent diabetic macular edema, an eye condition that causes blurred vision.

Alpha-lipoic acid and vitamin E supplements taken separately or in combination did not improve cholesterol levels or the body's response to insulin in a 2011 clinical trial of 102 people with type 2 diabetes.

Safety

High doses of alpha-lipoic acid supplements can cause gastrointestinal problems.

Chromium

Found in many foods, chromium is an essential trace mineral. If you have too little chromium in your diet, your body can't use glucose efficiently. Studies, including a 2007 systematic review, have found few or no benefits of chromium supplements for controlling diabetes or reducing the risk of developing it. Many of the studies used for the review were small or not high quality.

Safety
Chromium supplements may cause stomach pain and bloating, and there have been a few reports of kidney damage, muscular problems, and skin reactions following large doses.

Herbal supplements

There is no strong evidence that herbal supplements can help to control diabetes or its complications.

- Researchers have found some risks but no clear benefits of cinnamon for people with diabetes.

- A 2012 systematic review of 10 randomized controlled trials did not support using cinnamon for type 1 or type 2 diabetes.

- A trial of 59 people with type 2 diabetes found that a combination of cinnamon, calcium, and zinc didn't improve their blood pressure.

- When researchers tested samples of the common spice cassia cinnamon for sale at grocery stores in Europe, they found many samples contained coumarin, a substance that may cause or worsen liver disease in people who are sensitive. Also, eating large amounts of cinnamon containing coumarin may be especially risky for people taking blood-thinning drugs; the interaction of coumarin and blood thinners can increase the likelihood of bleeding.

- Researchers are studying whether Asian ginseng and American ginseng may help control glucose levels. Currently, research reviews and clinical trials show that there is not enough evidence to support their use.

- Other herbal supplements studied for diabetes include aloe vera, bitter melon, Chinese herbal medicines, fenugreek, garlic, Gymnema sylvestre, milk thistle, nettle, prickly pear cactus, and sweet potato. None have been proven to be effective.

Safety

Information on the safety of herbal supplements for people with diabetes is generally inconclusive or unavailable. Interactions between herbs and conventional diabetes drugs have not been well studied and could be a health risk. For example, in some people cinnamon might worsen liver disease and interact with blood thinners.

Magnesium

Found in many foods, including whole grains, nuts, and green leafy vegetables, magnesium is essential to the body's ability to process glucose. Magnesium deficiency may increase the risk of developing diabetes.

- There is no evidence from clinical trials that magnesium helps to manage diabetes.

- A 2011 meta-analysis reviewed the results of 13 studies that looked at how much magnesium people got in their diets, either through supplements or food, and their risk of diabetes. The review found that people who had lower magnesium intake had a greater risk of developing diabetes.

- One of the studies in the 2011 research review mentioned above, a large 2007 clinical trial, found that people who ate more cereal fiber and magnesium-rich food had a lower risk of developing type 2 diabetes.

- People who had a diet rich in magnesium had a 15 percent reduced risk of developing type 2 diabetes, according to a 2007 meta-analysis of studies that looked at magnesium from foods or supplements.

Safety

No serious side effects were reported in studies where people with diabetes were given magnesium supplements for up to 16 weeks. However, the long-term safety of magnesium supplements for people with diabetes has not been established. Large doses of magnesium in supplements can cause diarrhea and abdominal cramping. Very large doses—more than 5,000 mg/day per day—can be deadly.

Omega-3s

Omega-3s supplements don't help people with diabetes control their blood sugar levels, a 2008 systematic review found. A 2012 study that combined a meta-analysis and a systematic review looked at the possible link between eating seafood or plants with omega-3s and the risk of developing type 2 diabetes. The study found little evidence that these dietary sources of Omega-3s affected the risk of developing diabetes.

Safety

- Omega-3 supplements usually do not have negative side effects. When side effects do occur, they typically consist of minor gastrointestinal symptoms, such as belching, indigestion, or diarrhea.

- Omega-3 supplements may extend bleeding time (the time it takes for a cut to stop bleeding). People who take drugs that affect bleeding time, such as anticoagulants ("blood thinners") or nonsteroidal anti-inflammatory drugs (NSAIDs), should discuss the use of omega-3 fatty acid supplements with a health care provider.

Vitamins

- Studies (including a 2010 research review and 2009 clinical trial) have found no evidence that taking vitamin C supplements is helpful for diabetes.

- The research on diabetes and vitamin D and calcium supplements is not conclusive.

- Supplementing with vitamin D combined with calcium appears to lower the risk of developing type 2 diabetes, according to a 2007 systematic review and meta-analysis.

- In a 2008 clinical trial studying 33,951 post-menopausal women over 7 years, calcium plus vitamin D supplements did no better than a placebo at reducing the risk of developing diabetes.

- The lower risk seen in some studies in people who consume more calcium may be because those individuals are also getting more magnesium, a 2012 meta-analysis reported.

Safety

Getting too much calcium may interfere with the body's ability to absorb iron and zinc. Also, calcium supplements can interact with certain medicines.

Other supplements

- There is no strong evidence that supplements of the trace mineral vanadium improve blood sugar control in people with type 2 diabetes.

- The evidence is still preliminary on the effects on diabetes of supplements and foods rich in polyphenols—antioxidants found in fruits, grains, and vegetables, a 2010 research review concluded.

If you have diabetes and are thinking about using a dietary supplement

- Talk to a health care provider before considering any dietary supplement for yourself, particularly if you are pregnant or nursing, or for a child. Many supplements have not been tested in pregnant women, nursing mothers, or children.

- Do not replace scientifically proven treatments for diabetes with unproven health products or practices. The consequences of not following your prescribed medical regimen for diabetes can be very serious.

- Keep in mind that dietary supplements may interact with medications or other dietary supplements and may contain ingredients not listed on the label.

- Tell all your health care providers about any complementary health approaches you use. Give them a full picture of what you do to manage your health. This will help ensure coordinated and safe care.

6 Things to Know About Type 2 Diabetes and Dietary Supplements

Here are 6 things you should know about taking dietary supplements for type 2 diabetes.
1. A healthy diet, physical activity, and blood glucose testing are the basic tools for managing type 2 diabetes. Your health care providers will help you learn to manage your diabetes and track how well you are controlling it. It is very important not to replace proven conventional medical treatment for diabetes with an unproven health product or practice.

2. Some dietary supplements may have side effects, including interacting with your diabetes treatment or increasing your risk of kidney problems. This is of particular concern because diabetes is the leading cause of chronic kidney disease and kidney failure in the United States. Supplement use should be monitored closely in patients who have or are at risk for kidney disease.

3. Chromium (an essential trace mineral found in many foods) has been studied for preventing diabetes and controlling glucose levels, but research has found it has few or no benefits. There have been a few reports of kidney damage, muscular problems, and skin reactions following large doses of chromium.

4. There is no evidence that magnesium helps to manage diabetes; however research suggests that people with lower magnesium intake may have a greater risk of developing diabetes. A large 2007 study found an association between a higher intake of cereal fiber and magnesium and a reduced risk of developing type 2 diabetes. Large doses of magnesium in supplements can cause diarrhea and abdominal cramping, and very large doses—more than 5,000 mg/day per day—can be deadly.

5. There is no strong evidence that herbs and other dietary supplements, including cinnamon and omega-3s, can help to control diabetes or its complications. Researchers have found some risks but no clear benefits of cinnamon for people with diabetes. For example, a 2012 review of the scientific literature did not support using cinnamon for type 1 or type 2 diabetes.

6. Talk with your health care provider before considering any dietary supplement for yourself, particularly if you are pregnant or nursing, or for a child. Do not replace scientifically proven treatments for diabetes with unproven health products or practices. The consequences of not following your prescribed medical regimen for diabetes can be very serious.

Chapter 29

Smoking and Diabetes

What you need to know about smoking and diabetes

The 2014 Surgeon General's Report has found that smoking is a cause of type 2 diabetes, which is also known as adult-onset diabetes. Smokers have a greater risk of developing type 2 diabetes than do non-smokers. The risk of developing diabetes increases with the number of cigarettes smoked per day.

Diabetes is a disease that causes blood sugar levels in the body to be too high and puts the body at risk for many serious health conditions. More than 25 million adults suffer from diabetes in the United States, where the disease is the seventh leading cause of death. It is also a growing health crisis around the world.

How smoking causes type 2 diabetes

Smoking increases inflammation in the body. Inflammation occurs when chemicals in cigarette smoke injure cells, causing swelling and interfering with proper cell function. Smoking also causes oxidative stress, a condition that occurs as chemicals from cigarette smoke combine with oxygen in the body. This causes damage to cells.

Text in this chapter is excerpted from "Smoking and Diabetes," Centers for Disease Control and Prevention (CDC), October 15, 2014.

Evidence strongly suggests that both inflammation and oxidative stress may be related to an increased risk of diabetes. The evidence also shows that smoking is associated with a higher risk of abdominal obesity, or belly fat. Abdominal obesity is a known risk factor for diabetes because it encourages the production of cortisol, a hormone that increases blood sugar. Smokers tend to have higher concentrations of cortisol than nonsmokers.

What smoking means to people with diabetes

Studies have confirmed that when people with type 2 diabetes are exposed to high levels of nicotine, insulin (the hormone that lowers blood sugar levels) is less effective. People with diabetes who smoke need larger doses of insulin to control their blood sugar.

Smokers who have diabetes are more likely to have serious health problems, including:

- heart and kidney disease;
- poor blood flow in the legs and feet that can lead to foot infections, ulcers, and possible amputation of toes or feet;
- retinopathy (an eye disease that can cause blindness); and
- peripheral neuropathy (damaged nerves to the arms and legs that cause numbness, pain, weakness, and poor coordination).

Even though we don't know exactly which smokers will develop type 2 diabetes, we do know that all diabetic smokers should quit smoking or using any type of tobacco product immediately. The health benefits of quitting begin right away. People with diabetes who quit have better control of their blood sugar. Studies have shown that insulin can start to become more effective at lowering blood sugar levels eight weeks after a smoker quits. People who want to quit smoking can get help from their doctors. Free help is also available at 1-800-QUIT-NOW and at smokefree.gov and cdc.gov/tips.

Chapter 30

Weight Management and Diabetes

Chapter Contents

Section 30.1—Diabetic Patients and Weight
          Concerns 220
Section 30.2—Helping Your Child Manage Weight 223

Section 30.1

Diabetic Patients and Weight Concerns

Text in this section is excerpted from "Do You Know Some of the Health Risks of Being Overweight?" National Institute of Diabetes and Digestive and Kidney Diseases (NIDDK), National Institutes of Health (NIH), December 2012.

What kinds of health problems are linked to overweight and obesity?

Excess weight may increase the risk for many health problems, including:

- type 2 diabetes
- high blood pressure
- heart disease and strokes
- certain types of cancer
- sleep apnea
- osteoarthritis
- fatty liver disease
- kidney disease
- pregnancy problems, such as high blood sugar during pregnancy, high blood pressure, and increased risk for cesarean delivery (C-section)

How can I tell if I weigh too much?

Gaining a few pounds during the year may not seem like a big deal. But these pounds can add up over time. How can you tell if your weight could increase your chances of developing health problems? Knowing two numbers may help you understand your risk: your body mass index (BMI) score and your waist size in inches.

Weight Management and Diabetes

Body Mass Index

The BMI is one way to tell whether you are at a normal weight, are overweight, or have obesity. It measures your weight in relation to your height and provides a score to help place you in a category:

- normal weight: BMI of 18.5 to 24.9
- overweight: BMI of 25 to 29.9
- obesity: BMI of 30 or higher

Waist Size

Another important number to know is your waist size in inches. Having too much fat around your waist may increase health risks even more than having fat in other parts of your body. Women with a waist size of more than 35 inches and men with a waist size of more than 40 inches may have higher chances of developing diseases related to obesity.

Type 2 Diabetes

How is type 2 diabetes linked to overweight?

About 80 percent of people with type 2 diabetes are overweight or obese. It isn't clear why people who are overweight are more likely to develop this disease. It may be that being overweight causes cells to change, making them resistant to the hormone insulin. Insulin carries sugar from blood to the cells, where it is used for energy. When a person is insulin resistant, blood sugar cannot be taken up by the cells, resulting in high blood sugar. In addition, the cells that produce insulin must work extra hard to try to keep blood sugar normal. This may cause these cells to gradually fail.

How can weight loss help?

If you are at risk for type 2 diabetes, losing weight may help prevent or delay the onset of diabetes. If you have type 2 diabetes, losing weight and becoming more physically active can help you control your blood sugar levels and prevent or delay health problems. Losing weight and exercising more may also allow you to reduce the amount of diabetes medicine you take.

How can I lower my risk of having health problems related to overweight and obesity?

If you are considered to be overweight, losing as little as 5 percent of your body weight may lower your risk for several diseases, including heart disease and type 2 diabetes. If you weigh 200 pounds, this means losing 10 pounds. Slow and steady weight loss of 1/2 to 2 pounds per week, and not more than 3 pounds per week, is the safest way to lose weight.

Federal guidelines on physical activity recommend that you get at least 150 minutes a week of moderate aerobic activity (like biking or brisk walking). To lose weight, or to maintain weight loss, you may need to be active for up to 300 minutes per week. You also need to do activities to strengthen muscles (like push-ups or sit-ups) at least twice a week.

Federal dietary guidelines and the MyPlate website recommend many tips for healthy eating that may also help you control your weight. Here are a few examples:

- Make half of your plate fruits and vegetables.

- Replace unrefined grains (white bread, pasta, white rice) with whole-grain options (whole wheat bread, brown rice, oatmeal).

- Enjoy lean sources of protein, such as lean meats, seafood, beans and peas, soy, nuts, and seeds.

For some people who have obesity and related health problems, bariatric (weight-loss) surgery may be an option. Bariatric surgery has been found to be effective in promoting weight loss and reducing the risk for many health problems.

Section 30.2

Helping Your Child Manage Weight

Text in this section is excerpted from "How to Help Your Children Stay Healthy," National Diabetes Education Program (NDEP), July 2014.

This section is for parents who have kids that are 8 to 12 years old. It tells you about type 2 diabetes and why some kids have more chance of getting diabetes. It also gives you great ideas about how you can help your kids be active and eat healthy foods.

What makes some kids more likely to get type 2 diabetes than other kids?

- Having a mom, dad, sister, brother, or other family member with diabetes
- Being overweight
- Not being active
- Weighing 9 pounds or more at birth
- Being born to a mother who had diabetes during the pregnancy
- Being an American Indian, Alaska Native, African American,
- Asian American, Hispanic/Latino, or Pacific Islander

What can you do?

- Help your children be active each day.
- Make meals and snacks that are healthy and taste good.
- Take your kids grocery shopping. Teach them how to read food
- Labels to help find healthy foods.

- Limit portion sizes of foods high in fat, sugar, and salt.
- Limit your kids' play time in front of the computer, tablets,
- Smartphones, and TV to 2 hours per day.
- Ask the doctor if your kids are at a healthy weight and if they have
- A greater chance of getting type 2 diabetes.
- Be a good role model. Eat healthy foods and be active with your kids.

What can kids do to be healthy?

- Be more active.
- Eat well.

How can your kids be active?

Ask your kids how they like to be active. What is fun for them? If they don't have ideas, you can suggest that they:

- Ride a bike
- Dance
- Shoot hoops
- Skateboard
- Jump rope
- Swim
- Go for a walk or run with a parent or
- Older family member

How much activity should your kids get?

Your kids need about 60 minutes of activity a day. They don't have to do it all at once. For example, 20 minutes at a time, 3 times a day is fine.

How will being active help?

Being active can help your children:

- Build muscle and burn off extra fat.
- Grow strong bones and stay flexible.
- Feel good and sleep better.
- Be at a healthy weight.

How can your kids eat well?

They can:

- Make good food choices.
- Eat healthy snacks.
- Adopt healthy eating habits.

What are good food choices?

Talk with your kids about how they think they can eat healthier.

Make a list together. Here are some tips you might want to include:

- Eat foods that are high in fiber such as whole grain breads and cereals, brown rice, lentils, beans, fruits, and vegetables.
- Eat foods low in saturated and *trans* fats such as lean meat, chicken without the skin, fish, and non-fat or low-fat milk, yogurt, and cheese.
- Eat baked, broiled, or grilled foods instead of fried foods.
- Eat foods that are low in salt such as fruits, vegetables, and whole grains. Do not add salt to your foods.
- Eat lots of vegetables. For example, make a salad with leafy greens, carrots, tomatoes, and peppers. Use 2 tablespoons or less of a low-fat dressing.
- Drink water instead of sugary drinks such as soda, sport drinks, and fruit juice.

Have your kids start out slow. Support them. Let them know the important thing is to just keep moving! They can add more activity each week.

What are healthy snacks?

Here are some easy, healthy snacks:

- A piece of fruit such as an apple or banana
- A slice of toast with 1 tablespoon of peanut butter
- A cup of low-fat or non-fat yogurt
- Raw vegetables such as carrots or celery with salsa

What are healthy eating habits my family can try?

You can:

- Eat breakfast, lunch, and dinner every day.
- Limit portion sizes when eating a meal. Fill half of your plate with fruits and vegetables. Fill one quarter with a lean protein, such as chicken or turkey without the skin or beans. Fill one quarter with a whole grain, such as brown rice or whole wheat pasta. Drink a cup of low-fat or non-fat milk with your meal.
- Limit desserts such as cookies and ice cream to only 1 or 2 times a week.
- Turn the TV and other devices off during meals. Enjoy eating and talking with family members.

Chapter 31

Physical Activity and Diabetes

How can physical activity help me take care of my diabetes?

Physical activity and keeping a healthy weight can help you take care of your diabetes and prevent diabetes problems. Physical activity helps your blood glucose, also called blood sugar, stay in your target range.

Physical activity also helps the hormone insulin absorb glucose into all your body's cells, including your muscles, for energy. Muscles use glucose better than fat does. Building and using muscle through physical activity can help prevent high blood glucose. If your body doesn't make enough insulin, or if the insulin doesn't work the way it should, the body's cells don't use glucose. Your blood glucose levels then get too high, causing diabetes.

Starting a physical activity program can help you lose weight or keep a healthy weight and keep your blood glucose levels on target. Even without reaching a healthy weight, just a 10 or 15 pound weight loss makes a difference in reducing the risk of diabetes problems.

Text in this chapter is excerpted from "What I Need to Know about Physical Activity and Diabetes," National Institute of Diabetes and Digestive and Kidney Diseases (NIDDK), National Institutes of Health (NIH), May 2014.

What should I do before I start a physical activity program?

Before you start a physical activity program, you should:
- talk with your health care team
- plan ahead
- find an exercise buddy
- decide how you'll track your physical activity
- decide how you'll reward yourself

Talk with your health care team

Your health care team may include a doctor, nurse, dietitian, diabetes educator, and others. Always talk with your health care team before you start a new physical activity program. Your health care team will tell you a target range for your blood glucose levels.

People with diabetes who take insulin or certain diabetes medicines are more likely to have low blood glucose, also called hypoglycemia. If your blood glucose levels drop too low, you could pass out, have a seizure, or go into a coma. Physical activity can make hypoglycemia more likely or worse in people who take insulin or certain diabetes medicines, so planning ahead is key. It's important to stay active. Ask your health care team how to stay active safely.

Physical activity works together with healthy eating and diabetes medicines to prevent diabetes problems. Studies show that people with type 2 diabetes who lose weight with physical activity and make healthy changes to their eating plan are less likely to need diabetes and heart medicines. Ask your health care team about your healthy eating plan and all your medicines. Ask if you need to change the amount of medicine you take or the food you eat before any physical activity.

Talk with your health care team about what types of physical activity are safe for you, such as walking, weightlifting, or housework. Certain activities may be unsafe for people who have low vision or have nerve damage to their feet.

Make copies of the table of questions and topics in the "My Physical Activity Planning Tools" section to take with you when you visit your health care team. Write down the answers on the table of questions and topics.

Physical Activity and Diabetes

Plan ahead

Decide in advance what type of physical activity you'll do. Before you start, also choose,

- the days and times you'll be physically active
- the length of each physical activity session
- your plan for warming up, stretching, and cooling down for each physical activity session
- a backup plan, such as where you'll walk if the weather is bad
- how you will measure your progress

To make sure you stay active, find activities you like to do. If you keep finding excuses not to be physically active, think about why:

- Are your goals realistic?
- Do you need a change in activity?
- Would another time be more convenient?

Find an exercise buddy

Many people find they are more likely to be physically active if someone joins them. Ask a friend or family member to be your exercise buddy. When you do physical activities with a buddy you may find that you:

- enjoy the company
- stick to the physical activity plan
- are more eager to do physical activities

Being active with your family may help everyone stay at a healthy weight. Keeping a healthy weight may prevent them from developing diabetes or prediabetes. Prediabetes is when the amount of glucose in your blood is above normal yet not high enough to be called diabetes.

Decide how you'll track your physical activity

Write down your blood glucose levels and when and how long you are physically active in a record book. You'll be able to track your progress and see how physical activity affects your blood glucose.

Decide how you'll reward yourself

Reward yourself with a nonfood item or activity when you reach your goals. For example, treat yourself to a movie or buy a new plant for the garden.

What kinds of physical activity can help me?

Many kinds of physical activity can help you take care of your diabetes. Even small amounts of physical activity can help. You can measure your physical activity level by how much effort you use.

Doctors suggest that you aim for 30 to 60 minutes of moderate to vigorous physical activity most days of the week. Children and adolescents with type 2 diabetes who are 10 to 17 years old should aim for 60 minutes of moderate to vigorous activity every day.

Your health care team can tell you more about what kind of physical activity is best for you. They can also tell you when and how much you can increase your physical activity level.

Light physical activity

Light activity is easy. Your physical activity level is light if you:

- are breathing normally
- are not sweating
- can talk normally or even sing

Moderate physical activity

Moderate activity feels somewhat hard. Your physical activity level is moderate if you:

- are breathing quickly, yet you're not out of breath
- are lightly sweating after about 10 minutes of activity
- can talk normally, yet you can't sing

Vigorous physical activity

Vigorous, or intense, activity feels hard. Your physical activity level is vigorous if you:

- are breathing deeply and quickly

Physical Activity and Diabetes

- are sweating after a few minutes of activity
- can't talk normally without stopping for a breath

Not all physical activity has to take place at the same time. You might take a walk for 20 minutes, lift hand weights for 10 minutes, and walk up and down the stairs for 5 minutes.

Breaking the physical activity into different groups can help. You can:

- do aerobic exercise
- do strength training to build muscle
- do stretching exercises
- add extra activity to your daily routine

Do Aerobic Exercise

Aerobic exercise is activity that uses large muscles, makes your heart beat faster, and makes you breathe harder. Doing moderate to vigorous aerobic exercise for 30 to 60 minutes a day most days of the week provides many benefits. You can even split up these minutes into several parts.

Doing moderate to vigorous aerobic exercise for 30 to 60 minutes a day most days of the week provides many benefits.

Talk with your health care team about how to warm up and cool down before and after you exercise. Start slowly, with 5 to 10 minutes a day, and add a little more time each week. Try:

- walking briskly
- hiking
- climbing stairs
- swimming or taking a water-aerobics class
- dancing
- riding a bicycle outdoors or a stationary bicycle indoors
- taking an exercise class
- playing basketball, tennis, or other sports
- in-line skating, ice skating, or skateboarding

When is the best time of day for me to do physical activity?

Your health care team can help you decide the best time of day for you to do physical activity based on your daily schedule, healthy eating plan, and diabetes medicines.

If you have type 1 diabetes, try not to do vigorous physical activity when you have ketones in your blood or urine. Ketones are chemicals your body might make when your blood glucose levels are too high and your insulin level is too low. If you are physically active when you have ketones in your blood or urine, your blood glucose levels may go even higher.

Light or moderate physical activity can help lower blood glucose if you have type 2 diabetes and you don't have ketones. Ketones are rare in people with type 2 diabetes. Ask your health care team whether you should be physically active when your blood glucose levels are high.

Part Five

Complications of Diabetes and Co-Occurring Disorders

Chapter 32

Complications Associated with Diabetes

Diabetes can affect any part of your body. The good news is that you can prevent most of these problems by keeping your blood glucose (blood sugar) under control, eating healthy, being physical active, working with your health care provider to keep your blood pressure and cholesterol under control, and getting necessary screening tests.

How can diabetes affect cardiovascular health?

Cardiovascular disease is the leading cause of early death among people with diabetes. Adults with diabetes are two to four times more likely than people without diabetes to die of heart disease or experience a stroke. Also, about 70% of people with diabetes have high blood pressure, a risk factor for cardiovascular disease.

How are cholesterol, triglyceride, weight, and blood pressure problems related to diabetes?

People with type 2 diabetes have high rates of cholesterol and triglyceride abnormalities, obesity, and high blood pressure, all of which are major contributors to higher rates of cardiovascular disease. Many people with diabetes have several of these conditions at the same time.

Text in this chapter is excerpted from "Prevent Complications," Centers for Disease Control and Prevention (CDC), September 25, 2015.

This combination of problems is often called metabolic syndrome (formerly known as Syndrome X). The metabolic syndrome is often defined as the presence of any three of the following conditions:

- excess weight around the waist;
- high levels of triglycerides;
- low levels of HDL, or "good," cholesterol;
- high blood pressure; and
- high fasting blood glucose levels.

If you have one or more of these conditions, you are at an increased risk for having one or more of the others. The more conditions that you have, the greater the risk to your health.

How can diabetes affect the eyes?

In diabetic eye disease, high blood glucose and high blood pressure cause small blood vessels to swell and leak liquid into the retina of the eye, blurring the vision and sometimes leading to blindness. People with diabetes are also more likely to develop cataracts—a clouding of the eye's lens, and glaucoma—optic nerve damage. Laser surgery can help these conditions.

How can diabetes affect the kidneys?

In diabetic kidney disease (also called diabetic nephropathy), cells and blood vessels in the kidneys are damaged, affecting the organs' ability to filter out waste. Waste builds up in your blood instead of being excreted. In some cases this can lead to kidney failure. When the kidneys fail, a person has to have his or her blood filtered through a machine (a treatment called dialysis) several times a week, or has to get a kidney transplant.

How can diabetes affect nerve endings?

Having high blood glucose for many years can damage the blood vessels that bring oxygen to some nerves, as well as the nerve coverings. Damaged nerves may stop sending messages, or send messages too slowly or at the wrong times. Numbness, pain, and weakness in the hands, arms, feet, and legs may develop. Problems may also occur in various organs, including the digestive tract, heart, and sex organs.

Complications Associated with Diabetes

Diabetic neuropathy is the medical term for damage to the nervous system from diabetes. The most common type is peripheral neuropathy, which affects the arms and legs.

An estimated 50% of those with diabetes have some form of neuropathy, but not all with neuropathy have symptoms. People with diabetes can develop nerve problems at any time, but the longer a person has diabetes, the greater the risk. The highest rates of neuropathy are among people who have had the disease for at least 25 years.

Diabetic neuropathy also appears to be more common in people who have had problems controlling their blood glucose levels, in those with high levels of blood fat and blood pressure, in overweight people, and in people over the age of 40.

Why is it especially important to take care of my feet if I have diabetes?

Nerve damage, circulation problems, and infections can cause serious foot problems for people with diabetes. Sometimes nerve damage can deform or misshape your feet, causing pressure points that can turn into blisters, sores, or ulcers. Poor circulation can make these injuries slow to heal. Sometimes this can lead to amputation of a toe, foot, or leg.

How can diabetes affect the digestion?

Gastroparesis, otherwise known as delayed gastric emptying, is a disorder where, due to nerve damage, the stomach takes too long to empty itself. It frequently occurs in people with either type 1 or type 2 diabetes.

Symptoms of gastroparesis include heartburn, nausea, vomiting of undigested food, an early feeling of fullness when eating, weight loss, abdominal bloating, erratic blood glucose levels, lack of appetite, gastroesophageal reflux, and spasms of the stomach wall.

How can diabetes affect oral health?

Because of high blood glucose, people with diabetes are more likely to have problems with their teeth and gums. And like all infections, dental infections can make your blood glucose go up. Sore, swollen, and red gums that bleed when you brush your teeth are a sign of a dental problem called gingivitis. Another problem, called periodontitis, happens when your gums shrink or pull away from your teeth.

People with diabetes can have tooth and gum problems more often if their blood glucose stays high. Also, smoking makes it more likely for you to get a bad case of gum disease, especially if you have diabetes and are age 45 or older.

People with diabetes are also prone to other mouth problems, like fungal infections, poor post-surgery healing, and dry mouth.

How can diabetes affect my sexual response?

Many people with diabetic nerve damage have trouble having sex. For example, men can have trouble maintaining an erection and ejaculating. Women can have trouble with sexual response and vaginal lubrication. Both men and women with diabetes can get urinary tract infections and bladder problems more often than average.

How can diabetes affect my mood?

Several studies suggest that diabetes doubles the risk of depression, although it's still unclear why. The psychological stress of having diabetes may contribute to depression, but diabetes' metabolic effect on brain function may also play a role. At the same time, people with depression may be more likely to develop diabetes.

The risk of depression increases as more diabetes complications develop. When you are depressed, you do not function as well, physically or mentally; this makes you less likely to eat properly, exercise, and take your medication regularly.

Psychotherapy, medication, or a combination of both can treat depression effectively. In addition, studies show that successful treatment for depression also helps improve blood glucose control.

How does diabetes affect how I respond to a cold or flu?

Being sick by itself can raise your blood glucose. Moreover, illness can prevent you from eating properly, which further affects blood glucose.

In addition, diabetes can make the immune system more vulnerable to severe cases of the flu. People with diabetes who come down with the flu may become very sick and may even have to go to a hospital. You can help keep yourself from getting the flu by getting a flu shot every year. Everyone with diabetes—even pregnant women—should get a yearly flu shot. The best time to get one is between October and mid-November, before the flu season begins.

Chapter 33

Diabetes-Related Bone Disease

What Is Osteoporosis?

Osteoporosis is a condition in which the bones become less dense and more likely to fracture. Fractures from osteoporosis can result in pain and disability. In the United States, more than 53 million people either already have osteoporosis or are at high risk due to low bone mass.

Risk factors for developing osteoporosis include:

- being thin or having a small frame
- having a family history of the disease
- for women, being postmenopausal, having an early menopause, or not having menstrual periods (amenorrhea)
- using certain medications, such as glucocorticoids
- not getting enough calcium

Text in this chapter is excerpted from "What People with Diabetes Need to Know about Osteoporosis," National Institute of Arthritis and Musculoskeletal and Skin Diseases (NIAMS), National Institutes of Health (NIH), April 2015.

- not getting enough physical activity
- smoking
- drinking too much alcohol.

Osteoporosis is a disease that often can be prevented. If undetected, it can progress for many years without symptoms until a fracture occurs.

The Diabetes–Osteoporosis link

Type 1 diabetes is linked to low bone density, although researchers don't know exactly why. Insulin, which is deficient in type 1 diabetes, may promote bone growth and strength. The onset of type 1 diabetes typically occurs at a young age when bone mass is still increasing. It is possible that people with type 1 diabetes achieve lower peak bone mass, the maximum strength and density that bones reach. People usually reach their peak bone mass by age 30. Low peak bone mass increases one's risk of developing osteoporosis later in life. Some people with type 1 diabetes also have celiac disease, which is associated with reduced bone mass. It is also possible that cytokines, substances produced by various cells in the body, play a role in the development of both type 1 diabetes and osteoporosis.

Recent research also suggests that women with type 1 diabetes may have an increased fracture risk, since vision problems and nerve damage associated with the disease have been linked to an increased risk of falls and related fractures. Hypoglycemia, or low blood sugar reactions, may also contribute to falls.

Increased body weight can reduce one's risk of developing osteoporosis. Since excessive weight is common in people with type 2 diabetes, affected people were long believed to be protected against osteoporosis. However, although bone density is increased in people with type 2 diabetes, fractures are increased. As with type 1 diabetes, this may be due to increased falls because of vision problems and nerve damage. Moreover, the sedentary lifestyle common in many people with type 2 diabetes also interferes with bone health.

Osteoporosis management strategies

Strategies to prevent and treat osteoporosis in people with diabetes are the same as for those without diabetes.

Diabetes-Related Bone Disease

Nutrition

A diet rich in calcium and vitamin D is important for healthy bones. Good sources of calcium include low-fat dairy products; dark green, leafy vegetables; and calcium-fortified foods and beverages. Many low-fat and low-sugar sources of calcium are available. Also, supplements can help you meet the daily requirements of calcium and other important nutrients.

Vitamin D

plays an important role in calcium absorption and bone health. It is synthesized in the skin through exposure to sunlight. Although many people are able to obtain enough vitamin D naturally, older individuals are often deficient in this vitamin due, in part, to limited time spent outdoors. They may require vitamin D supplements to ensure an adequate daily intake.

Exercise

Like muscle, bone is living tissue that responds to exercise by becoming stronger. The best exercise for your bones is weight-bearing exercise that forces you to work against gravity. Some examples include walking, stair climbing, and dancing. Regular exercise can help prevent bone loss and, by enhancing balance and flexibility, reduce the likelihood of falling and breaking a bone. Exercise is especially important for people with diabetes since exercise helps insulin lower blood glucose levels.

Healthy lifestyle

Smoking is bad for bones as well as for the heart and lungs. Women who smoke tend to go through menopause earlier, triggering earlier bone loss. In addition, smokers may absorb less calcium from their diets. Alcohol can also negatively affect bone health. Heavy drinkers are more prone to bone loss and fracture because of poor nutrition as well as an increased risk of falling. Avoiding smoking and alcohol can also help with managing diabetes.

Bone density test

Specialized tests known as bone mineral density (BMD) tests measure bone density in various parts of the body. These tests can detect osteoporosis before a bone fracture occurs and predict one's chances of fracturing in the future. The most widely recognized bone mineral density test is called a dual-energy x-ray absorptiometry or DXA test. It is painless: a bit like having an x-ray, but with much less exposure to radiation. It can measure bone density at your hip and spine. People with diabetes should talk to their doctors about whether they might be candidates for a bone density test.

Medication

Like diabetes, there is no cure for osteoporosis. However, several medications are approved by the Food and Drug Administration for the prevention and treatment of osteoporosis in postmenopausal women and men. Medications are also approved for use in both women and men with glucocorticoid-induced osteoporosis.

Chapter 34

Diabetes-Related Eye Diseases

What is diabetic eye disease?

Diabetic eye disease is a group of eye conditions that can affect people with diabetes.

- **Diabetic retinopathy** affects blood vessels in the light-sensitive tissue called the retina that lines the back of the eye. It is the most common cause of vision loss among people with diabetes and the leading cause of vision impairment and blindness among working-age adults.

- **Diabetic macular edema (DME)**. A consequence of diabetic retinopathy, DME is swelling in an area of the retina called the macula.

Diabetic eye disease also includes cataract and glaucoma:

- **Cataract** is a clouding of the eye's lens. Adults with diabetes are 2-5 times more likely than those without diabetes to develop

---

Text in this chapter is excerpted from "Facts about Diabetic Eye Disease," National Eye Institute (NEI), National Institutes of Health (NIH), September 2015.

cataract. Cataract also tends to develop at an earlier age in people with diabetes.

- **Glaucoma** is a group of diseases that damage the eye's optic nerve—the bundle of nerve fibers that connects the eye to the brain. Some types of glaucoma are associated with elevated pressure inside the eye. In adults, diabetes nearly doubles the risk of glaucoma.

All forms of diabetic eye disease have the potential to cause severe vision loss and blindness.

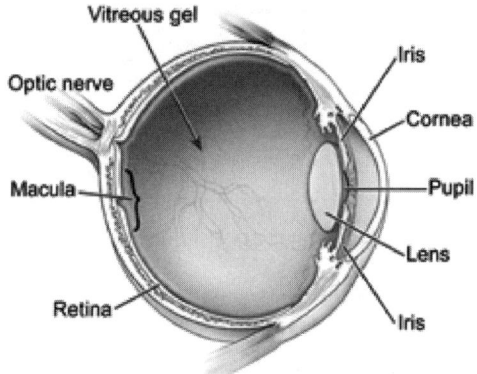

Figure 34.1. *Parts of the eye*

What causes diabetic retinopathy?

Chronically high blood sugar from diabetes is associated with damage to the tiny blood vessels in the retina, leading to diabetic retinopathy. The retina detects light and converts it to signals sent through the optic nerve to the brain. Diabetic retinopathy can cause blood vessels in the retina to leak fluid or hemorrhage (bleed), distorting vision. In its most advanced stage, new abnormal blood vessels proliferate (increase in number) on the surface of the retina, which can lead to scarring and cell loss in the retina.

Diabetic retinopathy may progress through four stages:

1. **Mild nonproliferative retinopathy**. Small areas of balloon-like swelling in the retina's tiny blood vessels, called

microaneurysms, occur at this earliest stage of the disease. These microaneurysms may leak fluid into the retina.

2. **Moderate nonproliferative retinopathy**. As the disease progresses, blood vessels that nourish the retina may swell and distort. They may also lose their ability to transport blood. Both conditions cause characteristic changes to the appearance of the retina and may contribute to DME.

3. **Severe nonproliferative retinopathy**. Many more blood vessels are blocked, depriving blood supply to areas of the retina. These areas secrete growth factors that signal the retina to grow new blood vessels.

4. **Proliferative diabetic retinopathy (PDR)**. At this advanced stage, growth factors secreted by the retina trigger the proliferation of new blood vessels, which grow along the inside surface of the retina and into the vitreous gel, the fluid that fills the eye. The new blood vessels are fragile, which makes them more likely to leak and bleed. Accompanying scar tissue can contract and cause retinal detachment—the pulling away of the retina from underlying tissue, like wallpaper peeling away from a wall. Retinal detachment can lead to permanent vision loss.

What is diabetic macular edema (DME)?

DME is the build-up of fluid (edema) in a region of the retina called the macula. The macula is important for the sharp, straight-ahead vision that is used for reading, recognizing faces, and driving. DME is the most common cause of vision loss among people with diabetic retinopathy. About half of all people with diabetic retinopathy will develop DME. Although it is more likely to occur as diabetic retinopathy worsens, DME can happen at any stage of the disease.

Who is at risk for diabetic retinopathy?

People with all types of diabetes (type 1, type 2, and gestational) are at risk for diabetic retinopathy. Risk increases the longer a person has diabetes. Between 40 and 45 percent of Americans diagnosed with diabetes have some stage of diabetic retinopathy, although only about half are aware of it. Women who develop or have diabetes during pregnancy may have rapid onset or worsening of diabetic retinopathy.

What are the symptoms of diabetic retinopathy and DME?

The early stages of diabetic retinopathy usually have no symptoms. The disease often progresses unnoticed until it affects vision. Bleeding from abnormal retinal blood vessels can cause the appearance of "floating" spots. These spots sometimes clear on their own. But without prompt treatment, bleeding often recurs, increasing the risk of permanent vision loss. If DME occurs, it can cause blurred vision.

How are diabetic retinopathy and DME detected?

Diabetic retinopathy and DME are detected during a comprehensive dilated eye exam that includes:

1. **Visual acuity testing**. This eye chart test measures a person's ability to see at various distances.
2. **Tonometry**. This test measures pressure inside the eye.
3. **Pupil dilation**. Drops placed on the eye's surface dilate (widen) the pupil, allowing a physician to examine the retina and optic nerve.

Optical coherence tomography (OCT). This technique is similar to ultrasound but uses light waves instead of sound waves to capture images of tissues inside the body. OCT provides detailed images of tissues that can be penetrated by light, such as the eye.

A comprehensive dilated eye exam allows the doctor to check the retina for:

1. Changes to blood vessels
2. Leaking blood vessels or warning signs of leaky blood vessels, such as fatty deposits
3. Swelling of the macula (DME)
4. Changes in the lens
5. Damage to nerve tissue

If DME or severe diabetic retinopathy is suspected, a fluorescein angiogram may be used to look for damaged or leaky blood vessels. In this test, a fluorescent dye is injected into the bloodstream, often into an arm vein. Pictures of the retinal blood vessels are taken as the dye reaches the eye.

How can people with diabetes protect their vision?

Vision lost to diabetic retinopathy is sometimes irreversible. However, early detection and treatment can reduce the risk of blindness by 95 percent. Because diabetic retinopathy often lacks early symptoms, people with diabetes should get a comprehensive dilated eye exam at least once a year. People with diabetic retinopathy may need eye exams more frequently. Women with diabetes who become pregnant should have a comprehensive dilated eye exam as soon as possible. Additional exams during pregnancy may be needed.

Studies such as the Diabetes Control and Complications Trial (DCCT) have shown that controlling diabetes slows the onset and worsening of diabetic retinopathy. DCCT study participants who kept their blood glucose level as close to normal as possible were significantly less likely than those without optimal glucose control to develop diabetic retinopathy, as well as kidney and nerve diseases. Other trials have shown that controlling elevated blood pressure and cholesterol can reduce the risk of vision loss among people with diabetes.

Treatment for diabetic retinopathy is often delayed until it starts to progress to PDR, or when DME occurs. Comprehensive dilated eye exams are needed more frequently as diabetic retinopathy becomes more severe. People with severe nonproliferative diabetic retinopathy have a high risk of developing PDR and may need a comprehensive dilated eye exam as often as every 2 to 4 months.

How is diabetic macular edema (DME) treated?

DME can be treated with several therapies that may be used alone or in combination.

Anti-VEGF Injection Therapy

Anti-VEGF drugs are injected into the vitreous gel to block a protein called vascular endothelial growth factor (VEGF), which can stimulate abnormal blood vessels to grow and leak fluid. Blocking VEGF can reverse abnormal blood vessel growth and decrease fluid in the retina. Available anti-VEGF drugs include Avastin (bevacizumab), Lucentis (ranibizumab), and Eylea (aflibercept). Lucentis and Eylea are approved by the U.S. Food and Drug Administration (FDA) for treating DME. Avastin was approved by the FDA to treat cancer, but is commonly used to treat eye conditions, including DME.

The NEI-sponsored Diabetic Retinopathy Clinical Research Network compared Avastin, Lucentis, and Eylea in a clinical trial. The study found all three drugs to be safe and effective for treating most people with DME. Patients who started the trial with 20/40 or better vision experienced similar improvements in vision no matter which of the three drugs they were given. However, patients who started the trial with 20/50 or worse vision had greater improvements in vision with Eylea.

Most people require monthly anti-VEGF injections for the first six months of treatment. Thereafter, injections are needed less often: typically three to four during the second six months of treatment, about four during the second year of treatment, two in the third year, one in the fourth year, and none in the fifth year. Dilated eye exams may be needed less often as the disease stabilizes.

Avastin, Lucentis, and Eylea vary in cost and in how often they need to be injected, so patients may wish to discuss these issues with an eye care professional.

Focal/grid macular laser surgery

In focal/grid macular laser surgery, a few to hundreds of small laser burns are made to leaking blood vessels in areas of edema near the center of the macula. Laser burns for DME slow the leakage of fluid, reducing swelling in the retina. The procedure is usually completed in one session, but some people may need more than one treatment. Focal/grid laser is sometimes applied before anti-VEGF injections, sometimes on the same day or a few days after an anti-VEGF injection, and sometimes only when DME fails to improve adequately after six months of anti-VEGF therapy.

Corticosteroids

Corticosteroids, either injected or implanted into the eye, may be used alone or in combination with other drugs or laser surgery to treat DME. The Ozurdex (dexamethasone) implant is for short-term use, while the Iluvien (fluocinolone acetonide) implant is longer lasting. Both are biodegradable and release a sustained dose of corticosteroids to suppress DME. Corticosteroid use in the eye increases the risk of cataract and glaucoma. DME patients who use corticosteroids should be monitored for increased pressure in the eye and glaucoma.

How is proliferative diabetic retinopathy (PDR) treated?

For decades, PDR has been treated with scatter laser surgery, sometimes called panretinal laser surgery or panretinal photocoagulation.

Diabetes-Related Eye Diseases

Treatment involves making 1,000 to 2,000 tiny laser burns in areas of the retina away from the macula. These laser burns are intended to cause abnormal blood vessels to shrink. Although treatment can be completed in one session, two or more sessions are sometimes required. While it can preserve central vision, scatter laser surgery may cause some loss of side (peripheral), color, and night vision. Scatter laser surgery works best before new, fragile blood vessels have started to bleed. Recent studies have shown that anti-VEGF treatment not only is effective for treating DME, but is also effective for slowing progression of diabetic retinopathy, including PDR, so anti-VEGF is increasingly used as a first-line treatment for PDR.

Chapter 35

Diabetes-Related Foot Problems

How can diabetes affect my feet?

Too much glucose, also called sugar, in your blood from diabetes can cause nerve damage and poor blood flow, which can lead to serious foot problems.

Nerve Damage

Damaged nerves may stop sending signals, or they may send signals too slowly or at the wrong times. Nerve damage can cause you to lose feeling in your feet. You may not feel pain, heat, or cold in your legs and feet. You may not feel a pebble inside your sock that is causing a sore. You may not feel a blister caused by poorly fitting shoes.

Sores on your feet can become infected. If your blood glucose is high, the extra glucose feeds the infection in those sores and the infection gets worse. Nerve damage can also cause pain and lead to foot deformities, or changes in the muscles, bones, and shape of your feet.

Text in this chapter is excerpted from "Prevent Diabetes Problems: Keep Your Feet Healthy," National Institute of Diabetes and Digestive and Kidney Diseases (NIDDK), National Institutes of Health (NIH), February 2014.

Poor Blood Flow

Poor blood flow means not enough blood flows to your legs and feet through your blood vessels. Poor blood flow makes it hard for a sore or an infection to heal. This problem is called peripheral artery disease, also called PAD.

Sometimes, a bad infection never heals. The infection might cause gangrene. If you have gangrene, the skin and tissue around the sore die. The area becomes black and smelly.

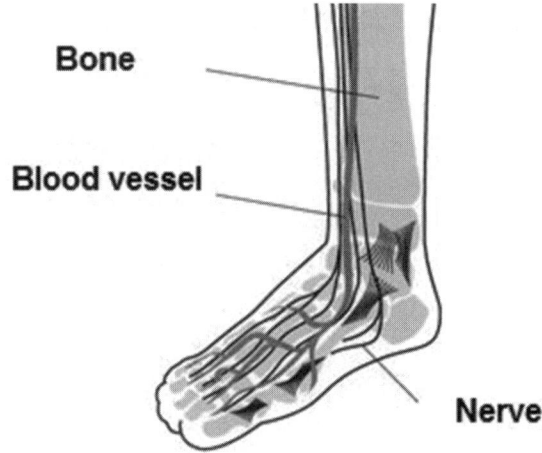

Figure 35.1. *Blood Vessels*

Prompt attention to any sore or infection on your toe or foot can prevent gangrene. Your doctor may decide to cut away the infected tissue or give you antibiotics. Your doctor also may perform tests to see how well blood is reaching your legs and feet. Sometimes, your doctor may be able to clear blocked blood vessels to improve the blood flow.

If these treatments don't work, or if you have severe pain or infection, a doctor may have to perform an amputation—surgery to cut off a body part—of your toe, foot, or part of your leg. A surgeon performs this operation in a hospital. You will receive anesthesia and be asleep during the operation.

What common foot problems can lead to pain or infections?

If you have diabetes, the common foot problems below can lead to pain or infections that make it hard to walk. If you have any of these problems, make sure you get prompt treatment from your doctor.

Diabetes-Related Foot Problems

Table 35.1. Common Foot Problems

Corn and callus Corns and calluses are thick layers of skin.	• Corns and calluses are caused by too much rubbing or pressure on the same spot. They often form where the first and second toes overlap. • You can gently rub a pumice stone on a corn or callus after you take a bath or shower to wear it down. A pumice stone is a type of rock used to smooth the skin. However, check with your doctor about the best way to care for a corn or callus. • If an infection occurs in an area of a corn or callus, your doctor may need to remove the unhealthy tissue and give you antibiotics.
Blisters Blisters are areas of skin that are raised and filled with fluid.	• A blister can form if your shoe always rubs the same spot on yor foot. • Wearing shoes that do not fit or wearing shoes without socks also can cause blisters. • To prevent a blister, use socks or a bandage over the spot being rubbed. Wear shoes that fit properly. • Cover small blisters with a bandage, and cover large ones with a gauze pad held with adhesive or paper tape. You also can buy special blister bandages in different sizes at a drugstore. • If your blister is infected, your doctor may need to drain the fluid from the blister and give you antibiotics.
Ingrown toenail Ingrown toenails happen when the edges of your toenails grow into your skin.	• Ingrown toenails can form if you wear shoes that are too tight or cut into the corners of your toenails when you trim them. • To prevent ingrown toenails, wear shoes that fit properly. • If your toenail edges are sharp, smooth them with a nail file or emery board instead of cutting them. • If you go to a salon for a pedicure, make sure they do not cut into the corners of your toenails. Never treat ingrown toenails at home. Your doctor may remove part of your toenail to help it heal or keep it from growing back into your skin. If your toe is infected, you may need antibiotics.

Table 35.1. Continued

Bunion at the outside edge of your big toe. As the bump gets worse, it can be filled with extra bone and fluid.	• Bunions form when your big toe slants toward your small toes. High heels, pointed shoes, or shoes that are too tight or narrow may cause bunions. Bunions often run in families. • To prevent bunions, wear shoes that fit well. • Your doctor may suggest using padded shoe inserts to prevent a bunion from getting worse and using medicine to reduce pain and swelling. You may need surgery to remove a bunion that causes frequent pain.
Plantar warts Plantar warts are small, flesh-colored growths on the bottoms of your feet. Sometimes you see tiny, black dots in the warts.	• Plantar warts are caused by a virus that enters your feet through small breaks in your skin. The warts can be painful and make it hard to walk. • To prevent plantar warts from spreading, avoid contact with your warts and wash your hands after touching them. • Keep your feet clean and dry. • Don't go barefoot in public areas. • Your doctor may remove plantar warts with minor surgery, laser treatment, liquid nitrogen, or medicines.
Hammertoe **Hammertoes are toes that curl under your feet.**	• Hammertoes form when one or both joints of the small toes bend from weakness in your foot muscle. Diabetic nerve damage may cause the weakness. • You may get sores on the bottoms of your feet and on the tops of your toes that can become infected. • The shape of your feet may change. • You can have problems walking and finding shoes that fit well. • Avoid high heels or shoes with pointed toes. • Your doctor may give you an orthotic, or insert, to place in your shoe. Medicines can reduce pain and swelling. If your hammertoe becomes rigid and painful, or if an open sore has formed, you may need surgery to correct your toe.

Diabetes-Related Foot Problems

Table 35.1. Continued

Dry and cracked skin Dry and cracked skin is rough, scaly, and flaking. Your skin may be gray if you have dark skin. Your skin may be red or itch.	• Dry and cracked skin can be caused by high blood glucose, nerve damage, or poor blood flow. • Cracks allow infection to start. • Keep your feet moist with lotion or petroleum jelly. • Do not soak your feet because your skin could become drier. • If you cannot treat your dry and cracked skin at home, see your doctor. You may need a prescription ointment or cream.
Athlete's Foot Athlete's foot is a fungus that causes itching, burning, redness, and cracking of your skin. The fungus grows on the soles of your feet and in between your toes.	• To prevent athlete's foot, keep your feet as dry as you can. • Try not to wear the same shoes all the time. Try to wear socks that do not trap moisture, such as cotton or wool socks. • Wear waterproof shoes or flip-flops in public showers. • If you go to a salon for a pedicure, ensure the tools are sterilized or bring your own tools. • See your doctor to make sure you have athlete's foot. You can buy sprays and creams to treat fungus at a drugstore; however, your doctor may prescribe a stronger oral medicine.
Fungal Infection Fungal infection of the toenails makes them thick, hard to cut, and appear yellow, green, brown, or black. A nail may also fall off.	• To prevent a fungal infection of the toenails, keep your feet as dry as you can. • Try not to wear the same shoes all the time. Try to wear socks that do not trap moisture, such as cotton or wool socks. • Wear waterproof shoes or flip-flops in public showers. • If you go to a salon for a pedicure, ensure the tools are sterilized or bring your own tools. • See your doctor to make sure you have a fungal infection of the toenails. Your doctor may prescribe an oral medicine to treat them. Sometimes, a doctor may remove the nail surgically or chemically or perform laser treatment. A laser beam can go deep into the nail tissue and kill the fungus; however, doctors are still studying how well this treatment works.

How can diabetes change the shape of my feet?

Nerve damage from diabetes can lead to changes in the shape of your feet. The damaged nerves cannot send messages to your foot muscles about movement. Your foot muscles become weak and imbalanced. The bones of your feet and toes may shift.

Nerve damage from diabetes also causes Charcot's foot, a problem in which the joints and soft tissue in your foot are destroyed.

In the early stages of Charcot's foot, your joints are stiff and collect fluid. The problem can quickly worsen. Your bones can slip out of place, making your foot look deformed.

You might not sense pain, so you may keep walking on your foot, making the problem worse. Without knowing it, you could injure and damage the joints or break a bone in your foot.

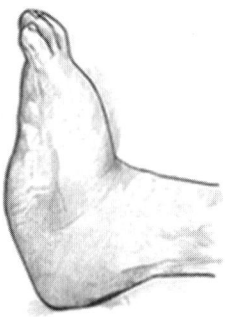

Figure 35.2. *Charcot's foot*

The symptoms of Charcot's foot appear quickly and include:

- warm, red skin
- swelling
- pain

Your doctor may first treat Charcot's foot by placing your foot in a cast and asking you to walk only with crutches or use a wheelchair. You may need surgery to correct the placement of the bones.

How often should I have a foot exam?

See your doctor at least once a year for a foot exam, or more often if you have foot problems. During the exam, your doctor will:

- look at your feet for signs of problems, especially if you have nerve damage

Diabetes-Related Foot Problems

- test the sense of feeling in your feet
- test how well blood is flowing to your legs and feet
- show you how to care for your feet
- decide if special shoes or shoe inserts would help your feet stay healthy
- trim your toenails if you cannot trim your own

Help your doctor care for your feet during every checkup. Start every checkup by taking off your shoes and socks. Tell your doctor about any foot problems you are having. If needed, your doctor may send you to a foot doctor, called a podiatrist.

Chapter 36

Diabetes and the Flu

If you have diabetes, you are three times more likely to be hospitalized from the flu and its complications than other people. The flu may also interfere with your blood glucose levels.

- But there are steps you can take to protect yourself.
- Get a flu shot! It's the single best way to protect yourself against the flu.
- Take prescription flu medicine when your health care provider prescribes it.
- Follow special sick day rules for people with diabetes.
- Take everyday steps to protect your health.

People with diabetes should talk with their health care provider now to discuss preventing and treating the flu. People infected with the flu can pass it on to others a day or two before any symptoms appear. That's why it is important to make sure the people around you get a flu shot as well.

Symptoms of Flu

Talk with your doctor now about how to reach him or her quickly by telephone if you think you have the flu. Symptoms of influenza can include:

Text in this chapter is excerpted from "Stay Well in Flu Season," Centers for Disease Control and Prevention (CDC), September 25, 2015.

- fever
- cough
- sore throat
- runny or stuffy nose
- body aches
- headache
- chills
- fatigue
- some people may also have vomiting and diarrhea.

People may be infected with the flu and have some symptoms without a fever.

Sick Day Guidelines for People with Diabetes

If you have diabetes, even if your blood sugars are in good control, and are sick with flu-like illness, you should follow these additional steps.

- Be sure to continue taking your diabetes pills or insulin. Don't stop taking them even if you can't eat. Your health care provider may even advise you to take more insulin during sickness.
- Test your blood glucose every four hours, and keep track of the results.
- Drink extra (calorie-free) liquids, and try to eat as you normally would. If you can't, try to have soft foods and liquids containing the equivalent amount of carbohydrates that you usually consume.
- Weigh yourself every day. Losing weight without trying is a sign of high blood glucose.
- Check your temperature every morning and evening. A fever may be a sign of infection.

Call your health care provider or go to an emergency room if any of the following happen to you:

- You feel too sick to eat normally and are unable to keep down food for more than 6 hours.

Diabetes and the Flu

- You're having severe diarrhea.
- You lose 5 pounds or more.
- Your temperature is over 101 degrees F.
- Your blood glucose is lower than 60 mg/dL or remains over 250 mg/dL on 2 checks.
- You have moderate or large amounts of ketones in your urine.
- You're having trouble breathing.
- You feel sleepy or can't think clearly.

How does diabetes affect how I respond to a cold or flu?

- Being sick can cause changes in your blood sugars. Also, illness can prevent you from eating properly, which further affects blood glucose.

- In addition, sometimes diabetes can make it more difficult for you to handle an infection like the flu. People with diabetes who come down with the flu may become very sick and may even have to go to a hospital. You can help keep yourself from getting the flu by getting a flu shot every year. Everyone with diabetes (type 1 OR type 2)—even pregnant women—should get a yearly flu shot. The best time to get one is now. The flu season often doesn't peak until February or even later. It takes several weeks for the shot offers its best protection, so don't delay . . . get your flu shot now!

Chapter 37

Diabetes and Gastroparesis

What is gastroparesis?

Gastroparesis, also called delayed gastric emptying, is a disorder that slows or stops the movement of food from the stomach to the small intestine. Normally, the muscles of the stomach, which are controlled by the vagus nerve, contract to break up food and move it through the gastrointestinal (GI) tract. The GI tract is a series of hollow organs joined in a long, twisting tube from the mouth to the anus. The movement of muscles in the GI tract, along with the release of hormones and enzymes, allows for the digestion of food. Gastroparesis can occur when the vagus nerve is damaged by illness or injury and the stomach muscles stop working normally. Food then moves slowly from the stomach to the small intestine or stops moving altogether.

What causes gastroparesis?

Most people diagnosed with gastroparesis have idiopathic gastroparesis, which means a health care provider cannot identify the cause, even with medical tests. Diabetes is the most common known cause of gastroparesis. People with diabetes have high levels of blood glucose, also called blood sugar. Over time, high blood glucose levels

---

Text in this chapter is excerpted from "Gastroparesis," National Institute of Diabetes and Digestive and Kidney Diseases (NIDDK), National Institutes of Health (NIH), June 2012.

can damage the vagus nerve. Other identifiable causes of gastroparesis include intestinal surgery and nervous system diseases such as Parkinson's disease or multiple sclerosis. For reasons that are still unclear, gastroparesis is more commonly found in women than in men.

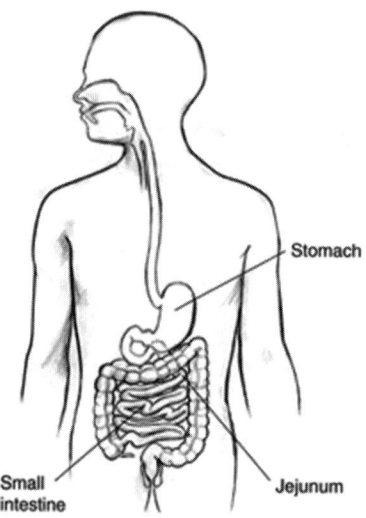

Figure 37.1. *The movement of food from the stomach to the small intestine*

What are the problems of gastroparesis?

The problems of gastroparesis can include:

- severe dehydration due to persistent vomiting
- gastroesophageal reflux disease (GERD), which is GER that occurs more than twice a week for a few weeks; GERD can lead to esophagitis—irritation of the esophagus
- bezoars, which can cause nausea, vomiting, obstruction, or interfere with absorption of some medications in pill form
- difficulty managing blood glucose levels in people with diabetes
- malnutrition due to poor absorption of nutrients or a low calorie intake
- decreased quality of life, including work absences due to severe symptoms

What are the symptoms of gastroparesis?

The most common symptoms of gastroparesis are nausea, a feeling of fullness after eating only a small amount of food, and vomiting undigested food—sometimes several hours after a meal. Other symptoms of gastroparesis include:

- gastroesophageal reflux (GER), also called acid reflux or acid regurgitation—a condition in which stomach contents flow back up into the esophagus, the organ that connects the mouth to the stomach
- pain in the stomach area
- abdominal bloating
- lack of appetite

Symptoms may be aggravated by eating greasy or rich foods, large quantities of foods with fiber—such as raw fruits and vegetables—or drinking beverages high in fat or carbonation. Symptoms may be mild or severe, and they can occur frequently in some people and less often in others. The symptoms of gastroparesis may also vary in intensity over time in the same individual. Sometimes gastroparesis is difficult to diagnose because people experience a range of symptoms similar to those of other diseases.

health care provider to calculate how fast the stomach is emptying.

How is gastroparesis treated?

Treatment of gastroparesis depends on the severity of the person's symptoms. In most cases, treatment does not cure gastroparesis, which is usually a chronic, or long-lasting, condition. Gastroparesis is also a relapsing condition—the symptoms can come and go for periods of time. Treatment helps people manage the condition so they can be as comfortable and active as possible.

How is gastroparesis treated if a person has diabetes?

An elevated blood glucose level directly interferes with normal stomach emptying, so good blood glucose control in people with diabetes is important. However, gastroparesis can make blood glucose control difficult. When food that has been delayed in the stomach finally enters the small intestine and is absorbed, blood glucose levels rise. Gastric emptying is unpredictable with gastroparesis, causing a person's blood glucose levels to be erratic and difficult to control.

The primary treatment goals for gastroparesis related to diabetes are to improve gastric emptying and regain control of blood glucose levels. In addition to the dietary changes and treatments already described, a health care provider will likely adjust the person's insulin regimen.

To better control blood glucose, people with diabetes and gastroparesis may need to:

- take insulin more often or change the type of insulin they take
- take insulin after meals, instead of before
- check blood glucose levels frequently after eating and administer insulin when necessary

A health care provider will give specific instructions for taking insulin based on the individual's needs and the severity of gastroparesis.

In some cases, the dietitian may suggest eating several liquid or puréed meals a day until gastroparesis symptoms improve and blood glucose levels are more stable.

Chapter 38

Diabetes, Heart Disease, and Stroke

What is the connection among diabetes, heart disease, and stroke?

If you have diabetes, you are at least twice as likely as someone who does not have diabetes to have heart disease or a stroke. People with diabetes also tend to develop heart disease or have strokes at an earlier age than other people. If you are middle-aged and have type 2 diabetes, some studies suggest that your chance of having a heart attack is as high as someone without diabetes who has already had one heart attack. Women who have not gone through menopause usually have less risk of heart disease than men of the same age. But women of all ages with diabetes have an increased risk of heart disease because diabetes cancels out the protective effects of being a woman in her child-bearing years.

People with diabetes who have already had one heart attack run an even greater risk of having a second one. In addition, heart attacks in people with diabetes are more serious and more likely to result in death. High blood glucose levels over time can lead to increased deposits of fatty materials on the insides of the blood vessel walls. These

---

Text in this chapter is excerpted from "Diabetes, Heart Disease, and Stroke," National Institute of Diabetes and Digestive and Kidney Diseases (NIDDK), National Institutes of Health (NIH), August 2013.

deposits may affect blood flow, increasing the chance of clogging and hardening of blood vessels (atherosclerosis).

What are the risk factors for heart disease and stroke in people with diabetes?

Diabetes itself is a risk factor for heart disease and stroke. Also, many people with diabetes have other conditions that increase their chance of developing heart disease and stroke. These conditions are called risk factors. One risk factor for heart disease and stroke is having a family history of heart disease. If one or more members of your family had a heart attack at an early age (before age 55 for men or 65 for women), you may be at increased risk.

You can't change whether heart disease runs in your family, but you can take steps to control the other risk factors for heart disease listed here:

- **Having central obesity.** Central obesity means carrying extra weight around the waist, as opposed to the hips. A waist measurement of more than 40 inches for men and more than 35 inches for women means you have central obesity. Your risk of heart disease is higher because abdominal fat can increase the production of LDL (bad) cholesterol, the type of blood fat that can be deposited on the inside of blood vessel walls.

- **Having abnormal blood fat (cholesterol) levels.**
  - LDL cholesterol can build up inside your blood vessels, leading to narrowing and hardening of your arteries—the blood vessels that carry blood from the heart to the rest of the body. Arteries can then become blocked. Therefore, high levels of LDL cholesterol raise your risk of getting heart disease.
  - Triglycerides are another type of blood fat that can raise your risk of heart disease when the levels are high.
  - HDL (good) cholesterol removes deposits from inside your blood vessels and takes them to the liver for removal. Low levels of HDL cholesterol increase your risk for heart disease.

- **Having high blood pressure.** If you have high blood pressure, also called hypertension, your heart must work harder to pump blood. High blood pressure can strain the heart, damage blood vessels, and increase your risk of heart attack, stroke, eye problems, and kidney problems.

- **Smoking.** Smoking doubles your risk of getting heart disease. Stopping smoking is especially important for people with diabetes because both smoking and diabetes narrow blood vessels. Smoking also increases the risk of other long-term complications, such as eye problems. In addition, smoking can damage the blood vessels in your legs and increase the risk of amputation.

How will I know whether my diabetes treatment is working?

You can keep track of the ABCs of diabetes to make sure your treatment is working. Talk with your health care provider about the best targets for you.

A stands for A1C (a test that measures blood glucose control). Have an A1C test at least twice a year. It shows your average blood glucose level over the past 3 months. Talk with your doctor about whether you should check your blood glucose at home and how to do it.

A1C Target: Below 7 percent, unless your doctor sets a different target

Blood Glucose Targets:

- Before Meals: 90 to 130 mg/dL
- 1 to 2 hours after the start of a meal: Less than 180 mg/dL

B is for blood pressure. Have it checked at every office visit.

Blood Pressure Target: Below 140/80 mm Hg, unless your doctor sets a different target

C is for cholesterol. Have it checked at least once a year.

Table 38.1. Blood fat targets

Blood fat (cholesterol) targets	
LDL (bad) cholesterol	Under 100 mg/dL
Triglycerides	Under 150 mg/dL
HDL (good) cholesterol **For men**: above 40 mg/dL **For women**: above 50 mg/dL	

Control of the ABCs of diabetes can reduce your risk for heart disease and stroke. If your blood glucose, blood pressure, and cholesterol levels aren't on target, ask your doctor what changes in diet, activity, and medications can help you reach these goals.

What types of heart and blood vessel disease occur in people with diabetes?

Two major types of heart and blood vessel disease, also called cardiovascular disease, are common in people with diabetes: coronary artery disease (CAD) and cerebral vascular disease. People with diabetes are also at risk for heart failure. Narrowing or blockage of the blood vessels in the legs, a condition called peripheral arterial disease, can also occur in people with diabetes.

Chapter 39

Diabetes and Hepatitis B

What is hepatitis B?

Hepatitis B is a contagious liver disease that results from infection with the hepatitis B virus. When first infected, a person can develop an "acute" infection, which can range in severity from a very mild illness with few or no symptoms to a serious condition requiring hospitalization. **Acute** hepatitis B refers to the first 6 months after someone is infected with the hepatitis B virus. Some people are able to fight the virus and clear the infection. For others, the infection remains and leads to a "chronic," or lifelong, illness. **Chronic** hepatitis B refers to the illness that occurs when the hepatitis B virus remains in a person's body. Over time, the infection can cause serious damage to the liver and lead to complications such as liver failure or liver cancer.

How is hepatitis B spread?

The hepatitis B virus is usually spread when blood or other body fluids from a person infected with the hepatitis B virus enters the body of someone who is not infected. Hepatitis B can be spread through sharing needles, syringes, or other injection equipment. In addition,

---

Text in this chapter is excerpted from "Diabetes and Hepatitis B Vaccination," Centers for Disease Control and Prevention (CDC), October 2012.

the hepatitis B virus can spread through sexual contact and from an infected mother to her baby during childbirth.

Why is hepatitis B relevant to people with diabetes?

Among people living with diabetes, the hepatitis B virus has been spread through contact with infectious blood. People living with diabetes are at increased risk for hepatitis B if they share blood glucose meters, fingerstick devices or other diabetes-care equipment such as syringes or insulin pens.

How infectious is the hepatitis B virus?

The hepatitis B virus is 50 – 100 times more infectious than HIV which makes it easily transmitted. The hepatitis B virus can survive outside the body at least a week. During that time, the virus can still cause infection if it enters the body of a person who is not infected.

What should diabetes educators tell their patients about hepatitis B?

Diabetes educators should provide their clients or patients with the following information on how to protect themselves from getting the hepatitis B virus:

- Prevent exposure to hepatitis B and other blood borne pathogens by not sharing equipment such as blood glucose monitors or other diabetes care equipment.
- The best way to prevent hepatitis B is by getting vaccinated. CDC recommends hepatitis B vaccination for all unvaccinated adults with diabetes younger than 60 years of age.
- If you think you have already been vaccinated, confirm with your doctor.
- The hepatitis B vaccine is given as a series of 3 shots over a period of 6 months (0, 1, 6 month schedule). The entire series is needed for long-term protection.

If you have not received the hepatitis B vaccine series talk to your doctor about getting vaccinated.

Chapter 40

Diabetic Kidney Disease

What are the kidneys and what do they do?

The kidneys are two bean-shaped organs, each about the size of a fist. They are located just below the rib cage, one on each side of the spine. Every day, the two kidneys filter about 120 to 150 quarts of blood to produce about 1 to 2 quarts of urine, composed of wastes and extra fluid. The urine flows from the kidneys to the bladder through tubes called ureters. The bladder stores urine. When the bladder empties, urine flows out of the body through a tube called the urethra, located at the bottom of the bladder. In men the urethra is long, while in women it is short.

What is diabetic kidney disease?

Diabetic kidney disease, also called diabetic nephropathy, is kidney disease caused by diabetes. Even when well controlled, diabetes can lead to chronic kidney disease (CKD) and kidney failure, described as endstage kidney disease or ESRD when treated with a kidney transplant or blood-filtering treatments called dialysis.

Text in this chapter is excerpted from "Diabetic Kidney Disease," National Institute of Diabetes and Digestive and Kidney Diseases (NIDDK), National Institutes of Health (NIH), August 2014.

Diabetes affects 25.8 million people of all ages in the United States. As many as 40 percent of people who have diabetes are expected to develop CKD. Diabetes, the most common cause of kidney failure in the United States, accounts for nearly 44 percent of new cases of kidney failure.

Kidneys work at the microscopic level. The kidney is not one large filter. Each kidney is made up of about a million filtering units called nephrons. Each nephron filters a small amount of blood. The nephron includes a filter, called the glomerulus, and a tubule. The nephrons work through a two-step process. The glomerulus lets fluid and waste products pass through it; however, it prevents blood cells and large molecules, mostly proteins, from passing. The filtered fluid then passes through the tubule, which sends needed minerals back to the bloodstream and removes wastes. The final product becomes urine.

How does diabetes lead to kidney disease?

Diabetes leads to kidney disease in several ways. At the onset of diabetes, blood flow into the kidneys increases, which may strain the glomeruli and lessen their ability to filter blood. Higher levels of blood glucose lead to the buildup of extra material in the glomeruli, which increases the force of the blood moving through the kidneys and creates stress in the glomeruli. This stress leads to gradual and progressive scarring of the glomeruli, eventually reducing the kidneys' ability to filter blood properly. Other factors—including heredity, diet, lifestyle, and other medical conditions—are also involved in the development of kidney disease, though scientists cannot fully explain how the interaction of these factors leads to diabetic kidney disease.

Many people with diabetes can develop high blood pressure, another factor in the development of kidney disease. High blood pressure, also called hypertension, is an increase in the amount of force that blood places on blood vessels as it moves through the entire body. When the force of blood flow is high, blood vessels stretch so blood flows more easily. Eventually, this stretching scars and weakens blood vessels throughout the body, including those in the kidneys.

What are the symptoms of diabetic kidney disease?

People with diabetic kidney disease do not have symptoms in the early stages. As kidney disease progresses, a person can develop

Diabetic Kidney Disease

edema, or swelling. Edema happens when the kidneys cannot get rid of the extra fluid and salt in the body. Edema can occur in the legs, feet, or ankles and less often in the hands or face. Once kidney function decreases further, symptoms may include:

- appetite loss
- nausea
- vomiting
- drowsiness, or feeling tired
- trouble concentrating
- sleep problems
- increased or decreased urination
- generalized itching or numbness
- dry skin
- headaches
- weight loss
- darkened skin
- muscle cramps
- shortness of breath
- chest pain

How can people prevent or slow the progression of diabetic kidney disease?

People can prevent or slow the progression of diabetic kidney disease by:

- taking medications to control high blood pressure
- managing blood glucose levels
- making changes in their eating, diet, and nutrition
- losing weight if they are overweight or obese
- getting regular physical activity

People with diabetes should see a health care provider who will help them learn to manage their diabetes and monitor their diabetes control. Most people with diabetes get care from primary care providers, including internists, family practice doctors, or pediatricians. However, having a team of health care providers can often improve diabetes care. In addition to a primary care provider, the team can include:

- an endocrinologist—a doctor with special training in diabetes
- a nephrologist—a doctor who specializes in treating people who have kidney problems or related conditions
- diabetes educators such as a nurse or dietitian
- a podiatrist—a doctor who specializes in foot care
- an ophthalmologist or optometrist for eye care
- a pharmacist
- a dentist
- a mental health counselor for emotional support and access to community resources

The team can also include other health care providers and specialists.

Blood Pressure Medications

Medications that lower blood pressure can also significantly slow the progression of kidney disease. Two types of blood pressure-lowering medications, angiotensin-converting enzyme (ACE) inhibitors and angiotensin receptor blockers (ARBs), have been shown to slow the progression of kidney disease. Many people require two or more medications to control their blood pressure. In addition to an ACE inhibitor or an ARB, a health care provider may prescribe a diuretic—a medication that helps the kidneys remove fluid from the blood. A person may also need beta-blockers, calcium channel blockers, and other blood pressure medications. People should talk with their health care provider about their individual blood pressure goals and how often they should have their blood pressure checked.

Managing Blood Glucose Levels

- People manage blood glucose levels by testing blood glucose throughout the day
- Following a diet and physical activity plan

Diabetic Kidney Disease

- Taking insulin throughout the day based on food and liquid intake and physical activity

People with diabetes need to talk with their health care team regularly and follow their directions closely. The goal is to keep blood glucose levels within the normal range or within a range set by the person's health care team.

Eating, Diet, and Nutrition

Following a healthy eating plan can help lower blood pressure and control blood sugar. A health care provider may recommend the Dietary Approaches to Stop Hypertension (DASH) eating plan. DASH focuses on fruits, vegetables, whole grains, and other foods that are heart healthy and lower in sodium, which often comes from salt. The DASH eating plan:

- is low in fat and cholesterol

- features fat-free or low-fat milk and dairy products, fish, poultry, and nuts

- suggests less red meat, and fewer sweets, added sugars, and sugar containing beverages

- is rich in nutrients, protein, and fiber

People with diabetic kidney disease may need to limit sodium and salt intake to help reduce edema and lower blood pressure. A dietitian may also recommend a diet low in saturated fat and cholesterol to help control high levels of lipids, or fats, in the blood.

Health care providers may recommend that people with CKD eat moderate or reduced amounts of protein, though the benefits of reducing protein in a person's diet are still being researched. Proteins break down into waste products the kidneys must filter from the blood. Eating more protein than the body needs may burden the kidneys and cause kidney function to decline faster. However, protein intake that is too low may lead to malnutrition, a condition that occurs when the body does not get enough nutrients.

How is kidney failure due to diabetic kidney disease treated?

A health care provider may treat kidney failure due to diabetic kidney disease with dialysis or a kidney transplant. In some cases, people with diabetic kidney disease receive kidney and pancreas transplants. In most cases, people with diabetic kidney disease start dialysis earlier than people with kidney failure who do not have diabetes.

People with diabetic end-stage kidney disease who receive a kidney transplant have a much better survival rate than those people on dialysis, although survival rates for those on dialysis have increasingly improved over time. However, people who receive a kidney transplant and do not have diabetes have a higher survival rate than people with diabetic kidney disease who receive a transplant.

Chapter 41

Diabetes-Related Mouth Problems

What happens if I have plaque?

Plaque that is not removed hardens over time into tartar and collects above your gum line. Tartar makes it more difficult to brush and clean between your teeth. Your gums become red and swollen, and bleed easily—signs of unhealthy or inflamed gums, called gingivitis.

When gingivitis is not treated, it can advance to gum disease called periodontitis. In periodontitis, the gums pull away from the teeth and form spaces, called pockets, which slowly become infected. This infection can last a long time. Your body fights the bacteria as the plaque spreads and grows below the gum line. Both the bacteria and your body's response to this infection start to break down the bone and the tissue that hold the teeth in place. If periodontitis is not treated, the gums, bones, and tissue that support the teeth are destroyed. Teeth may become loose and might need to be removed. If you have periodontitis, your dentist may send you to a periodontist, an expert in treating gum disease.

Text in this chapter is excerpted from "Prevent Diabetes Problems: Keep Your Mouth Healthy," National Institute of Diabetes and Digestive and Kidney Diseases (NIDDK), National Institutes of Health (NIH), July 2014.

What are the most common mouth problems from diabetes?

The following chart shows the most common mouth problems from diabetes.

Table 41.1. Common mouth problems from Diabetes

Problem	What it is	Symptoms	Treatment
gingivitis	• unhealthy or inflamed gums	• red, swollen, and bleeding gums	• daily brushing and flossing
			• regular cleanings at the dentist
periodontitis	• gum disease, which can change from mild to severe	• red, swollen, and bleeding gums	• deep cleaning at your dentist
		• gums that have pulled away from the teeth	• medicine that your dentist prescribes
		• long-lasting infection between the teeth and gums	• gum surgery in severe cases
		• bad breath that won't go away	
		• permanent teeth that are loose or moving away from one another	
		• changes in the way your teeth fit together when you bite	
		• sometimes pus between the teeth and gums	
		• changes in the fit of dentures, which are teeth you can remove	

Table 41.1. Continued

Problem	What it is	Symptoms	Treatment
thrush, called candidiasis	• the growth of a naturally occurring fungus that the body is unable to control	• sore, white—or sometimes red—patches on your gums, tongue, cheeks, or the roof of your mouth	• medicine that your doctor or dentist prescribes to kill the fungus
		• patches that have turned into open sores	• cleaning dentures
			• removing dentures for part of the day or night, and soaking them in medicine that your doctor or dentist prescribes
dry mouth, called xerostomia	• a lack of saliva in your mouth, which raises your risk for tooth decay and gum disease	• dry feeling in your mouth, often or all of the time	• taking medicine to keep your mouth wet that your doctor or dentist prescribes
		• dry, rough tongue	• rinsing with a fluoride mouth rinse to prevent cavities
		• pain in the mouth cracked lips	• using sugarless gum or mints to increase saliva flow
		• mouth sores or infection	• taking frequent sips of water
		• problems chewing, eating, swallowing, or talking	• avoiding tobacco, caffeine, and alcoholic beverages

Table 41.1. Continued

Problem	What it is	Symptoms	Treatment
oral burning	• a burning sensation inside the mouth caused by uncontrolled blood glucose levels	• burning feeling in the mouth	• seeing your doctor, who may change your diabetes medicine
		• dry mouth • bitter taste • symptoms may worsen throughout the day	• once your blood glucose is under control, the oral burning will go away

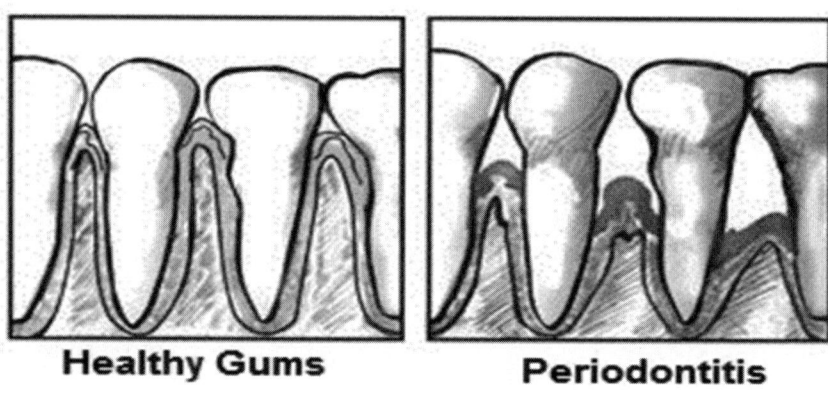

Figure 41.1. *Healthy Gums and Gums with Problems*

Chapter 42

Diabetes-Related Nerve Damage

What is my nervous system and what does it do?

Your nervous system carries signals between your brain and other parts of your body through your spinal cord. Nerves are bundles of special tissues that transmit these signals.

The signals share information between your brain and body about how things feel. The signals also send information between your brain and body to control automatic body functions, such as breathing and digestion, and to move your body parts.

The nerves in your spinal cord branch out to all of your organs and body parts. All your nerves together make up your nervous system.

Your nervous system is composed of the:

- central nervous system—your brain and spinal cord
- cranial nerves—nerves that connect your brain to your head, neck, and face

---

Text in this chapter is excerpted from "Prevent Diabetes Problems: Keep Your Nervous System Healthy," National Institute of Diabetes and Digestive and Kidney Diseases (NIDDK), National Institutes of Health (NIH), February 2014.

- peripheral nervous system—nerves that connect your spinal cord to your entire body, including your organs and your arms, hands, legs, and feet

How can diabetes affect my nervous system?

Over time, too much fat and glucose, also called sugar, in your blood from diabetes can damage your nerves. High blood glucose also can damage the small blood vessels that nourish your nerves with oxygen and nutrients. Without enough oxygen and nutrients, nerves cannot function well. Damaged nerves may stop sending signals, or they may send signals too slowly or at the wrong times.

Nerve damage from diabetes is called diabetic neuropathy.

If you have diabetes, you can develop nerve damage at any time; however, you are more likely to have it the older you are and the longer you have diabetes. Nerve damage is also more likely if you:

- have high cholesterol and blood fat
- have high blood pressure
- are overweight
- have kidney disease
- smoke
- drink too many alcoholic beverages

What are the symptoms of nerve damage?

Nerve damage symptoms depend on which nerves have damage. Some people have no symptoms or mild symptoms. Other people have painful and long-lasting symptoms. As most nerve damage develops over many years, a person may not notice mild cases for a long time. In some people, the onset of pain may be sudden and severe.

What are the types of nerve damage from diabetes?

Peripheral Neuropathy

Peripheral neuropathy is the most common type of diabetic neuropathy, and it affects the sensory nerves of your feet, legs, hands, and arms. These areas of your body may feel:

- numb
- weak

Diabetes-Related Nerve Damage

- cold
- burning or tingling, like "pins and needles"

You may feel extreme pain in these areas of your body, even when they are touched lightly. You also may feel pain in your legs and feet when walking.

These feelings are often worse at night and can make it hard to sleep. Most of the time, you will have these feelings on both sides of your body, such as in both feet; however, they can occur just on one side.

You might have other problems, such as:

- swollen feet
- loss of balance
- loss of muscle tone in your hands and feet
- a deformity or shape change in your toes and feet
- calluses or open sores on your feet

Autonomic Neuropathy

Autonomic neuropathy can affect your:

- digestive system
- sex organs
- bladder
- sweat glands
- eyes
- heart rate and blood pressure
- ability to sense low blood glucose

Digestive system

Damage to nerves in your stomach, intestines, and other parts of your digestive system may:

- make it hard to swallow both solid food and liquids
- cause stomach pain, nausea, vomiting, constipation, or diarrhea
- make it hard to keep your blood glucose under control

Your doctor or dietitian may advise you to eat smaller, more frequent meals; avoid fatty foods; and eat less fiber.

Sex organs

Damage to nerves in the sex organs may:

- prevent a man's penis from getting firm when he wants to have sex, called erectile dysfunction or impotence. Many men who have had diabetes for several years have impotence.
- prevent a woman's vagina from getting wet when she wants to have sex. A woman might also have less feeling around her vagina.

Bladder

Damage to nerves in your bladder may make it hard to know when you need to urinate and when your bladder is empty. This damage can cause you to hold urine for too long, which can lead to bladder infections. You also might leak drops of urine.

Sweat glands

Damage to nerves in your sweat glands may prevent them from working properly. Nerve damage can cause you to sweat a lot at night or while eating.

Eyes

Damage to nerves in your pupils, the parts of your eyes that react to changes in light and darkness, may make them slow to respond to these changes. You may have trouble seeing the lights of other cars when driving at night. Your eyes may take longer to adjust when you enter a dark room.

Heart rate and blood pressure

Damage to nerves that control your heart rate and blood pressure may make these nerves respond more slowly to changes in position, stress, physical activity, sleep, and breathing patterns. You might feel dizzy or pass out when you go from lying down to standing up or when you do physical activity. You also might have shortness of breath or swelling in your feet.

Diabetes-Related Nerve Damage

Ability to sense low blood glucose

Autonomic nerves also let you know when your blood glucose is low. Damage to these nerves can prevent you from feeling the symptoms of low blood glucose, also called hypoglycemia. This kind of nerve damage is more likely to happen if you have had diabetes for a long time or if your blood glucose has often been too low. Low blood glucose can make you:

- hungry
- dizzy or shaky
- confused
- pale
- sweat more
- weak
- anxious or cranky
- have headaches
- have a fast heartbeat

Severe hypoglycemia can cause you to pass out. If that happens, you'll need help bringing your blood glucose level back to normal. Your health care team can teach your family members and friends how to give you an injection of glucagon, a hormone that raises blood glucose levels quickly. If glucagon is not available, someone should call 911 to get you to the nearest emergency room for treatment.

> Consider wearing a diabetes medical alert identification bracelet or necklace. If you have hypoglycemia and are not able to communicate, the emergency team will know you have diabetes and get you the proper treatment. You can find these bracelets or necklaces at your pharmacy or on the Internet. You can also ask your doctor for information on available products.

Other Neuropathies

Other types of neuropathies from diabetes can cause:

- damage to the joint and bones of your foot, called Charcot's foot, in which you cannot sense pain or the position of your foot
- carpal tunnel syndrome, in which a nerve in your forearm is compressed at your wrist, causing numbness, swelling, and pain in your fingers

- paralysis on one side of your face, called Bell's palsy
- double vision or not being able to focus your eyes
- aching behind one eye

How does nerve damage affect my feet?

The nerves to your feet are the longest in your body and are the most affected by nerve damage. If you have damage to these nerves, you may not feel pain, heat, or cold in your legs and feet. You might not notice sores or injuries, which can become infected. If you have any sores on your feet, see your doctor right away. Prompt attention to any sore or infection on your toe or foot can prevent more serious problems with your toes, feet, or parts of your legs.

Remind your doctor to check your feet at every office visit. See your doctor at least once a year for a foot exam, or more often if you have foot problems.

Check your feet every day for problems. If you have problems with your feet, your doctor may send you to a foot doctor, called a podiatrist.

How does smoking affect my diabetes and nervous system?

Smoking can narrow and harden the blood vessels that nourish your nerves with oxygen and nutrients.

Smoking and diabetes are a dangerous mix. Smoking raises your risk for many diabetes problems. If you quit smoking,

- you will lower your risk for heart attack, stroke, nerve disease, kidney disease, and amputation
- your cholesterol and blood pressure levels might improve
- your blood circulation will improve

If you smoke, stop smoking. Ask for help so that you don't have to do it alone. You can start by calling 1–800–QUITNOW or 1–800–784–8669.

What is the treatment for nerve damage from diabetes?

The treatment for nerve damage from diabetes is based on your symptoms. No treatment can reverse nerve damage; however, it can help you feel better. Your doctor might suggest taking low doses of

Diabetes-Related Nerve Damage

medicines that both treat other health problems and help the pain of neuropathy. Some of these medicines include:

- antidepressants
- anticonvulsants, or anti-seizure medicines

Other treatment options include:

- creams or patches on your skin for burning pain
- over-the-counter pain medicines
- acupuncture, a form of pain treatment that uses needles inserted into your body at certain pressure points
- physical therapy, which helps with muscle weakness and loss of balance
- relaxation exercises, such as yoga
- special shoes to fit softly around sore feet or feet that have changed shape

Your doctor also can prescribe medicines to help with problems caused by nerve damage in other areas of your body, such as poor digestion, dizziness, sexual problems, and lack of bladder control.

Stopping smoking and drinking alcoholic beverages also may help with symptoms.

Chapter 43

Diabetes and Polycystic Ovary Syndrome

What is polycystic ovary syndrome (PCOS)?

Polycystic ovary syndrome (PCOS) is a health problem that can affect a woman's:

- Menstrual cycle
- Ability to have children
- Hormones
- Heart
- Blood vessels
- Appearance

With PCOS, women typically have:

- High levels of androgens. These are sometimes called male hormones, though females also make them.
- Missed or irregular periods (monthly bleeding)
- Many small cysts (sists) (fluid-filled sacs) in their ovaries

---

Text in this chapter is excerpted from "Polycystic Ovary Syndrome (PCOS) Fact Sheet," Office on Women's Health (OWH), December 23, 2014.

What causes PCOS?

The cause of PCOS is unknown. But most experts think that several factors, including genetics, could play a role. Women with PCOS are more likely to have a mother or sister with PCOS.

A main underlying problem with PCOS is a hormonal imbalance. In women with PCOS, the ovaries make more androgens than normal. Androgens are male hormones that females also make. High levels of these hormones affect the development and release of eggs during ovulation.

Researchers also think insulin may be linked to PCOS. Insulin is a hormone that controls the change of sugar, starches, and other food into energy for the body to use or store. Many women with PCOS have too much insulin in their bodies because they have problems using it. Excess insulin appears to increase production of androgen. High androgen levels can lead to:

- Acne
- Excessive hair growth
- Weight gain
- Problems with ovulation

What are the symptoms of PCOS?

The symptoms of PCOS can vary from woman to woman. Some of the symptoms of PCOS include:

- Infertility (not able to get pregnant) because of not ovulating. In fact, PCOS is the most common cause of female infertility.
- Infrequent, absent, and/or irregular menstrual periods
- Hirsutism—increased hair growth on the face, chest, stomach, back, thumbs, or toes
- Cysts on the ovaries
- Acne, oily skin, or dandruff
- Weight gain or obesity, usually with extra weight around the waist
- Male-pattern baldness or thinning hair
- Patches of skin on the neck, arms, breasts, or thighs that are thick and dark brown or black

Chapter 44

Diabetes and Proteinuria

What is proteinuria?

Proteinuria—also called albuminuria or urine albumin—is a condition in which urine contains an abnormal amount of protein. Albumin is the main protein in the blood. Proteins are the building blocks for all body parts, including muscles, bones, hair, and nails. Proteins in the blood also perform a number of important functions. They protect the body from infection, help blood clot, and keep the right amount of fluid circulating throughout the body.

As blood passes through healthy kidneys, they filter out the waste products and leave in the things the body needs, like albumin and other proteins. Most proteins are too big to pass through the kidneys' filters into the urine. However, proteins from the blood can leak into the urine when the filters of the kidney, called glomeruli, are damaged.

Proteinuria is a sign of chronic kidney disease (CKD), which can result from diabetes, high blood pressure, and diseases that cause inflammation in the kidneys. For this reason, testing for albumin in the urine is part of a routine medical assessment for everyone. Kidney disease is sometimes called renal disease. If CKD progresses,

---

Text in this chapter is excerpted from "Proteinuria," National Institute of Diabetes and Digestive and Kidney Diseases (NIDDK), National Institutes of Health (NIH), February 2014.

it can lead to end-stage renal disease (ESRD), when the kidneys fail completely. A person with ESRD must receive a kidney transplant or regular blood-cleansing treatments called dialysis.

Who is at risk for proteinuria?

People with diabetes, hypertension, or certain family backgrounds are at risk for proteinuria. In the United States, diabetes is the leading cause of ESRD.

In both type 1 and type 2 diabetes, albumin in the urine is one of the first signs of deteriorating kidney function. As kidney function declines, the amount of albumin in the urine increases.

Another risk factor for developing proteinuria is hypertension, or high blood pressure. Proteinuria in a person with high blood pressure is an indicator of declining kidney function. If the hypertension is not controlled, the person can progress to full kidney failure.

African Americans are more likely than Caucasians to have high blood pressure and to develop kidney problems from it, even when their blood pressure is only mildly elevated. In fact, African Americans are six times more likely than Caucasians to develop hypertension-related kidney failure.

Other groups at risk for proteinuria are American Indians, Hispanics/Latinos, Pacific Islander Americans, older adults, and overweight people. These at-risk groups and people who have a family history of kidney disease should have their urine tested regularly.

What are the signs and symptoms of proteinuria?

Proteinuria has no signs or symptoms in the early stages. Large amounts of protein in the urine may cause it to look foamy in the toilet. Also, because protein has left the body, the blood can no longer soak up enough fluid, so swelling in the hands, feet, abdomen, or face may occur. This swelling is called edema. These are signs of large protein loss and indicate that kidney disease has progressed. Laboratory testing is the only way to find out whether protein is in a person's urine before extensive kidney damage occurs.

Several health organizations recommend regular urine checks for people at risk for CKD. A 1996 study sponsored by the National Institutes of Health determined that proteinuria is the best predictor of progressive kidney failure in people with type 2 diabetes. The American Diabetes Association recommends regular urine testing for proteinuria for people with type 1 or type 2 diabetes. The National Kidney

Foundation recommends that routine checkups include testing for excess protein in the urine, especially for people in high-risk groups.

What are the tests for proteinuria?

Until recently, an accurate protein measurement required a 24-hour urine collection. In a 24-hour collection, the patient urinates into a container, which is kept refrigerated between trips to the bathroom. The patient is instructed to begin collecting urine after the first trip to the bathroom in the morning. Every drop of urine for the rest of the day is to be collected in the container. The next morning, the patient adds the first urination after waking and the collection is complete.

In recent years, researchers have found that a single urine sample can provide the needed information. In the newer technique, the amount of albumin in the urine sample is compared with the amount of creatinine, a waste product of normal muscle breakdown. The measurement is called a urine albumin-to-creatinine ratio (UACR). A urine sample containing more than 30 milligrams of albumin for each gram of creatinine (30 mg/g) is a warning that there may be a problem. If the laboratory test exceeds 30 mg/g, another UACR test should be done 1 to two weeks later. If the second test also shows high levels of protein, the person has persistent proteinuria, a sign of declining kidney function, and should have additional tests to evaluate kidney function.

What should a person with proteinuria do?

If a person has diabetes, hypertension, or both, the first goal of treatment will be to control blood glucose, also called blood sugar, and blood pressure. People with diabetes should test their blood glucose often, follow a healthy eating plan, take prescribed medicines, and get the amount of exercise recommended by their doctor. A person with diabetes and high blood pressure may need a medicine from a class of drugs called angiotensin-converting enzyme (ACE) inhibitors or a similar class called angiotensin receptor blockers (ARBs). These drugs have been found to protect kidney function even more than other drugs that provide the same level of blood pressure control. Many patients with proteinuria but without hypertension may also benefit from ACE inhibitors or ARBs.

Part Six

Diabetes in Specific Populations

Chapter 45

Diabetes in Children and Adolescents

Type 1 Diabetes

Type 1 diabetes accounts for approximately 5 percent of all diagnosed cases of diabetes, but is the leading cause of diabetes in children of all ages. Type 1 diabetes accounts for almost all diabetes in children less than 10 years of age. Type 1 diabetes is an autoimmune disease in which the immune system destroys the insulin-producing beta cells of the pancreas that help regulate blood glucose levels.

Onset: Type 1 diabetes mostly has an acute onset, with children and adolescents usually able to pinpoint when symptoms began. Onset can occur at any age. Children and adolescents may present with ketoacidosis as the first indication of type 1 diabetes. Others may have post-meal hyperglycemia, or modest fasting hyperglycemia that rapidly progresses to severe hyperglycemia and/or ketoacidosis in the presence of infection or other stress.

Symptoms: The immunologic process that leads to type 1 diabetes can begin years before the symptoms of type 1 diabetes develop. Symptoms become apparent when most of the beta-cell population

---

Text in this chapter is excerpted from "Overview of Diabetes in Children and Adolescents," National Diabetes Education Program (NDEP), July 2014.

is destroyed and usually develop over a short period of time. Early symptoms, which are mainly due to hyperglycemia, include increased thirst and urination, constant hunger, weight loss, and blurred vision. Children also may feel very tired.

As insulin deficiency worsens, ketones, which are formed from the breakdown of fat, build up in the blood and are excreted in the urine and breath. Increased ketones are associated with shortness of breath and abdominal pain, vomiting, and worsening dehydration. Elevation of blood glucose, acidosis, and dehydration comprise the condition known as diabetic ketoacidosis or DKA. If diabetes is not diagnosed and treated with insulin at this point, the individual can lapse into a life-threatening coma. Often, children with vomiting are mistakenly diagnosed as having gastroenteritis. New-onset diabetes can be differentiated from gastroenteritis by the frequent urination that accompanies continued vomiting, as opposed to decreased urination due to dehydration if the vomiting is caused by gastroenteritis.

Risk Factors: A combination of genetic and environmental factors put people at increased risk for type 1 diabetes. Researchers have identified many factors and continue working so that targeted treatments can be designed to stop the autoimmune process that destroys the pancreatic beta-cells.

Co-morbidities: Children with type 1 diabetes are at risk for the long-term complications of diabetes. Autoimmune diseases such as celiac disease and autoimmune thyroid disease are also associated with type 1 diabetes.

Type 2 Diabetes

Type 2 diabetes used to occur mainly in adults who were overweight and older than 40 years. Now, as more children and adolescents in the United States become overweight or obese and inactive, type 2 diabetes is occurring more often in young people aged 10 or older. Most children and adolescents diagnosed with type 2 diabetes are also insulin resistant, and have a family history of type 2 diabetes. Type 2 diabetes is more common in certain racial and ethnic groups such as African Americans, American Indians, Hispanic/Latino Americans, and some Asian and Pacific Islander Americans.

The increased incidence of type 2 diabetes in youth is a first consequence of the obesity epidemic among young people, and is a significant and growing public health problem.

Onset: The first stage in the development of type 2 diabetes is often insulin resistance, requiring increasing amounts of insulin to be produced by the pancreas to control blood glucose levels. Initially, the pancreas responds by producing more insulin, but after several years, insulin production may decrease and diabetes develops. Type 2 diabetes usually develops slowly and insidiously.

Type 2 Diabetes Risk Factors and Testing Criteria

Overweight (BMI >85th percentile for age and gender; weight for height >85th percentile; or weight >120 percent of ideal for height
Plus
Any two of the following risk factors:
- family history of type 2 diabetes in first- or second-degree relative
- race/ethnicity – American Indian, African American, Hispanic/Latino, Asian American, or Pacific Islander
- signs of insulin resistance or conditions associated with insulin resistance (acanthosis nigricans, hypertension, dyslipidemia, polycystic ovarian syndrome, or small-for-gestational-age birth weight)
- maternal history of diabetes or Gestational Diabetes Mellitus (GDM) during the child's gestation

Age to begin testing – 10 years old or at onset of puberty if puberty occurs earlier
Frequency of testing – every 3 years
Tests to use – fasting plasma glucose, A1C, 2-h oral glucose tolerance test
Clinical judgment should be used to perform testing in children and adolescents who do not meet the above criteria.

Symptoms: Some children or adolescents with type 2 diabetes may show no symptoms at all. In others, symptoms may be similar to those of type 1 diabetes. A youth may feel very tired, thirsty, or nauseated and have to urinate often. Other symptoms may include weight loss, blurred vision, frequent infections, and slow healing of wounds or sores. Some youth may present with vaginal yeast infection or burning on urination due to yeast infection. Some may have extreme elevation of the blood glucose level associated with severe dehydration and coma.

Because symptoms are varied, it is important for health care providers to identify and test youth who are at high risk for the disease.

Signs of Diabetes: Physical signs of insulin resistance include acanthosis nigricans, where the skin around the neck or in the armpits appears dark and thick, and feels velvety. Girls can have polycystic ovary syndrome with infrequent or absent periods, and excess hair and acne. Microalbuminuria and cardiovascular risk factors such as abnormal cholesterol and high blood pressure may be present at the time of diagnosis.

Diabetes Risk Factors and Testing Criteria: Current diabetes risk factors and testing criteria given below in the text box will help identify type 2 diabetes in children before the onset of complications.

Co-morbidities: Children with type 2 diabetes also are at risk for the long-term complications of diabetes and the comorbidities associated with insulin resistance (lipid abnormalities and hypertension). Recent studies show that the onset of complications and co-morbidities and the speed of progression is particularly aggressive in youth with type 2 diabetes.

Other Forms of Diabetes

Other types of diabetes result from specific genetic conditions (such as maturity-onset diabetes of youth or latent autoimmune diabetes in adults), surgery, medications, infections, pancreatic disease, and other illnesses. Such types of diabetes account for 1% to 5% of all diagnosed cases.

Chapter 46

Diabetes and Women

Who gets diabetes?

Type 1 diabetes usually develops in childhood, but it can happen at any age. It is more common in whites than in other racial or ethnic groups. About 5% of adults with diabetes have type 1 diabetes. Genes you inherit from your parents play an important role in the development of type 1 diabetes. However, where you live may also affect your risk. Type 1 diabetes develops more often in winter and in people who live in colder climates.

Type 2 diabetes is more common in adults, especially in people who are overweight and have a family history of diabetes. About 95% of adults with diabetes have type 2 diabetes. Type 2 diabetes is becoming more common in children and teens as more of them become overweight and obese.

Do women of color need to worry about diabetes?

Yes. Certain racial and ethnic groups have a higher risk for type 2 diabetes. These groups include:

- **African-Americans**. African-American women are twice as likely to develop diabetes as white women. African-Americans

---

Text in this chapter is excerpted from "Diabetes," Office on Women's Health in the Department of Health and Human Services (OWH), August 4, 2015.

are also more likely to have health problems caused by diabetes and excess weight.

- **Hispanics.** Hispanic women are twice as likely to develop diabetes as white women. Diabetes affects more than one in 10 Hispanics. Among Hispanic women, diabetes affects Mexican-Americans and Puerto Ricans most often.

- **American Indian/Alaskan Native.** Diabetes affects nearly 16% of American Indian/Alaskan Native adults.

- **Native Hawaiian/Pacific Islander.** Native Hawaiians/Pacific Islanders are about twice as likely to develop diabetes as whites.

- **Asian-Americans.** Diabetes is the fifth-leading cause of death for Asian-Americans. Asian-American women are also more likely to develop gestational diabetes than white women and usually develop gestational diabetes at a lower body weight.

How does diabetes affect women differently than men?

Diabetes affects women and men in almost equal numbers. However, diabetes affects women differently than men.

Compared with men with diabetes, women with diabetes have:

- A higher risk for heart disease. Heart disease is the most common complication of diabetes.

- Lower survival rates and a poorer quality of life after heart attack

- A higher risk for blindness

- *A higher risk for depression.* Depression, which affects twice as many women as men, also raises the risk for diabetes in women.

Does diabetes raise my risk for other health problems?

Yes. The longer you have type 2 diabetes, the higher your risk for developing serious medical problems from diabetes. Also, if you smoke and have diabetes, you are even more likely to develop serious medical problems from diabetes, compared with people who have diabetes and do not smoke.

The extra glucose in the blood that leads to diabetes can damage your nerves and blood vessels. Nerve damage from diabetes can lead to pain or a permanent loss of feeling in your hands, feet, and other parts of your body.

Blood vessel damage from diabetes can also lead to:
- Heart disease
- Stroke
- Blindness
- Kidney failure
- Leg or foot amputation
- Hearing loss

Women with diabetes are also at higher risk for:
- Problems getting pregnant
- Problems during pregnancy, including possible health problems for you and your baby
- Repeated urinary and vaginal infections

What are the signs and symptoms of diabetes?

Type 1 diabetes symptoms are usually more severe and may develop suddenly.

Type 2 diabetes may not cause any signs or symptoms at first. Symptoms can develop slowly over time. You may not notice them right away.

Common signs and symptoms of type 1 and type 2 diabetes include:
- Feeling more tired than usual
- Extreme thirst
- Urinating more than usual
- Blurry vision
- Feeling hungrier than usual
- Losing weight without trying
- Sores that are slow to heal
- Dry, itchy skin
- Tingling in the hands or feet

- More infections, such as urinary tract infections and vaginal yeast infections, than usual

Do I need to be tested for diabetes?

Maybe. The United States Preventive Services Task Force recommends getting tested for diabetes if your blood pressure is higher than 135/80 mmHg.

Talk to your doctor about diabetes testing if you have signs or symptoms of diabetes. Your doctor will use a blood test to see if you have diabetes.

Is it safe for women with diabetes to get pregnant?

Yes. If you have type 1 or type 2 diabetes, you can have a healthy pregnancy. If you have diabetes and you want to have a baby, you need to plan ahead, before you get pregnant.

Talk to your doctor before you get pregnant. He or she can talk to you about steps you can take to keep your baby healthy. This may include a diabetes education program to help you better understand your diabetes and how to control it during pregnancy.

Chapter 47

Diabetes and Pregnancy

Chapter Contents

Section 47.1—Diabetes and Pregnancy Preparation 308

Section 47.2—Gestational Diabetes and Pregnancy 315

Section 47.1

Diabetes and Pregnancy Preparation

> Text in this section is excerpted from "What I Need to Know about Preparing for Pregnancy if I Have Diabetes," National Institute of Diabetes and Digestive and Kidney Diseases (NIDDK), National Institutes of Health (NIH), August 2013.

If you have diabetes, the best time to control your blood glucose, also called blood sugar, is before you get pregnant. High blood glucose levels can be harmful to your baby during the first weeks of pregnancy—even before you know you are pregnant. Blood glucose targets are different for women who are trying to get pregnant. Targets are numbers you aim for.

Pregnancy and new motherhood are times of great excitement and change for any woman. If you have type 1 or type 2 diabetes and are hoping to get pregnant soon, you can learn what to do to have a healthy baby. You can also learn how to take care of yourself and your diabetes before, during, and after your pregnancy. If you have diabetes and are already pregnant, don't panic! Just make sure you are doing everything you can to take care of yourself and your diabetes during your pregnancy.

If you have diabetes, your pregnancy is considered high risk, which means you have an increased risk of problems during your pregnancy. You need to pay special attention to your health, and you may need to see doctors who specialize in treating diabetes or its complications. Millions of high-risk pregnancies, such as those in which women are older than 35 or carrying two or more babies, produce perfectly healthy babies without affecting the mother's health.

Taking care of your baby and yourself

Keeping your blood glucose as close to normal as possible before and during your pregnancy is the most important thing you can do to stay healthy and have a healthy baby. Your health care team can help you learn how to use meal planning, physical activity, and medicines

Diabetes and Pregnancy

to reach your blood glucose targets. Together, you'll create a plan for taking care of yourself and your diabetes.

Pregnancy causes a number of changes in your body, so you might need to change how you manage your diabetes. Even if you've had diabetes for years, you may need to change your meal plan, physical activity routine, and medicines. As you get closer to your delivery date, your needs might change again.

Your diabetes, before and during your pregnancy

As you know, in diabetes, blood glucose levels are above normal. Whether you have type 1 or type 2 diabetes, you can manage your blood glucose levels and lower the risk of health problems.

A baby's brain, heart, kidneys, and lungs form during the first 8 weeks of pregnancy. High blood glucose levels are especially harmful during this early stage. Yet many women don't realize they're pregnant until 5 or 6 weeks after conception. To protect your baby's health, work with your health care team to get your blood glucose under control before you get pregnant.

If you are already pregnant, see your doctor as soon as possible to make a plan for taking care of yourself and your baby. Even if you learn you're pregnant later in your pregnancy, you can still do a lot for your health and your baby's health.

My blood glucose levels

Daily Blood Glucose Levels before Pregnancy

If you are thinking about getting pregnant, talk with your doctor about what your blood glucose targets should be as you get ready to have a baby. Find out when and how often you should check your daily blood glucose levels with a blood glucose meter. If you already check your blood glucose levels, you may need to check them more often than you do now.

The following table shows target blood glucose numbers for women with diabetes who are planning to become pregnant.

Table 47.1. Target Blood Glucose Numbers for Women with Diabetes Planning to Become Pregnant

Target Blood Glucose Numbers (mg/dL) for Women with Diabetes Planning to Become Pregnant	
Before meals and when you wake up	80 to 110
1 to 2 hours after eating	100 to 155

Daily Blood Glucose Levels during Pregnancy

During your pregnancy, you'll check your blood glucose levels using a blood glucose meter several times a day. Most doctors recommend testing at least four times a day. Talk with your doctor about when you should check your blood glucose levels and glucose levels using "My Daily Blood Glucose Record." Write down the results every time you check your blood glucose.

Getting correct results from your meter is important. Follow the directions for using your meter and take care of your meter. Recheck your blood glucose level if a test result seems off. Ask your health care team for help if you have questions about using your meter or your test results.

The daily target blood glucose numbers recommended by the American Diabetes Association for most pregnant women are in the following table.

Table 47.2. Target Blood Glucose Numbers for Women with Diabetes who Became Pregnant

Target Blood Glucose Numbers (mg/dL) for Women with Diabetes who Became Pregnant	
Before meals, at bedtime, and overnight	60 to 99
1 to 2 hours after eating	100 to 129

Ask your doctor what targets are right for you.

You can keep track of your blood glucose levels using "My Daily Blood Glucose Record." Write down the results every time you check your blood glucose. Your blood glucose records can help you and your health care team decide whether your diabetes care plan is working. You also can use this form to make notes about your insulin and ketones.

The A1C Test

Another way to see whether you're meeting your targets is to have an A1C blood test. Results of the A1C test reflect your average blood glucose levels during the past 3 months. The American Diabetes Association now recommends that most women with diabetes should aim for an A1C target as close to normal as possible—below 7 percent, and ideally below 6 percent—before getting pregnant and during pregnancy. Your doctor can help you set an A1C target that is best for you. Write your target under "My Target Blood Glucose and A1C Numbers."

Diabetes and Pregnancy

Low Blood Glucose

When you're pregnant, you're at increased risk of having low blood glucose, also called hypoglycemia. When blood glucose levels are too low, your body can't get the energy it needs. Although hypoglycemia can happen suddenly, it is usually mild and can be treated quickly. Eating or drinking something with carbohydrates—sugars and starches found in many foods—can bring your blood glucose level back to normal. Left untreated, hypoglycemia can make you pass out.

Low blood glucose can make you:

- hungry
- dizzy or shaky
- confused
- pale
- sweat more
- weak
- anxious or cranky
- have headaches
- have a fast heartbeat

Low blood glucose can be caused by:

- meals or snacks that are too small, delayed, or skipped
- doses of insulin that are too high
- increased physical activity

Low blood glucose also can be caused by drinking too many alcoholic beverages. However, women who are trying to get pregnant or who are already pregnant should avoid drinking alcohol.

Using Glucagon for Severe Low Blood Glucose

If you have severe low blood glucose and pass out, you'll need help to quickly bring your blood glucose level back to normal. Your health care team can teach your family members and friends how to give you an injection of glucagon, a hormone that raises blood glucose levels right away. If glucagon is not available, someone should call 911 to get you to the nearest emergency room for treatment.

High Blood Glucose

High blood glucose, also called hyperglycemia, can happen when you don't have enough insulin or when your body isn't able to use insulin correctly. High blood glucose can result from:

- not taking your diabetes medicines
- eating more food than usual
- being less active than usual
- illness
- stress

Also, if your blood glucose level is already high and you have chemicals called ketones in your blood or urine, physical activity can make your blood glucose level go even higher. Symptoms of high blood glucose include:

- frequent urination
- thirst
- weight loss

Talk with your doctor about what to do when your blood glucose is too high. Your doctor might suggest a change in your insulin, meal plan, or physical activity routine.

My Ketone Levels

When your blood glucose is too high or if you're not eating enough, your body might make ketones. Ketones in your urine or blood mean your body is using fat for energy instead of glucose. Your body can't use glucose for energy if you don't have enough insulin or you aren't getting enough glucose from food, so it uses fat instead. Burning fat instead of glucose can be harmful to your health and your baby's health. Harmful ketones can pass from you to your baby. Your health care team can teach you how and when to test your urine or blood for ketones.

If ketones build up in your body, you can develop a condition called ketosis. Ketosis can quickly turn into diabetic ketoacidosis, which can be life threatening. Symptoms of ketoacidosis are:

- stomach pain
- nausea and vomiting

- frequent urination or frequent thirst, for a day or more
- fatigue
- muscle stiffness or aching
- feeling dazed or in shock
- rapid, deep breathing
- breath that smells fruity

Checking Your Urine or Blood Ketone Levels

Your doctor might recommend you test your urine or blood daily for ketones or when your blood glucose is above a certain level, such as 200 mg/dL. If you use an insulin pump, your doctor might recommend that you test for ketones when your blood glucose level is unexpectedly high. You can write down the times you should check for ketones in "My Plan to Check for Ketones."

You can prevent serious health problems by checking for ketones as recommended. Talk with your doctor about what to do if you have ketones. Your doctor might suggest making changes in the amount of insulin you take or when you take insulin.

Medicines for Diabetes

Some medicines are not safe during pregnancy and should be stopped before you get pregnant. Tell your doctor about all the medicines you currently take, such as those for high cholesterol and high blood pressure. Your doctor can tell you which medicines to stop taking.

During pregnancy, the safest diabetes medicine is insulin. If you're already taking insulin, you might need to change the kind, the amount, or how and when you take it. The amount of insulin you take is likely to increase as you go through pregnancy because your body becomes less able to respond to the action of insulin, a condition called insulin resistance. Your insulin needs may double or even triple as you get closer to your delivery date. Your doctor will work with you to make a personalized insulin routine.

If you've been taking medicines other than insulin to control your blood glucose levels, you'll need to stop taking them. Research studies have not yet proved that diabetes medicines other than insulin are safe for use during pregnancy.

Labor and delivery with diabetes

Your health care team will consider your health, your baby's health, and the state of your pregnancy in deciding how and when delivery should occur. Your doctor may recommend inducing labor before your due date or delivering the baby surgically using a cesarean section, or c-section. However, most women with diabetes have the option of delivering vaginally. You'll want to talk with your health care team about your options well ahead of time.

The factors your health care team will consider in deciding what type of delivery is best for you and your baby may include:

- your baby's size and position
- your baby's lung maturity
- your baby's movements
- your baby's heart rate
- the amount of amniotic fluid
- your blood glucose and blood pressure levels
- your general health

Blood Glucose Control during Labor and Delivery

Keeping your blood glucose levels under control helps ensure your baby won't have low blood glucose right after birth. You will be physically active when you're in labor, therefore you may not need much insulin. Hospital staff will check your blood glucose levels frequently. Some women take both insulin and glucose, as well as fluids, through an intravenous (IV) line during labor. Sending insulin and glucose directly into your bloodstream through a vein provides good control of blood glucose levels. If you are using an insulin pump, you might continue to use it throughout labor.

If you are having a c-section, your blood glucose levels may increase because of the stress of surgery. Your health care team will closely monitor your blood glucose levels and will likely use an IV for insulin and glucose to keep your levels under control.

Taking Care of Yourself

Remember, to be a good mom, you have to take good care of yourself. In addition to taking care of your diabetes and eating right, you can take care of yourself by taking the time for physical activity. Active moms provide a good example for their children to follow. Check with your health care team about how soon after delivery you can safely begin physical activity.

Section 47.2

Gestational Diabetes and Pregnancy

Text in this section is excerpted from "Gestational Diabetes and Pregnancy," Centers for Disease Control and Prevention (CDC), September 16, 2015.

Gestational diabetes is a type of diabetes that is first seen in a pregnant woman who did not have diabetes before she was pregnant. Some women have more than one pregnancy affected by gestational diabetes. Gestational diabetes usually shows up in the middle of pregnancy. Doctors most often test for it between 24 and 28 weeks of pregnancy.

Often gestational diabetes can be controlled through eating healthy foods and regular exercise. Sometimes a woman with gestational diabetes must also take insulin.

Problems of Gestational Diabetes in Pregnancy

Blood sugar that is not well controlled in a woman with gestational diabetes can lead to problems for the pregnant woman and the baby:

An Extra Large Baby

Diabetes that is not well controlled causes the baby's blood sugar to be high. The baby is "overfed" and grows extra large. Besides causing discomfort to the woman during the last few months of pregnancy, an extra large baby can lead to problems during delivery for both the mother and the baby. The mother might need a C-Section to deliver the baby. The baby can be born with nerve damage due to pressure on the shoulder during delivery.

C-Section (Cesarean Section)

A C-section is an operation to deliver the baby through the mother's belly. A woman who has diabetes that is not well controlled has a higher chance of needing a C-section to deliver the baby. When the baby is delivered by a C-section, it takes longer for the woman to recover from childbirth.

High Blood Pressure (Preeclampsia)

When a pregnant woman has high blood pressure, protein in her urine, and often swelling in fingers and toes that doesn't go away, she might have preeclampsia. It is a serious problem that needs to be watched closely and managed by her doctor. High blood pressure can cause harm to both the woman and her unborn baby. It might lead to the baby being born early and also could cause seizures or a stroke (a blood clot or a bleed in the brain that can lead to brain damage) in the woman during labor and delivery. Women with diabetes have high blood pressure more often than women without diabetes.

Low Blood Sugar (Hypoglycemia)

People with diabetes who take insulin or other diabetes medications can develop blood sugar that is too low. Low blood sugar can be very serious, and even fatal, if not treated quickly. Seriously low blood sugar can be avoided if women watch their blood sugar closely and treat low blood sugar early.

If a woman's diabetes was not well controlled during pregnancy, her baby can very quickly develop low blood sugar after birth. The baby's blood sugar must be watched for several hours after delivery.

Tips for Women with Gestational Diabetes

Eat Healthy Foods

Eat healthy foods from a meal plan made for a person with diabetes. A dietitian can help you create a healthy meal plan. A dietitian can also help you learn how to control your blood sugar while you are pregnant.

Exercise Regularly

Exercise is another way to keep blood sugar under control. It helps to balance food intake. After checking with your doctor, you can exercise regularly during and after pregnancy. Get at least 30 minutes of

Diabetes and Pregnancy

moderate-intensity physical activity at least five days a week. This could be brisk walking, swimming, or actively playing with children.

Monitor Blood Sugar Often

Because pregnancy causes the body's need for energy to change, blood sugar levels can change very quickly. Check your blood sugar often, as directed by your doctor.

Take Insulin, If Needed

Sometimes a woman with gestational diabetes must take insulin. If insulin is ordered by your doctor, take it as directed in order to help keep blood sugar under control.

Get Tested for Diabetes after Pregnancy

Get tested for diabetes 6 to 12 weeks after your baby is born, and then every 1 to 3 years.

For most women with gestational diabetes, the diabetes goes away soon after delivery. When it does not go away, the diabetes is called type 2 diabetes. Even if the diabetes does go away after the baby is born, half of all women who had gestational diabetes develop type 2 diabetes later. It's important for a woman who has had gestational diabetes to continue to exercise and eat a healthy diet after pregnancy to prevent or delay getting type 2 diabetes. She should also remind her doctor to check her blood sugar every 1 to 3 years.

Chapter 48

Diabetes in the Elderly

Diabetes is a serious disease. People get diabetes when their blood glucose level, sometimes called blood sugar, is too high. Diabetes can lead to dangerous health problems, such as having a heart attack or stroke. The good news is that there are things you can do to take control of diabetes and prevent its problems. And, if you are worried about getting diabetes, there are things you can do to lower your risk.

What Is Diabetes?

Our bodies change the food we eat into glucose. Insulin helps glucose get into our cells where it can be used to make energy. If you have diabetes, your body may not make enough insulin, may not use insulin in the right way, or both. That may cause too much glucose in the blood. Your family doctor may refer you to a doctor who specializes in taking care of people with diabetes, called an endocrinologist.

Types of Diabetes

There are two kinds of diabetes that can happen at any age. In type 1 diabetes, the body makes little or no insulin. This type of diabetes develops most often in children and young adults.

In type 2 diabetes, the body makes insulin, but doesn't use it the right way. It is the most common kind of diabetes. You may have heard it called

---

Text in this chapter is excerpted from "Diabetes in Older People—A Disease You Can Manage," National Institute on Aging (NIA), National Institutes of Health (NIH), October 20, 2015.

adult-onset diabetes. Your chance of getting type 2 diabetes is higher if you are overweight, inactive, or have a family history of diabetes.

Diabetes can affect many parts of your body. It's important to keep type 2 diabetes under control. Over time, it can cause problems like heart disease, stroke, kidney disease, blindness, nerve damage, and circulation problems that may lead to amputation. People with type 2 diabetes have a greater risk for Alzheimer's disease.

Prediabetes

Many people have "prediabetes." This means their glucose levels are higher than normal but not high enough to be called diabetes. Prediabetes is a serious problem because people with prediabetes are at high risk for developing type 2 diabetes. If your doctor says you have prediabetes, you may feel upset and worried. But, there are things you can do to prevent or delay actually getting type 2 diabetes. Losing weight may help. Healthy eating and being physically active for at least 30 minutes, 5 days a week is a small change that can make a big difference. Work with your doctor to set up a plan for good nutrition and exercise. Make sure to ask how often you should have your glucose levels checked.

Symptoms

Some people with type 2 diabetes may not know they have it. But, they may feel tired, hungry, or thirsty. They may lose weight without trying, urinate often, or have trouble with blurred vision. They may also get skin infections or heal slowly from cuts and bruises. See your doctor right away if you have one or more of these symptoms.

Tests for Diabetes

There are several blood tests doctors can use to help diagnosis of diabetes:

- Random glucose test—given at any time during the day
- Fasting glucose test—taken after you have gone without food for at least 8 hours
- Oral glucose tolerance test—taken after fasting overnight and then again 2 hours after having a sugary drink
- A1C blood test—shows your glucose level for the past 2–3 months

Diabetes in the Elderly

Your doctor may want you to be tested for diabetes twice before making a diagnosis.

Managing Diabetes

"Once you've been told you have type 2 diabetes, the doctor may prescribe diabetes medicines to help control blood glucose levels." help control blood glucose levels. There are many kinds of medication available. Your doctor will choose the best treatment based on the type of diabetes you have, your everyday routine, and other health problems.

In addition, you can keep control of your diabetes by:

- **Tracking your glucose levels.** Very high glucose levels or very low glucose levels (called hypoglycemia) can be risky to your health. Talk to your doctor about how to check your glucose levels at home.

- **Making healthy food choices.** Learn how different foods affect glucose levels. For weight loss, check out foods that are low in fat and sugar. Let your doctor know if you want help with meal planning.

- **Getting exercise.** Daily exercise can help improve glucose levels in older people with diabetes. Ask your doctor to help you plan an exercise program.

- **Keeping track of how you are doing.** Talk to your doctor about how well your diabetes care plan is working. Make sure you know how often to check your glucose levels.

Your doctor may want you to see other healthcare providers who can help manage some of the extra problems caused by diabetes. He or she can also give you a schedule for other tests that may be needed. Talk to your doctor about how to stay healthy.

Here are some things to keep in mind:

- **Have yearly eye exams.** Finding and treating eye problems early may keep your eyes healthy.

- **Check your kidneys yearly.** Diabetes can affect your kidneys. A urine and blood test will show if your kidneys are okay.

- **Get flu shots every year and the pneumonia vaccine.** A yearly flu shot will help keep you healthy. If you're over 65, make sure you have had the pneumonia vaccine. If you were younger than 65 when you had the pneumonia vaccine, you may need another one. Ask your doctor.

- **Check your cholesterol.** At least once a year, get a blood test to check your cholesterol and triglyceride levels. High levels may increase your risk for heart problems.
- **Care for your teeth and gums.** Your teeth and gums need to be checked twice a year by a dentist to avoid serious problems.
- **Find out your average blood glucose level.** At least twice a year, get a blood test called the A1C test. The result will show your average glucose level for the past 2 to 3 months.
- **Protect your skin.** Keep your skin clean and use skin softeners for dryness. Take care of minor cuts and bruises to prevent infections.
- **Look at your feet.** Take time to look at your feet every day for any red patches. Ask someone else to check your feet if you can't. If you have sores, blisters, breaks in the skin, infections, or build-up of calluses, see a foot doctor, called a podiatrist.
- **Watch your blood pressure.** Get your blood pressure checked often.

> **Be Prepared**
>
> It's a good idea to make sure you always have at least 3 days' worth of supplies on hand for testing and treating your diabetes in case of an emergency.

Medicare Can Help

Medicare will pay to help you learn how to care for your diabetes. It will also help pay for diabetes tests, supplies, special shoes, foot exams, eye tests, and meal planning. Be sure to check your Medicare plan to find more information.

Chapter 49

Diabetes in Minority Groups

Diabetes and African Americans

African Americans are almost twice as likely to be diagnosed with diabetes as non-Hispanic whites. In addition, they are more likely to suffer complications from diabetes, such as end-stage renal disease and lower extremity amputations. Although African Americans have the same or lower rate of high cholesterol as their non-Hispanic white counterparts, they are more likely to have high blood pressure.

- African American adults are 80 percent more likely than non-Hispanic white adults to have been diagnosed with diabetes by a physician.

- In 2010, non-Hispanic blacks were 3.4 times more likely to be diagnosed with end stage renal disease as compared to non-Hispanic whites.

This chapter includes excerpts from "Diabetes and African Americans," Office of Minority Health (OMH), June 16, 2015; text from "Diabetes and American Indians/Alaska Natives," Office of Minority Health (OMH), June 15, 2015; text from "Diabetes and Asians and Pacific Islanders," Office of Minority Health (OMH), May 20, 2015; text from "Diabetes and Hispanic Americans," Office of Minority Health (OMH), June 15, 2015; and text from "Diabetes and Native Hawaiians/Pacific Islanders," Office of Minority Health (OMH), May 22, 2015.

- In 2012, non-Hispanic blacks were 3.5 times more likely to be hospitalized for lower limb amputations as compared to non-Hispanic whites.

- In 2013, African Americans were twice as likely as non-Hispanic Whites to die from diabetes.

At a glance – Death Rate:
Age-Adjusted Diabetes Death Rates per 100,000 (2013)

Table 49.1. Age-Adjusted Diabetes Death Rates

	Non-Hispanic Black	Non-Hispanic White	Non-Hispanic Black/Non-Hispanic White Ratio
Male	45.1	23.1	2
Female	35.2	14.9	2.4
Total	39.5	18.6	2.1

Source: CDC, 2014. National Vital Statistic Report. Vol. 64, Num 2 Table 17.

Diabetes and American Indians/Alaska Natives

American Indians/Alaska Natives are more than twice as likely to be told by a physician that they have diabetes as their non-Hispanic white counterparts. They also are almost twice as likely to die from diabetes as non-Hispanic whites. Data is limited for this population.

- American Indian/Alaska Native adults are 2.5 times as likely as white adults to be diagnosed with diabetes.

- American Indians/Alaska Native women were 2.3 times more likely than non-Hispanic whites to die from diabetes in 2010.

- In 2010, American Indians/Native Americans were 2.7 times more likely to be diagnosed with end stage renal disease than non-Hispanic whites.

Diabetes and Asians and Pacific Islanders

Asian Americans are 20 percent less likely than non-Hispanic whites to die from diabetes, however they have additional risk factors.

- Asian Americans are 20 percent more likely to be diagnosed with diabetes than non-Hispanic whites.

- Asians are 60 percent more likely to be diagnosed with end stage renal disease than non-Hispanic whites.
- In 2009, Asian Americans were 10 percent less likely than non-Hispanic whites to have a retinal eye examination.

At a glance – Death Rate:
Age-Adjusted Diabetes Death Rates per 100,000 (2013)

Table 49.2. Age-Adjusted Diabetes Death Rates

	American Indian/ Native American	Non-Hispanic White	African Americans/Non-Hispanic White Ratio
Male	37.9	23.1	1.6
Female	30.9	14.9	2.1
Total	34.1	18.6	1.8

Source: CDC, 2014. National Vital Statistic Report. Vol. 64, Num 2 Table 17 and Table 16.

At a glance – Death Rate:
Age-Adjusted Diabetes Death Rates per 100,000 (2013)

Table 49.3. Age-Adjusted Diabetes Death Rates

	Asian American/ Pacific Islanders	Non-Hispanic White	Asian American/ Pacific Islanders/ Non-Hispanic White Ratio
Male	19.4	23.1	0.8
Female	13.1	14.9	0.9
Total	15.8	18.6	0.8

Source: CDC, 2014. National Vital Statistic Report. Vol. 64, Num 2 Table 17 and Table 16.

Diabetes and Hispanic Americans

According to national examination surveys, Hispanics are almost twice as likely as non-Hispanic whites to be diagnosed with diabetes by a physician. They have higher rates of end-stage renal disease, caused by diabetes, and they are 40% more likely to die from diabetes as non-Hispanic whites.

- Hispanic adults are 1.7 times more likely than non-Hispanic white adults to have been diagnosed with diabetes by a physician.

- In 2010, Hispanics were 2.6 times more likely to start treatment for end-stage renal disease related to diabetes, as compared to non-Hispanic whites.

- In 2010, Hispanics were 1.5 times as likely as non-Hispanic whites to die from diabetes.

At a glance—Death Rate

Age-Adjusted Diabetes Death Rates per 100,000 (2013)

Table 49.4. Age-Adjusted Diabetes Death Rates

	Hispanics	Non-Hispanic White	Hispanic/Non-Hispanic White Ratio
Male	30.4	23.1	1.3
Female	23.0	14.9	1.5
Total	26.3	18.6	1.4

Source: CDC, 2014. National Vital Statistic Report. Vol. 61, Num 4 Table 17.

Diabetes and Native Hawaiians/Pacific Islanders

Asian Americans, in general, have the same rate of diabetes as non-Hispanic whites. However, there are differences within the Native Hawaiian/Pacific Islander population.

- From a national survey, Native Hawaiians/Pacific Islanders are just as likely to be diagnosed with diabetes as the white population.

- However in the state of Hawaii, Native Hawaiians are 2.2 times more likely to be diagnosed with diabetes, as compared to the white population.

- In 2010, Native Hawaiians/Pacific Islanders were 30 percent more likely to have had a foot examination within the past 12 months than non-Hispanic whites.

Part Seven

Living with Diabetes

Chapter 50

Take Care of Your Diabetes Each Day

Do four things each day to help your blood glucose levels stay in your target range:

- Follow your healthy eating plan.
- Be physically active.
- Take your medicines as prescribed.
- Monitor your diabetes.

These things may seem like a lot to do at first. Just make small changes until these steps become a normal part of your day.

Follow your healthy eating plan

Ask your doctor to give you the name of someone trained to help you create a healthy eating plan, such as a dietitian. This plan, often called medical nutrition therapy, will include regular monitoring by

---

Text in this chapter is excerpted from "Take Care of Your Diabetes Each Day," National Institute of Diabetes and Digestive and Kidney Diseases (NIDDK), National Institutes of Health (NIH), February 12, 2014.

your dietitian and education about how to adjust your eating habits as the need occurs. Medical nutrition therapy is usually covered by insurance or Medicare as long as your doctor refers you. Your dietitian can help you plan meals that include foods that you and your family like and that are good for you.

Your healthy eating plan will include:

- breads, cereals, rice, and whole grains
- fruits and vegetables
- meat and meat substitutes
- dairy products
- healthy fats

Your plan will also help you learn how to eat the right amount, or portions, of food. Making good food choices will:

- help you reach and stay at a healthy weight
- keep your blood glucose, blood pressure, and cholesterol levels under control
- prevent heart and blood vessel disease

Action Steps – If You Take Insulin

- Follow your healthy eating plan.
- Don't skip meals, especially if you've already taken your insulin, because your blood glucose levels may drop too low.
- Learn more about how to handle low blood glucose, also called hypoglycemia

Action Steps – If You Don't Take Insulin

- Follow your healthy eating plan.
- Don't skip meals, especially if you take diabetes medicines, because your blood glucose levels may drop too low.
- Learn more about how to handle low blood glucose, also called hypoglycemia.
- Eat several small meals during the day instead of big meals.

Take Care of Your Diabetes Each Day

Be physically active

Physical activity helps you stay healthy. Physical activity is especially good if you have diabetes because it:

- helps you reach or stay at a healthy weight
- helps insulin work better to lower your blood glucose levels
- is good for your heart and lungs
- gives you more energy

Even small amounts of physical activity help manage diabetes, such as when you are physically active at work or home. People with diabetes should aim for 30 to 60 minutes of activity most days of the week. Children and adolescents with type 2 diabetes who are 10 to 17 years old should aim for 60 minutes of activity every day. Not all physical activity has to take place at the same time.

Increase daily activity by decreasing time spent watching TV or at the computer. Children and adolescents should limit screen time not related to school to less than 2 hours a day. Limiting screen time can help you meet your physical activity goal.

People with diabetes should:

- always talk with a doctor before starting a new physical activity program.
- do aerobic activities, such as brisk walking, which use the body's large muscles to make the heart beat faster. The large muscles are those of the upper and lower arms and legs and those that control head, shoulder, and hip movements.
- do activities to strengthen muscles and bone, such as sit-ups or lifting weights. Aim for two times a week.
- stretch to increase flexibility, lower stress, and help prevent muscle soreness after physical activity.

Many activities can help your child and your family stay active and have fun. Consider activities that they might enjoy and can stick with, such as:

- playing basketball
- dancing to music with friends
- taking a walk or a bike ride

Action Steps – If You Take Insulin

- See your doctor before becoming physically active.
- Check your blood glucose levels before, during, and after physical activity. Don't start a physical activity program when your blood glucose levels are high or if you have ketones in your blood or urine.
- Don't be physically active right before you go to bed because it could cause low blood glucose while you sleep.

Action Steps – If You Don't Take Insulin

- See your doctor before becoming physically active.
- Ask your doctor about whether you need to eat before you are physically active.

When you are being physically active, carry glucose tablets or a carbohydrate-rich snack or drink with you, such as fruit or juice, in case your blood glucose levels go too low.

Take your medicines as prescribed

If you have type 2 diabetes and are unable to reach your target blood glucose levels with a healthy eating plan and physical activity, diabetes medicines may help. Your doctor may prescribe you diabetes medicines that work best for you and your lifestyle.

If you have type 1 diabetes, you need insulin shots if your body has stopped making insulin or if it doesn't make enough. Some people with type 2 diabetes or gestational diabetes also need to take insulin shots.

Diabetes Medicines

Most people with type 2 diabetes use medicines other than insulin shots. People with type 2 diabetes use medicine to help their blood glucose levels stay in their target range. If your body makes insulin and the insulin doesn't lower your blood glucose levels enough, you may need to take one or more medicines.

Diabetes medicines come in pill and shot form. Some people take diabetes medicines once a day and other medicines more often. Ask your health care team when you should take your diabetes medicines. Sometimes, people who take diabetes medicines may also need insulin shots for a while.

Take Care of Your Diabetes Each Day

Be sure to tell your doctor if your medicines make you feel sick or if you have any other problems. If you get sick or have surgery, your diabetes medicines may no longer work to lower your blood glucose levels. Always check with your doctor before you stop taking your diabetes medicines.

Insulin Shots

Only a doctor can prescribe insulin. Your doctor can tell you how much insulin you should take and which of the following ways to take insulin is best for you:

- **Insulin shot**. You'll use a needle attached to a syringe—a hollow tube with a plunger—that you fill with a dose of insulin. Some people use an insulin pen, a penlike device with a needle and a cartridge of insulin. Never share insulin needles or insulin pens, even with family.

- **Insulin pump**. An insulin pump is a small device filled with insulin that you wear on your belt or keep in your pocket. The pump connects to a small, plastic tube and a small needle. You or your doctor inserts the needle under your skin. The needle can stay in for several days.

- **Insulin jet injector**. This device sends a fine spray of insulin through your skin with high-pressure air instead of a needle.

- **Insulin injection port**. You or your doctor inserts a small tube just beneath your skin, where it remains in place for several days. You can inject insulin into the end of the tube instead of through your skin.

Other Medicines

Your doctor may prescribe other medicines to help with problems related to diabetes, such as:

- aspirin for heart health
- cholesterol-lowering medicines
- medicines for high blood pressure

Remembering to take your medicines at the correct times each day can be challenging. Many people find that keeping a weekly pill box with separate boxes for each day, and even separate boxes for morning and evening, can help. Also ask your health care team to update your list of medicines at each visit so you always have an accurate list of what medicines to take and when.

Chapter 51

Monitor Your Diabetes

Check Your Blood Glucose Levels

Checking and recording your blood glucose levels can help you monitor and better manage your diabetes. If your blood has too much or too little glucose, you may need a change in your healthy eating plan, physical activity plan, or medicines.

A member of your health care team will show you how to check your blood glucose levels using a blood glucose meter. Your health care team can teach you how to:

- prick your finger to get a drop of blood for testing
- use your meter to find out your blood glucose level from your drop of blood

Your health insurance or Medicare may pay for the blood glucose meter and test strips you need.

Ask your doctor how often you should check your blood glucose levels. You may need to check before and after eating, before and after physical activity, before bed, and sometimes in the middle of the night. Make sure to keep a record of your blood glucose self-checks.

This chapter includes excerpts from "Monitor Your Diabetes," National Institute of Diabetes and Digestive and Kidney Diseases (NIDDK), National Institutes of Health (NIH), February 12, 2014; and text from "Your Diabetes Care Records," National Institute of Diabetes and Digestive and Kidney Diseases (NIDDK), National Institutes of Health (NIH), February 12, 2014.

Target range for blood glucose levels

Most people with diabetes should try to keep their blood glucose levels as close as possible to the level of someone who doesn't have diabetes. This normal target range is about 70 to 130. The closer to normal your blood glucose levels are, the lower your chance of developing serious health problems.

Ask your doctor what your target levels are and when you should check your blood glucose levels with a meter. Make copies of the chart "Your Diabetes Care Records" to take with you when you visit your doctor.

Reaching your target range all of the time can be hard. Remember, the closer you get to your target range, the better you will feel.

The A1C Test

Another test for blood glucose, the A1C—also called the hemoglobin A1C test, HbA1C, or glycohemoglobin test—is a blood test that reflects the average level of glucose in your blood during the past 2 to 3 months.

You should have the A1C test at least twice a year. If your result is not on target, your doctor may have you take the test more often to see if your A1C improves.

For the test, your doctor will draw a sample of your blood during an office visit or send you to a lab to have your blood drawn. Your A1C test result is given as a percentage. Your A1C result plus the record of your blood glucose numbers show whether your blood glucose levels are under control.

If your A1C result is too high, you may need to change your diabetes treatment plan. Your health care team can help you decide what part of your plan to change.

If your A1C result is on target, then your diabetes treatment plan is working. The lower your A1C result, the lower your chance of having diabetes problems.

Talk with your doctor about what your A1C target should be. Your personal target may be above or below the target shown in the chart.

Table 51.1. A1C Targets

A1C Targets	
Target for most people with diabetes	Below 7 percent
Target for most people with diabetes	8 percent or above

Monitor Your Diabetes

A1C targets can also depend on:
- how long you have had diabetes
- whether or not you have other health problems

Tests for ketones

You may need to check your blood or urine for ketones if you're sick or if your blood glucose levels are above 240. Your body makes ketones when you burn fat instead of glucose for energy. If you have too many ketones, you are more likely to have a serious condition called ketoacidosis. If not treated, ketoacidosis can cause death.

Signs of ketoacidosis are:
- vomiting
- weakness
- fast breathing
- sweet-smelling breath

Ketoacidosis is more likely in people with type 1 diabetes.

Your doctor or diabetes educator will show you how to test for ketones.

Keep daily records

Make copies of the daily diabetes record at the end of this publication. Then, write down the results of your blood glucose checks each day. You may also want to record what you ate, how you felt, and whether you were physically active.

Bring your blood glucose records to all visits with your health care team

They can use your records to see whether you need changes in your diabetes medicines or in your healthy eating plan.

Action Steps – If You Take Insulin

- Keep a daily record of
- your blood glucose levels

- the times of day you take insulin
- the amount and type of insulin you take
- what types of physical activity you do and for how long
- when and what you eat
- whether you have ketones in your blood or urine
- when you are sick

Action Steps – If You Don't Take Insulin

- Keep a daily record of
- your blood glucose levels
- the times of day you take your medicines
- what types of physical activity you do and for how long

Learn about high and low blood glucose levels

Sometimes, no matter how hard you try to keep your blood glucose levels in your target range, they will be too high or too low. Blood glucose that's too high or too low can make you feel sick. If you try to control your high or low blood glucose and can't, you may become even sicker and need help. Talk with your doctor to learn how to handle these emergencies.

Learn about high blood glucose levels

If your blood glucose levels stay above 180 for more than 1 to 2 hours, they may be too high. High blood glucose, also called hyperglycemia, means you don't have enough insulin in your body. High blood glucose can happen if you:

- miss taking your diabetes medicines
- eat too much
- don't get enough physical activity
- have an infection
- get sick
- are stressed
- take medicines that can cause high blood glucose

Monitor Your Diabetes

Be sure to tell your doctor about other medicines you take. When you're sick, be sure to check your blood glucose levels and keep taking your diabetes medicines.

Signs that your blood glucose levels may be too high are the following:
- feeling thirsty
- feeling weak or tired
- headaches
- urinating often
- having trouble paying attention
- blurry vision
- yeast infections

Very high blood glucose may also make you feel sick to your stomach.
If your blood glucose levels are high much of the time, or if you have symptoms of high blood glucose, call your doctor. You may need a change in your healthy eating plan, physical activity plan, or medicines.

Learn about low blood glucose levels

If your blood glucose levels drop below 70, you have low blood glucose, also called hypoglycemia. Low blood glucose can come on fast and can be caused by:
- taking too much diabetes medicine
- missing or delaying a meal
- being more physically active than usual
- drinking alcoholic beverages

Sometimes, medicines you take for other health problems can cause your blood glucose levels to drop.

Signs your blood glucose levels may be too low are the following:
- hunger
- dizziness or shakiness
- confusion
- being pale

- sweating more
- weakness
- anxiety or moodiness
- headaches
- a fast heartbeat

If your blood glucose levels drop lower, you could have severe hypoglycemia, where you pass out or have a seizure. A seizure occurs when cells in the brain release a rush of energy that can cause changes in behavior or muscle contractions. Some seizures are life threatening.

If you have any of these symptoms, check your blood glucose levels. If your blood glucose levels are less than 70, have one of the following right away:

- three or four glucose tablets
- one serving of glucose gel—the amount equal to 15 grams of carbohydrates
- 1/2 cup, or 4 ounces, of fruit juice
- 1/2 cup, or 4 ounces, of a regular—nondiet—soft drink
- 1 cup, or 8 ounces, of milk
- five or six pieces of hard candy
- 1 tablespoon of sugar, syrup, or honey

After 15 minutes, check your blood glucose levels again. Repeat these steps until your blood glucose levels are 70 or above. If it will be at least 1 hour before your next meal, eat a snack.

If you take diabetes medicines that can cause low blood glucose, always carry food for emergencies. You should also wear a medical identification bracelet or necklace that says you have diabetes.

If you take insulin, keep a prescription glucagon kit at home and at other places where you often go. A glucagon kit has a vial of glucagon, a syringe, and a needle to inject the glucagon. Given as a shot, the glucagon quickly raises blood glucose. If you have severe hypoglycemia, you'll need someone to help bring your blood glucose levels back to normal by giving you a glucagon shot. Show your family, friends, and coworkers how to give you a glucagon shot when you have severe hypoglycemia. Someone should call 911 for help if a glucagon kit is not available.

Monitor Your Diabetes

Action Steps – If You Take Insulin

- Tell your doctor if you have low blood glucose, especially at the same time of the day or night, several times in a row.
- Tell your doctor if you've passed out from low blood glucose.
- Ask your doctor about glucagon. Glucagon is a medicine that raises blood glucose.
- Show your family, friends, and coworkers how to give you a glucagon shot when you have severe hypoglycemia.
- When you have severe hypoglycemia, someone should call 911 for help if a glucagon shot is not available.

Action Steps – If You Don't Take Insulin

- Tell your doctor if you have low blood glucose, especially at the same time of the day or night, several times in a row.
- Tell your doctor about other medicines you are taking.
- Ask your doctor whether your diabetes medicines might cause low blood glucose.

Your Diabetes Care Records

The following pages in this section will have the charts with the things you can talk about with your health care team. The information such as your blood glucose levels, body weight, blood pressure, the medicines you consume, diet, smoking habits, etc. can be discussed with your health care team. Making copies of these charts will be very much helpful to you during your discussion with your doctor at each visit.

Things to Discuss with Your Health Care Team at Each Visit

Date: _____
Whom you visited: _____

Table 51.2. Details to be discussed with health care team

Your information	Things to remember	Check off what you covered, or write the result of your visit.
Your blood glucose levels	• Share your blood glucose records. Your doctor will ask how you are checking your blood glucose levels to make sure you are doing it right.	• Shared blood glucose records?
	• Mention if you often have low or high blood glucose.	• ☐ Checked meter?
		• ☐ Practiced blood glucose reading?
		• ☐ Shared high or low blood glucose?
Your weight	• Talk about how much you should weigh.	• My weight now is ____.
	• Talk about ways to reach your target weight that will work for you.	• ☐ My target weight is ____.
	• Ask about ways to reach your target.	• ☐ Steps to take:
Your blood pressure	• The target for most people with diabetes is below 140/80 unless your doctor helps you set a different target.	• ☐ My blood pressure now is ____.
		• ☐ My target blood pressure is ____.
		• ☐ Steps to take:

Monitor Your Diabetes

Table 51.2. Continued

Your medicines	• Talk about any problems you have had with your medicines.	• ☐ Shared medicine problems?
	• Ask if you should take a low-dose aspirin every day to lower your chance of getting heart disease.	• ☐ Take aspirin?
		Yes____
		No____
		• ☐ Steps to take:
Your feet	• Ask to have your feet checked for problems.	• Checked feet?
	• Talk about any problems you are having with your feet, such as numbness, tingling, or sores that heal slowly.	• ☐ Shared problems?
		• ☐ Steps to help with my feet:
Your physical activity plan	• Talk about how often you are physically active, the type of physical activity you do, and any problems you have when being physically active.	• ☐ Shared activities?
• ☐ Steps to take:
Your healthy eating plan	• Talk about what you eat, how much you eat, and when you eat.	• Shared eating habits?
• ☐ Steps to take:
Your feelings	• If you feel stressed, ask about ways to cope	• Shared stress and problems?
	• Talk about whether you are feeling sad.	• ☐ Steps to take:
Your smoking	• If you smoke, ask for help with quitting.	• Shared smoking habits?
• ☐
• Steps to take:

This chart lists important tests, exams, and vaccines to get at least once or twice a year.

Table 51.3. Tests, Exams, and Vaccines to Get at Least Once or Twice a Year

Tests	Instructions	Results or Dates
A1C test	• Have this blood test at least twice a year. Your result will tell you what your average blood glucose level was for the past 2 to 3 months.	Date: ___ A1C: ___ Next test: ___
Blood lipid (fats) lab tests	• Get a blood test to check your	Date: ___
	• total cholesterol—aim for below 200	Total cholesterol: ___
	• LDL, or bad, cholesterol—aim for below 100	
	• HDL, or good, cholesterol—men: aim for above 40; women: aim for above 50	LDL: ___ HDL: ___
	• triglycerides—aim for below 150	Triglycerides: ___ Next test: ___
Kidney function tests	• Once a year, get a urine test to check for protein.	Date: ___
	• At least once a year, get a blood test to check for creatinine.	
	•	Urine protein: ___
	•	Creatinine: ___
	•	Next test: ___

Monitor Your Diabetes

Table 51.3. Continued

Tests	Instructions	Results or Dates
Dilated eye exam	• See your dentist twice a year for a cleaning and checkup.	Date: ___ Result: ___ Next test: ___
Pneumonia vaccine (recommended by the Centers for Disease Control and Prevention [CDC])	• Get the vaccine if you are younger than 64. • If you're older than 64 and your shot was more than 5 years ago, get another vaccine.	Date received: ___
Flu vaccine (recommended by the CDC)	• Get a flu shot each year.	Date received: ___
Hepatitis B vaccine (recommended by the CDC)	• Get this vaccine if you are age 19 to 59 and have not had this vaccine. • Consider getting this vaccine if you are 60 or older and have not had this vaccine.	Date of 1st dose: ___ Date of 2nd dose: ___ Date of 3rd dose: ___

Chapter 52

Be Active!

Why is it important for people with diabetes to be physically active?

Physical activity can help you control your blood glucose, weight, and blood pressure, as well as raise your "good" cholesterol and lower your "bad" cholesterol. It can also help prevent heart and blood flow problems, reducing your risk of heart disease and nerve damage, which are often problems for people with diabetes.

How much and how often should people with diabetes exercise?

Experts recommend moderate-intensity physical activity for at least 30 minutes on 5 or more days of the week. Some examples of moderate-intensity physical activity are walking briskly, mowing the lawn, dancing, swimming, or bicycling.

If you are not accustomed to physical activity, you may want to start with a little exercise, and work your way up. As you become stronger, you can add a few extra minutes to your physical activity. Do some

---

This chapter includes excerpts from "Be Active," Centers for Disease Controland Prevention (CDC) September 25, 2015

physical activity every day. It's better to walk 10 or 20 minutes each day than one hour once a week.

Talk to your health care provider about a safe exercise plan. He or she may check your heart and your feet to be sure you have no special problems. If you have high blood pressure, eye, or foot problems, you may need to avoid some kinds of exercise.

What are some good types of physical activity for people with diabetes?

Walking vigorously, hiking, climbing stairs, swimming, aerobics, dancing, bicycling, skating, skiing, tennis, basketball, volleyball, or other sports are just some examples of physical activity that will work your large muscles, increase your heart rate, and make you breathe harder – important goals for fitness.

In addition, strength training exercises with hand weights, elastic bands, or weight machines can help you build muscle. Stretching helps to make you flexible and prevent soreness after other types of exercise.

Do physical activities you really like. The more fun you have, the more likely you will do it each day. It can be helpful to exercise with a family member or friend.

Are there any safety considerations for people with diabetes when they exercise?

Exercise is very important for people with diabetes to stay healthy, but there are a few things to watch out for.

You should avoid some kinds of physical activity if you have certain diabetes complications. Exercise involving heavy weights may be bad for people with blood pressure, blood vessel, or eye problems. Diabetes-related nerve damage can make it hard to tell if you've injured your feet during exercise, which can lead to more serious problems. If you do have diabetes complications, your health care provider can tell you which kinds of physical activity would be best for you. Fortunately, there are many different ways to get exercise.

Physical activity can lower your blood glucose too much, causing hypoglycemia, especially in people who take insulin or certain oral medications. Hypoglycemia can happen at the time you're exercising, just afterward, or even up to a day later. You can get shaky, weak, confused, irritable, anxious, hungry, tired, or sweaty. You can get a headache, or even lose consciousness.

Be Active!

To help prevent hypoglycemia during physical activity, check your blood glucose before you exercise. If it's below 100, have a small snack. In addition, bring food or glucose tablets with you when you exercise just in case. It is not good for people with diabetes to skip meals at all, but especially not prior to exercise. After you exercise, check to see how it has affected your blood glucose level. If you take insulin, ask your health care provider if there is a preferable time of day for you to exercise, or whether you should change your dosage before physical activity, before beginning an exercise regimen.

On the other hand, you should not exercise when your blood glucose is very high because your level could go even higher. Do not exercise if your blood glucose is above 300, or your fasting blood glucose is above 250 and you have ketones in your urine.

When you exercise, wear cotton socks and athletic shoes that fit well and are comfortable. After you exercise, check your feet for sores, blisters, irritation, cuts, or other injuries.

Drink plenty of fluids during physical activity, since your blood glucose can be affected by dehydration.

How can physical activity help me take care of my diabetes?

Physical activity and keeping a healthy weight can help you take care of your diabetes and prevent diabetes problems. Physical activity helps your blood glucose, also called blood sugar, stay in your target range.

Physical activity also helps the hormone insulin absorb glucose into all your body's cells, including your muscles, for energy. Muscles use glucose better than fat does. Building and using muscle through physical activity can help prevent high blood glucose. If your body doesn't make enough insulin, or if the insulin doesn't work the way it should, the body's cells don't use glucose. Your blood glucose levels then get too high, causing diabetes.

Starting a physical activity program can help you lose weight or keep a healthy weight and keep your blood glucose levels on target. Even without reaching a healthy weight, just a 10 or 15 pound weight loss makes a difference in reducing the risk of diabetes problems.

When is the best time of day for me to do physical activity?

Your health care team can help you decide the best time of day for you to do physical activity based on your daily schedule, healthy eating plan, and diabetes medicines.

If you have type 1 diabetes, try not to do vigorous physical activity when you have ketones in your blood or urine. Ketones are chemicals your body might make when your blood glucose levels are too high and your insulin level is too low. If you are physically active when you have ketones in your blood or urine, your blood glucose levels may go even higher.

Light or moderate physical activity can help lower blood glucose if you have type 2 diabetes and you don't have ketones. Ketones are rare in people with type 2 diabetes. Ask your health care team whether you should be physically active when your blood glucose levels are high.

Chapter 53

Stay Healthy!

It's very important for you to take your diabetes medicines exactly as directed. Not taking medications correctly may lower the level of glucose and cause the insulin your body to go up. The medicines then become less effective when taken. Some people report not feeling well as a reason for stopping their medication or not taking it as prescribed. Tell your doctor if your medicines are making you sick. He or she may be able to help you deal with side effects so you can feel better. Don't just stop taking your medicines, because your health depends on it.

This chapter provides information about staying healthy with your diabetes.

What routine medical examinations and tests are needed for people with diabetes?

Your doctors should:

- Measure your blood pressure at every visit.

- Check your feet for sores at every visit, and give a thorough foot exam at least once a year.

- Give you a hemoglobin A1C test at least twice a year to determine what your average blood glucose level was for the past 2 to 3 months.

Text in this chapter is excerpted from "Stay Healthy," Centers for Disease Control and Prevention (CDC), September 25, 2015.

- Test your urine and blood to check your kidney function at least once a year.

- Test your blood lipids (fats)—total cholesterol; LDL, or low-density lipoprotein ("bad" cholesterol); HDL, or high-density lipoprotein ("good" cholesterol); and triglycerides at least once a year.

You should also get a dental checkup twice a year, a dilated eye exam once a year, an annual flu shot, and a pneumonia shot.

How does maintaining healthy blood glucose levels help people with diabetes stay healthy?

Research studies in the United States and other countries have shown that controlling blood glucose benefits people with either type 1 or type 2 diabetes. In general, for every 1% reduction in results of A1C blood tests (e.g., from 8.0% to 7.0%), the risk of developing eye, kidney, and nerve disease is reduced by 40%.

How does maintaining a healthy body weight help people with diabetes stay healthy?

Most people newly diagnosed with type 2 diabetes are overweight. Excess weight, particularly in the abdomen, makes it difficult for cells to respond to insulin, resulting in high blood glucose. Often, people with type 2 diabetes are able to lower their blood glucose by losing weight and increasing physical activity. Losing weight also helps lower the risk for other health problems that especially affect people with diabetes, such as cardiovascular disease.

How does maintaining a healthy blood pressure level help people with diabetes stay healthy?

About 70% of adults with diabetes have high blood pressure or use prescription medications to reduce high blood pressure. Maintaining normal blood pressure—less than 130/80 millimeters of mercury (mm Hg) helps to prevent damage to the eyes, kidneys, heart, and blood vessels. Blood pressure measurements are written like a fraction, with the two numbers separated by a slash. The first number represents the pressure in your blood vessels when your heart beats (systolic pressure); the second number represents the pressure in the vessels when your heart is at rest (diastolic pressure).

Stay Healthy!

In general, for every 10 mm Hg reduction in systolic blood pressure (the first number in the fraction), the risk for any complication related to diabetes is reduced by 12%. Maintaining normal blood pressure control can reduce the risk of eye, kidney, and nerve disease (microvascular disease) by approximately 33%, and the risk of heart disease and stroke (cardiovascular disease) by approximately 33% to 50%. Healthy eating, medications, and physical activity can help you bring high blood pressure down.

How does exercise help people with diabetes stay healthy?

Physical activity can help you control your blood glucose, weight, and blood pressure, as well as raise your "good" cholesterol and lower your "bad" cholesterol. It also can help prevent heart and blood flow problems.

Experts recommend moderate-intensity physical activity for at least 30 minutes on 5 or more days of the week. Talk to your health care provider about a safe exercise plan. He or she may check your heart and your feet to be sure you have no special problems. If you have high blood pressure, eye, or foot problems you may need to avoid some kinds of exercise.

How does maintaining healthy cholesterol levels help people with diabetes stay healthy?

Several things, including having diabetes, can make your blood cholesterol level too high. When cholesterol is too high, the insides of large blood vessels become narrowed, even clogged, which can lead to heart disease and stroke, the biggest health problems for people with diabetes. Maintaining normal cholesterol levels will help prevent these diseases and can help prevent circulation problems—an issue for people with diabetes. Have your cholesterol checked at least once a year. Total cholesterol should be less than 200; LDL ("bad" cholesterol) should be less than 100; HDL ("good" cholesterol) should be more than 40 in men and more than 50 in women; and triglycerides should be less than 150. Healthy eating, medications, and physical activity can help you reach your cholesterol targets. Keeping cholesterol levels under control can reduce the risk of cardiovascular complications of diabetes by 20% to 50%.

How does quitting smoking help people with diabetes stay healthy?

Smoking puts people with diabetes at particular risk. Smoking raises your blood glucose, cholesterol, and blood pressure, all of which people with diabetes need to be especially concerned about. When you have diabetes and use tobacco, the risk of heart and blood vessel problems is even greater. If you quit smoking, you'll lower your risk for heart attack, stroke, nerve disease, kidney disease, and oral disease.

Why is it important for people with diabetes to get an annual flu shot?

Diabetes can make the immune system more vulnerable to severe cases of the flu. People with diabetes who come down with the flu may become very sick and may die. You can help keep yourself from getting the flu by getting a flu shot every year. Everyone with diabetes—even pregnant women—should get a yearly flu shot. The best time to get one is between October and mid-November, before the flu season begins.

Chapter 54

Managing Diabetes during Sick Days

Sick days can make blood sugars hard to control. Here are some things you can do to speed up your recovery.

Ahead of time

Ask your medical team about handling sick days before you get ill. Also train one or two family members or friends in blood glucose monitoring and other ways to help when you are sick.

Keep a box filled with medicines and easy-to-fix foods. If you wait until you are sick, you may not have the energy to collect all the things you need.

Good choices are:

- Milk of magnesia
- A pain reliever
- Medicine to control diarrhea
- A thermometer
- Antacids
- Suppositories for vomiting

Text in this chapter is excerpted from "Sick Days," Centers for Disease Control and Prevention (CDC), September 25, 2015.

If you cannot eat meals, you will need about 50 grams of carbohydrate every 4 hours.

Foods you may want to keep on hand are:

- Sports drinks
- Instant cooked cereals
- Small juice containers
- Crackers
- Canned soup
- Instant pudding
- Regular gelatin
- Canned applesauce
- Regular soft drinks

You can add other, more perishable, foods like toast, yogurt, ice cream, or milk when you are sick.

While you are sick

Even if you cannot eat normally, you will need to take your diabetes medicine. In fact, you may need to increase or change your medicine because your blood sugar may go higher. While you are sick, your medical team may ask you to test your blood sugar more often. Keep good written records about your blood sugar levels, medicines, temperature, and weight. You may need to test your urine for ketones if your blood sugar goes very high.

Drink plenty of fluids to prevent dehydration. Keep a pitcher of water or other non-caloric drink by your bed, so that you can drink 4 to 6 ounces every half hour. You may also need to drink beverages with sugar if you cannot get 50 grams of carbohydrate through other food choices. The portions of these sweet beverages must be controlled, as you don't want your blood sugar to get too high.

When to call the doctor

Call your health care provider if any of the following occurs:

- You have moderate to high ketone levels in your urine.
- You have not eaten normally for more than 24 hours.

Managing Diabetes during Sick Days

- You have a fever over 101 degrees for 24 hours.
- You can't keep any liquids down for more than 4 hours.
- You have vomiting and/or diarrhea for more than 6 hours.
- You lose 5 pounds or more during the illness.
- Your blood glucose reading is under 60 mg/dl or over 300 mg/dl.
- You have trouble breathing.
- You can't stay awake or think clearly.

If you cannot think clearly or feel too sleepy, have someone else call your health care provider or take you to the emergency room.

Questions to ask

- Do I have a written plan from my medical team to guide me on sick days?
- Have I made a sick day box with needed medicines and foods?
- Have I trained at least two persons who can help me if I am sick?

Chapter 55

Managing Your Diabetes during Special Times

Diabetes is part of your life. You can learn how to take care of yourself and your diabetes, when you're at school or work, when you're away from home, when an emergency or a natural disaster happens, or when you're thinking about having a baby or are pregnant.

When you're at school or work

Take care of your diabetes when you're at school or at work:

- Follow your healthy eating plan.
- Take your medicines and check your blood glucose levels as usual.
- Tell your teachers, friends, or close coworkers that you have diabetes and teach them about the signs of low blood glucose. You may need their help if your blood glucose levels drop too low.
- Keep snacks nearby and carry some with you at all times to treat low blood glucose.

Text in this chapter is excerpted from "Take Care of Your Diabetes during Special Times or Events," National Institute of Diabetes and Digestive and Kidney Diseases (NIDDK), National Institutes of Health (NIH), February 12, 2014.

- If you have trained diabetes staff at your school or work, tell them that you have diabetes.
- Wear or carry an identification tag or card that says you have diabetes.

When you're away from home

These tips can help you when you're away from home:

- Get all your vaccines and immunizations, or shots, before you travel. Find out what shot you need for where you're going, and make sure you get the right shots on time.
- Follow your healthy eating plan as much as possible when you eat out. Always carry a snack with you in case you have to wait for a waiter to serve you.
- Limit alcoholic beverages. Ask your health care team how many alcoholic beverages you can safely drink. Eat something when you drink to prevent low blood glucose.
- If you're taking a long trip by car, check your blood glucose levels before driving. Stop and check your blood glucose levels every 2 hours.
- Always carry your diabetes medicines and supplies in the car where you can reach them in case your blood glucose levels drop too low.
- In case you can't leave for home on time, bring twice the amount of diabetes supplies and medicines you normally need.
- Take comfortable, well-fitting shoes on vacation. You'll probably be walking more than usual. Keep your medical insurance card, emergency phone numbers, and a first aid kit handy.
- Wear or carry an identification tag or card that says you have diabetes.
- If you're going to be away for a long time, ask your doctor for a written prescription for your diabetes medicines and the name of a doctor in the place you're going to visit.
- Don't count on buying extra supplies when you're traveling, especially if you're going to another country. Different countries use different kinds of diabetes medicines.

Managing Your Diabetes during Special Times

When you're flying on a plane

These tips can help you when you're flying on a plane:

- Ask your health care team in advance how to adjust your medicines, especially your insulin, if you're traveling across time zones.
- Take a letter from your doctor stating you have diabetes. The letter should include a list of all the medical supplies and medicines you need on the plane. In the letter, the doctor should also include a list of any devices that shouldn't go through an x-ray machine.
- Carry your diabetes medicines and your blood testing supplies with you on the plane. Never put these items in your checked baggage.
- Bring food for meals and snacks on the plane.
- If you use an insulin pump, ask airport security to check the device by hand. X-ray machines can damage insulin pumps, whether the pump is on your body or in your luggage.
- When on a plane, get up from your seat and walk around when possible.

Action Steps – If You Take Insulin

- When you travel,
- take a special insulated bag to carry your insulin to keep it from freezing or getting too hot
- bring extra supplies for taking insulin and testing your blood glucose levels in case of loss or breakage
- ask your doctor for a letter saying you have diabetes and need to carry supplies for taking insulin and testing blood glucose

Action Steps – If You Don't Take Insulin

- When you travel,
- ask your health care team in advance how to adjust your medicines if you're traveling across time zones
- carry your diabetes medicines and your blood testing supplies with you on the plane

- ask your doctor for a letter saying you have diabetes and need to carry supplies for testing blood glucose

When an emergency or a natural disaster happens

Everyone with diabetes should be prepared for emergencies and natural disasters, such as power outages or hurricanes. Always have a disaster kit ready. Include everything you need to take care of your diabetes, such as:

- a blood glucose meter, lancets, and testing strips
- your diabetes medicines
- insulin, syringes, and an insulated bag to keep insulin cool, if you take insulin
- a glucagon kit if you take insulin or if recommended by your doctor
- glucose tablets and other food or drinks to treat low blood glucose
- antibiotic cream or ointment
- a copy of your medical information, including a list of your conditions, medicines, and recent lab test results
- a list of your prescription names with dosage information and prescription numbers from your pharmacy
- phone numbers for the American Red Cross and other disaster relief groups

You also might want to include some food that doesn't spoil, such as canned or dried food, along with bottled water.

If you're a woman and planning a pregnancy

Keeping your blood glucose levels near normal before and during pregnancy helps protect both you and your baby. Even before you become pregnant, your blood glucose levels should be close to the normal range.

Your health care team can work with you to get your blood glucose levels under control before you try to get pregnant. If you're already pregnant and you have diabetes, see your doctor right away. You can take steps to bring your blood glucose levels close to normal.

Managing Your Diabetes during Special Times

Your insulin needs may change when you're pregnant. Your doctor may want you to take more insulin and check your blood glucose levels more often.

If you plan to have a baby,

- work with your health care team to get your blood glucose levels as close to the normal range as possible
- see a doctor who has experience taking care of pregnant women with diabetes
- don't smoke, drink alcoholic beverages, or use harmful drugs
- follow your healthy eating plan

Be sure to have your eyes, heart and blood vessels, blood pressure, and kidneys checked. Your doctor should also check for nerve damage. Pregnancy can make some health problems worse.

Chapter 56

Managing Your Diabetes during the Holidays

Prepare to manage your diabetes during the holidays. Stay on track by taking medications on schedule and choosing healthy versions of favorite dishes. Remember to plan daily physical activities like walking after meals and dancing at festivities.

Having diabetes shouldn't stop you from enjoying holiday celebrations and travel. With some planning and a little preparation, you can stay healthy on the road and at holiday gatherings with friends and family.

Preparation is the most important step in managing diabetes during holiday travel and festivities. Know what you'll be eating, how to enjoy a few traditional favorites while sticking with a healthy meal plan, how to pack necessary supplies for a trip, and you're ready to celebrate!

Feasts and parties

Before you go, take these steps to ensure you stick to your healthy meal plan.

Text in this chapter is excerpted from "Managing Your Diabetes during the Holidays," Centers for Disease Control and Prevention (CDC), November 17, 2014.

- Eat a healthy snack early to avoid overeating at the party.
- Ask what food will be served, so you can see how it fits into your meal plan.
- Bring a nutritious snack

You don't have to give up all of your holiday favorites if you make healthy choices and limit portion sizes. At a party or holiday gathering, follow these tips to avoid overeating and to choose healthy foods.

- If you're at a buffet, fix your plate and move to another room away from the food, if possible. Choose smaller portions.
- Choose low-calorie drinks such as sparkling water, unsweetened tea or diet beverages. If you choose to drink alcohol, limit the amount, and have it with food. Talk with your health care team about whether alcohol is safe for you. Limit it to one drink a day for women, two for men, and drink only with a meal.
- Watch out for heavy holiday favorites such as hams with a honey glaze, turkey swimming in gravy and side dishes loaded with butter, sour cream, cheese, or mayonnaise. Instead, choose skinless turkey without gravy, or other lean meats.
- Look for side dishes and vegetables that are light on butter, dressing, and other extra fats and sugars, such as marshmallows or fried vegetable toppings.
- Watch the salt. Some holiday dishes are made with prepared foods high in sodium. Choose fresh or frozen vegetables with no sauce to keep your sodium intake down.
- Select fruit instead of pies, cakes and other desserts high in fat, cholesterol, and sugar.

Focus on friends, family, and activities instead of food. Take a walk after a meal, or join in the dancing at a party.

Traveling for the holidays

Leaving home to visit friends and family means changing routines. Take care of your diabetes while traveling. Check your blood glucose (sugar) more often than usual, because changing your schedule can affect levels.

Managing Your Diabetes during the Holidays

Remember your medication

- Pack twice the amount of diabetes supplies you expect to need in your carry-on bag, in case of travel delays.
- Keep snacks, glucose gel, or tablets with you in case your blood glucose drops.
- Make sure you keep your health insurance card and emergency phone numbers handy, including your doctor's name and phone number.
- Carry medical identification that says you have diabetes and wear medical identification jewelry.
- Keep time zone changes in mind so you'll know when to take medication.
- If you use insulin, make sure you also pack a glucagon emergency kit.
- Keep your insulin cool by packing it in an insulated bag with refrigerated gel packs.
- Get an influenza vaccination before traveling, unless your medical provider instructs otherwise.

Healthy routines

- Wash your hands often with soap and water. Try to avoid contact with sick people.
- Reduce your risk for blood clots by moving around every hour or two.
- Pack a small cooler of foods that may be difficult to find while traveling, such as fresh fruit and sliced raw vegetables. Pack dried fruit, nuts, and seeds as snacks. Since these foods can be high in calories, measure out small portions (¼ cup) in advance.
- If you're driving, bring a few bottles of water instead of sweetened soda or juice. If you're flying, choose unsweetened beverages on-board.
- If you're flying and don't want to walk through the metal detector with your insulin pump, tell a security officer that you're wearing an insulin pump and ask them to visually inspect the pump and do a full-body pat-down.

- Place all diabetes supplies in carry-on luggage. Keep medications and snacks at your seat for easy access. Don't store them in overhead bins.

- Have all syringes and insulin delivery systems (including vials of insulin) clearly marked with the pharmaceutical preprinted label that identifies the medications, in the original pharmacy labeled packaging.

- If a meal will be served during your flight, call ahead for a diabetic, low fat, or low cholesterol meal. If the airline doesn't offer a meal, bring a nutritious meal yourself. Wait until your food is about to be served before you take your insulin.

- When drawing up your dose of insulin, don't inject air into the bottle (the air on your plane will probably be pressurized).

- Stick with your routine for staying active. Get at least 150 minutes of physical activity every week. Ten minutes at a time is fine.

Chapter 57

Diabetes and Employee Rights

The Americans with Disabilities Act (ADA), which was amended by the ADA Amendments Act of 2008 ("Amendments Act" or "ADAAA"), is a federal law that prohibits discrimination against qualified individuals with disabilities. Individuals with disabilities include those who have impairments that substantially limit a major life activity, have a record (or history) of a substantially limiting impairment, or are regarded as having a disability.

Title I of the ADA covers employment by private employers with 15 or more employees as well as state and local government employers. Section 501 of the Rehabilitation Act provides similar protections related to federal employment. In addition, most states have their own laws prohibiting employment discrimination on the basis of disability. Some of these state laws may apply to smaller employers and may provide protections in addition to those available under the ADA.

The U.S. Equal Employment Opportunity Commission (EEOC) enforces the employment provisions of the ADA. This document, which is one of a series of question-and-answer documents addressing particular disabilities in the workplace, explains how the ADA applies to

---

Text in this chapter is excerpted from "Questions & Answers about Diabetes in the Workplace and the Americans with Disabilities Act (ADA)," U.S. Equal Employment Opportunity Commission (EEOC), May 15, 2013.

job applicants and employees who have or had diabetes. In particular, this document explains:

- when an employer may ask an applicant or employee questions about her diabetes and how it should treat voluntary disclosures;

- what types of reasonable accommodations employees with diabetes may need;

- how an employer should handle safety concerns about applicants and employees with diabetes; and

- how an employer can ensure that no employee is harassed because of diabetes or any other disability.

General information about diabetes

With nearly two million new cases diagnosed each year, diabetes is becoming more prevalent in the United States and is the most common endocrine disease. Today, an estimated 18.8 million adults in the United States have diabetes.

As a result of changes made by the ADAAA, individuals who have diabetes should easily be found to have a disability within the meaning of the first part of the ADA's definition of disability because they are substantially limited in the major life activity of endocrine function. Additionally, because the determination of whether an impairment is a disability is made without regard to the ameliorative effects of mitigating measures, diabetes is a disability even if insulin, medication, or diet controls a person's blood glucose levels. An individual with a past history of diabetes (for example, gestational diabetes) also has a disability within the meaning of the ADA. Finally, an individual is covered under the third ("regarded as") prong of the definition of disability if an employer takes a prohibited action (for example, refuses to hire or terminates the individual) because of diabetes or because the employer believes the individual has diabetes.

Obtaining, using, and disclosing medical information

Title I of the ADA limits an employer's ability to ask questions related to diabetes and other disabilities and to conduct medical examinations at three stages: pre-offer, post-offer, and during employment.

Diabetes and Employee Rights

Job Applicants

Before an Offer of Employment Is Made

May an employer ask a job applicant whether she has or had diabetes or about her treatment related to diabetes before making a job offer?

No. An employer may not ask questions about an applicant's medical condition or require an applicant to have a medical examination before it makes a conditional job offer. This means that an employer cannot legally ask an applicant questions such as:

- whether she has diabetes or has been diagnosed with diabetes (for example, gestational diabetes) in the past;
- whether she uses insulin or other prescription drugs or has ever done so in the past; or,
- whether she ever has taken leave for medical treatment, or how much sick leave she has taken in the past year.

Of course, an employer may ask questions pertaining to the qualifications for, or performance of, the job, such as:

- whether the applicant has a commercial driver's license; or
- whether she can work rotating shifts.

Does the ADA require an applicant to disclose that she has or had diabetes or some other disability before accepting a job offer?

No. The ADA does not require applicants to voluntarily disclose that they have or had diabetes or another disability unless they will need a reasonable accommodation for the application process (for example, a break to eat a snack or monitor their glucose levels). Some individuals with diabetes, however, choose to disclose their condition because they want their co-workers or supervisors to know what to do if they faint or experience other symptoms of hypoglycemia (low blood sugar), such as weakness, shakiness, or confusion.

Sometimes, the decision to disclose depends on whether an individual will need a reasonable accommodation to perform the job (for example, breaks to take medication or a place to rest until blood sugar levels become normal). A person with diabetes, however, may request an accommodation after becoming an employee even if she did not do so when applying for the job or after receiving the job offer.

May an employer ask any follow-up questions if an applicant voluntarily reveals that she has or had diabetes?

No. An employer generally may not ask an applicant who has voluntarily disclosed that she has diabetes any questions about her diabetes, its treatment, or its prognosis. However, if an applicant voluntarily discloses that she has diabetes **and the employer reasonably believes that she will require an accommodation to perform the job because of her diabetes or treatment**, the employer may ask whether the applicant will need an accommodation and what type. The employer must keep any information an applicant discloses about her medical condition confidential.

After an Offer of Employment Is Made

After making a job offer, an employer may ask questions about the applicant's health (including questions about the applicant's disability) and may require a medical examination, as long as all applicants for the same type of job are treated equally (that is, all applicants are asked the same questions and are required to take the same examination). After an employer has obtained basic medical information from all individuals who have received job offers, it may ask specific individuals for more medical information if it is medically related to the previously obtained medical information. For example, if an employer asks all applicants post-offer about their general physical and mental health, it can ask individuals who disclose a particular illness, disease, or impairment for more medical information or require them to have a medical examination related to the condition disclosed.

What may an employer do when it learns that an applicant has or had diabetes after she has been offered a job but before she starts working?

When an applicant discloses after receiving a conditional job offer that she has diabetes, an employer may ask the applicant additional questions such as how long she has had diabetes; whether she uses insulin or oral medication; whether and how often she experiences hypoglycemic episodes; and/or whether she will need assistance if her blood sugar level drops while at work. The employer also may send the applicant for a follow-up medical examination or ask her to submit documentation from her doctor answering questions specifically designed to assess her ability to perform the job's functions safely. Permissible follow-up questions at this stage differ from those at the pre-offer stage when an employer only may ask an applicant who voluntarily discloses a disability whether she needs an accommodation to perform the job and what type.

An employer may not withdraw an offer from an applicant with diabetes if the applicant is able to perform the essential functions of the job, with or without reasonable accommodation, without posing a direct threat (that is, a significant risk of substantial harm) to the health or safety of himself or others that cannot be eliminated or reduced through reasonable accommodation.

Employees

The ADA strictly limits the circumstances under which an employer may ask questions about an employee's medical condition or require the employee to have a medical examination. Once an employee is on the job, her actual performance is the best measure of ability to do the job.

When may an employer ask an employee whether diabetes, or some other medical condition, may be causing her performance problems?

Generally, an employer may ask disability-related questions or require an employee to have a medical examination when it knows about a particular employee's medical condition, has observed performance problems, and reasonably believes that the problems are related to a medical condition. At other times, an employer may ask for medical information when it has observed symptoms, such as extreme fatigue or irritability, or has received reliable information from someone else (for example, a family member or co-worker) indicating that the employee may have a medical condition that is causing performance problems. Often, however, poor job performance is unrelated to a medical condition and generally should be handled in accordance with an employer's existing policies concerning performance.

May an employer require an employee on leave because of diabetes to provide documentation or have a medical examination before allowing her to return to work?

Yes. If the employer has a reasonable belief that the employee may be unable to perform her job or may pose a direct threat to herself or others, the employer may ask for medical information. However, the employer may obtain only the information needed to make an assessment of the employee's present ability to perform her job and to do so safely.

Are there any other instances when an employer may ask an employee with diabetes about his condition?

Yes. An employer also may ask an employee about diabetes when it has a reasonable belief that the employee will be unable to safely perform the essential functions of his job because of diabetes. In addition, an employer may ask an employee about his diabetes to the extent the information is necessary:

- to support the employee's request for a reasonable accommodation needed because of his diabetes;
- to verify the employee's use of sick leave related to his diabetes if the employer requires all employees to submit a doctor's note to justify their use of sick leave; or
- to enable the employee to participate in a voluntary wellness program.

Keeping Medical Information Confidential

With limited exceptions, an employer must keep confidential any medical information it learns about an applicant or employee. Under the following circumstances, however, an employer may disclose that an employee has diabetes:

- to supervisors and managers in order to provide a reasonable accommodation or to meet an employee's work restrictions;
- to first aid and safety personnel if an employee may need emergency treatment or require some other assistance because, for example, her blood sugar level is too low;
- to individuals investigating compliance with the ADA and similar state and local laws; and
- where needed for workers' compensation or insurance purposes (for example, to process a claim).

May an employer tell employees who ask why their co-worker is allowed to do something that generally is not permitted (such as eat at his desk or take more breaks) that she is receiving a reasonable accommodation?

No. Telling co-workers that an employee is receiving a reasonable accommodation amounts to a disclosure that the employee has a disability. Rather than disclosing that the employee is receiving a reasonable accommodation, the employer should focus on the importance of maintaining the privacy of all employees and emphasize that its policy is to refrain from discussing the work situation of any employee with co-workers. Employers may be able to avoid many of these kinds of questions by training all employees on the requirements of equal employment opportunity laws, including the ADA.

Additionally, an employer will benefit from providing information about reasonable accommodations to all of its employees. This can be done in a number of ways, such as through written reasonable accommodation procedures, employee handbooks, staff meetings, and periodic training. This kind of proactive approach may lead to fewer questions from employees who misperceive co-worker accommodations as "special treatment."

If an employee experiences an insulin reaction at work, may an employer explain to other employees or managers that the employee has diabetes?

No. Although the employee's co-workers and others in the workplace who witness the reaction naturally may be concerned, an employer may not reveal that the employee has diabetes. Rather, the employer should assure everyone present that the situation is under control. An employee, however, may voluntarily choose to tell her co-workers that she has diabetes and provide them with helpful information, such as how to recognize when her blood sugar may be low, what to do if she faints or seems shaky or confused (for example, offer a piece of candy or gum), or where to find her glucose monitoring kit. However, even when an employee voluntarily discloses that she has diabetes, the employer must keep this information confidential consistent with the ADA. An employer also may not explain to other employees why an employee with diabetes has been absent from work if the absence is related to her diabetes or another disability.

Accommodating Employees with Diabetes

The ADA requires employers to provide adjustments or modifications—called reasonable accommodations—to enable applicants and employees with disabilities to enjoy equal employment opportunities unless doing so would be an undue hardship (that is, a significant difficulty or expense). Accommodations vary depending on the needs of the individual with a disability. Not all employees with diabetes will need an accommodation or require the same accommodations, and most of the accommodations a person with diabetes might need will involve little or no cost. An employer must provide a reasonable accommodation that is needed because of the diabetes itself, the effects of medication, or both. For example, an employer may have to accommodate an employee who is unable to work while learning to manage her diabetes or adjusting to medication. An employer, however, has no obligation to monitor an employee to make sure that she is regularly checking her blood sugar levels, eating, or taking medication as prescribed.

What other types of reasonable accommodations may employees with diabetes need?

Some employees may need one or more of the following accommodations:

- a private area to test their blood sugar levels or to administer insulin injections
- a place to rest until their blood sugar levels become normal
- breaks to eat or drink, take medication, or test blood sugar levels

How does an employee with diabetes request a reasonable accommodation?

There are no "magic words" that a person has to use when requesting a reasonable accommodation. A person simply has to tell the employer that she needs an adjustment or change at work because of her diabetes. A request for a reasonable accommodation also can come from a family member, friend, health professional, or other representative on behalf of a person with diabetes.

May an employer request documentation when an employee who has diabetes requests a reasonable accommodation?

Yes. An employer may request reasonable documentation where a disability or the need for reasonable accommodation is not known or obvious. An employer, however, is entitled only to documentation sufficient to establish that the employee has diabetes and to explain why an accommodation is needed. A request for an employee's entire medical record, for example, would be inappropriate as it likely would include information about conditions other than the employee's diabetes.

Does an employer have to grant every request for a reasonable accommodation?

Diabetes and Employee Rights

No. An employer does not have to provide an accommodation if doing so will be an undue hardship. Undue hardship means that providing the reasonable accommodation will result in significant difficulty or expense. An employer also does not have to eliminate an essential function of a job as a reasonable accommodation, tolerate performance that does not meet its standards, or excuse violations of conduct rules that are job-related and consistent with business necessity and that the employer applies consistently to all employees (such as rules prohibiting violence, threatening behavior, theft, or destruction of property).

If more than one accommodation will be effective, the employee's preference should be given primary consideration, although the employer is not required to provide the employee's first choice of reasonable accommodation. If a requested accommodation is too difficult or expensive, an employer may choose to provide an easier or less costly accommodation as long as it is effective in meeting the employee's needs.

May an employer be required to provide more than one accommodation for the same employee with diabetes?

Yes. The duty to provide a reasonable accommodation is an ongoing one. Although some employees with diabetes may require only one reasonable accommodation, others may need more than one. For example, an employee with diabetes may require leave to attend a class on how to administer insulin injections and later may request a part-time or modified schedule to better control his glucose levels. An employer must consider each request for a reasonable accommodation and determine whether it would be effective and whether providing it would pose an undue hardship.

May an employer automatically deny a request for leave from someone with diabetes because the employee cannot specify an exact date of return?

No. Granting leave to an employee who is unable to provide a fixed date of return may be a reasonable accommodation. Although diabetes can be successfully treated, some individuals experience serious complications that may be unpredictable and do not permit exact timetables. An employee requesting leave because of diabetes or resulting complications (for example, a foot or toe amputation), therefore, may be able to provide only an approximate date of return (e.g., "in six to eight weeks," "in about three months"). In such situations, or in situations in which a return date must be postponed because of unforeseen medical developments, employees should stay in regular communication with their employers to inform them of their progress and discuss the need for continued leave beyond what originally was granted. The employer also has the right to require that the employee provide periodic updates on his condition and possible date of return. After receiving these updates, the employer may reevaluate whether continued leave constitutes an undue hardship.

Concerns about Safety

When it comes to safety concerns, an employer should be careful not to act on the basis of myths, fears, or stereotypes about diabetes. Instead, the employer should evaluate each individual on her skills, knowledge, experience and how having diabetes affects her.

When may an employer refuse to hire, terminate, or temporarily restrict the duties of a person who has diabetes because of safety concerns?

An employer only may exclude an individual with diabetes from a job for safety reasons when the individual poses a direct threat. A "direct threat" is a significant risk of substantial harm to the individual or others that cannot be eliminated or reduced through reasonable accommodation. This determination must be based on objective, factual evidence, including the best recent medical evidence and advances in the treatment of diabetes.

In making a direct threat assessment, the employer must evaluate the individual's present ability to safely perform the job. The employer also must consider:

- the duration of the risk;
- the nature and severity of the potential harm;
- the likelihood that the potential harm will occur; and
- the imminence of the potential harm.

The harm must be serious and likely to occur, not remote or speculative. Finally, the employer must determine whether any reasonable accommodation (for example, temporarily limiting an employee's duties, temporarily reassigning an employee, or placing an employee on leave) would reduce or eliminate the risk.

May an employer require an employee who has had an insulin reaction at work to submit periodic notes from his doctor indicating that his diabetes is under control?

Yes, but only if the employer has a reasonable belief that the employee will pose a direct threat if he does not regularly see his doctor. In determining whether to require periodic documentation, the employer should consider the safety risks associated with the position the employee holds, the consequences of the employee's inability or impaired ability to perform his job, how long the employee has had diabetes, and how many insulin reactions the employee has had on the job.

What should an employer do when another federal law prohibits it from hiring anyone who uses insulin?

If a federal law prohibits an employer from hiring a person who uses insulin, the employer is not be liable under the ADA. The employer should be certain, however, that compliance with the law actually is required, not voluntary. The employer also should be sure that the law does not contain any exceptions or waivers. For example, the Department of Transportation's Federal Motor Carrier Safety Administration (FMCSA) issues exemptions to certain individuals with diabetes who wish to drive commercial motor vehicles (CMVs).

Harassment

The ADA prohibits harassment, or offensive conduct, based on disability just as other federal laws prohibit harassment based on race, sex, color, national origin, religion, age, and genetic information. Offensive conduct may include, but is not limited to, offensive jokes, slurs, epithets or name calling, physical assaults or threats, intimidation, ridicule or mockery, insults or put-downs, offensive objects or pictures, and interference with work performance. Although the law does not prohibit simple teasing, offhand comments, or isolated incidents that are not very serious, harassment is illegal when it is so frequent or severe that it creates a hostile or offensive work environment or when it results in an adverse employment decision (such as the victim being fired or demoted).

What should employers do to prevent and correct harassment?

Employers should make clear that they will not tolerate harassment based on disability or on any other basis. This can be done in a number of ways, such as through a written policy, employee handbooks, staff meetings, and periodic training. The employer should emphasize that harassment is prohibited and that employees should promptly report such conduct to a manager. Finally, the employer should immediately conduct a thorough investigation of any report of harassment and take swift and appropriate corrective action. For more information on the standards governing harassment under all of the EEO laws, see www.eeoc.gov/policy/docs/harassment.html.

Retaliation

The ADA prohibits retaliation by an employer against someone who opposes discriminatory employment practices, files a charge of employment discrimination, or testifies or participates in any way in an investigation, proceeding, or litigation related to a charge of employment discrimination. It is also unlawful for an employer to retaliate against someone for requesting a reasonable accommodation. Persons who believe that they have experienced retaliation may file a charge of retaliation as described below.

How to file a charge of employment discrimination

Against Private Employers and State/Local Governments

Any person who believes that his or her employment rights have been violated on the basis of disability and wants to make a claim against an employer must file a charge of discrimination with the EEOC. A third party may also file a charge on behalf of another person who believes he or she experienced discrimination. For example, a family member, social worker, or other representative can file a charge on behalf of someone who is incapacitated because of diabetes. The charge must be filed by mail or in person with the local EEOC office within 180 days from the date of the alleged violation. The 180-day filing deadline is extended to 300 days if a state or local anti-discrimination agency has the authority to grant or seek relief as to the challenged unlawful employment practice.

The EEOC will send the parties a copy of the charge and may ask for responses and supporting information. Before formal investigation, the EEOC may select the charge for EEOC's mediation program. Both parties have to agree to mediation, which may prevent a time consuming investigation of the charge. Participation in mediation is free, voluntary, and confidential.

If mediation is unsuccessful, the EEOC investigates the charge to determine if there is "reasonable cause" to believe discrimination has occurred. If reasonable cause is found, the EEOC will then try to resolve the charge with the employer. In some cases, where the charge cannot be resolved, the EEOC will file a court action. If the EEOC finds no discrimination, or if an attempt to resolve the charge fails and the EEOC decides not to file suit, it will issue a notice of a "right to sue," which gives the charging party 90 days to file a court action. A charging party can also request a notice of a "right to sue" from the EEOC 180 days after the charge was first filed with the Commission, and may then bring suit within 90 days after receiving the notice. For a detailed description of the process, you can visit our website at www.eeoc.gov/employees/howtofile.cfm.

Against the Federal Government

If you are a federal employee or job applicant and you believe that a federal agency has discriminated against you, you have a right to file a complaint. Each agency is required to post information about how to contact the agency's EEO Office. You can contact an EEO Counselor by calling the office responsible for the agency's EEO complaints program. Generally, you must contact the EEO Counselor within 45 days from the day the discrimination occurred. In most cases the EEO Counselor will give you the choice of participating either in EEO counseling or in an alternative dispute resolution (ADR) program, such as a mediation program.

If you do not settle the dispute during counseling or through ADR, you can file a formal discrimination complaint against the agency with the agency's EEO Office. You must file within 15 days from the day you receive notice from your EEO Counselor about how to file.

Once you have filed a formal complaint, the agency will review the complaint and decide whether or not the case should be dismissed for a procedural reason (for example, your claim was filed too late). If the agency doesn't dismiss the complaint, it will conduct an investigation. The agency has 180 days from the day you filed your complaint to finish the investigation. When the investigation is finished, the agency will issue a notice giving you two choices: either request a hearing before an EEOC Administrative Judge or ask the agency to issue a decision as to whether the discrimination occurred.

Part Eight

Research and Clinical Trials on Diabetes

Chapter 58

Ongoing Research in Diabetes Care

Chapter Contents

Section 58.1—Research on Diabetes at CDC 386
Section 58.2—Research on Diabetes at NIDDK 388
Section 58.3—Pancreatic Islet Transplantation 390
Section 58.4—Stem Cell Research 396

Section 58.1

Research on Diabetes at CDC

Text in this section is excerpted from "Research Projects," Centers for Disease Control and Prevention (CDC), September 16, 2015.

CDC has researched several diabetes prevention interventions that have proven effective in helping to prevent diabetes in certain populations and communities. CDC is continuing to collaborate with local departments of health, public health partners, community-based organizations in research and also creating effective programs, in both prevention and control to help prevent further cases of diabetes.

Surveillance, Natural History, Quality of Care, and Outcomes of Diabetes Mellitus with Onset in Childhood and Adolescence

This 5-year program is expected to provide estimates of trends in the incidence of diabetes for ages 0–19 years by type and race/ethnicity and support research aimed at assessing the incidence of diabetes-related complications, quality of care, quality of life, and mortality by diabetes type and race/ethnicity.

The program will achieve this goal by building on a 10-year collaborative multicenter research project called SEARCH for Diabetes in Youth, grantees will use sentinel surveillance network of diabetes registries in racial/ethnic, socio-economic, and geographically diverse populations to document trends in diabetes incidence in youth population 20 years old or younger by type and race-ethnicity. Grantees will also conduct a multicenter 5-year study to assess the incidence of both acute and chronic diabetes-related complications and their biological and socio-cultural risk factors, quality of life, and mortality in a diverse population of youth with diabetes.

Natural Experiments for Translation in Diabetes (NEXT-D) Study

Overall Objectives

To rigorously evaluate health policies and interventions coming from health care systems, businesses, communities, and health care legislation that may reduce diabetes risk, its complications, and health inequalities across broad segments of the United States population.

Funding Agencies

This cooperative agreement is jointly funded by the Centers for Disease Control and Prevention (CDC) and the National Institute of Diabetes and Digestive and Kidney Diseases (NIDDK) under CDC Funding Opportunity Announcement (FOA) Number: RFA- DP10-002, entitled Natural Experiments and Effectiveness Studies to Identify the Best Policy and System Level Practices to Prevent Diabetes and Its Complications.

Project Period

The NEXT-D Study is a 5-year research project that started in September 2010.

Study Outcomes

The NEXT-D study aims to understand how population-targeted policies affect preventive behaviors and diabetes outcomes, quantity and quality of care used, morbidity, costs, and unintended consequences.

Participating Federal Agencies

CDC and NIDDK, agencies with a history of work related to translating diabetes prevention and control, are supporting each site to ensure high-quality scientific delivery, synergies between sites yielding cross-cutting metrics and methods, and multi-site deliverables such as policy frameworks, briefs, and analysis.

Section 58.2

Research on Diabetes at NIDDK

Text in this section is excerpted from "Diabetes," National Institute of Diabetes and Digestive and Kidney Diseases (NIDDK), National Institutes of Health (NIH), May 10, 2013.

Diabetes affects an estimated 29.1 million people in the United States. It is the seventh leading cause of death, and the leading cause of kidney failure, non-traumatic lower limb amputations, and, in working-age adults, blindness.

The NIDDK supports basic, clinical, and translational research to combat diabetes and its associated complications. For example, NIDDK researchers are:

- identifying new methods to improve blood glucose monitoring and insulin delivery in type 1 diabetes;

- examining behavioral approaches to prevent type 2 diabetes and to enhance diabetes self-management;

- conducting clinical trials testing new prevention and treatment strategies for diabetes and its complications, such as a trial comparing different type 2 diabetes medications and trials testing ways to prevent type 1 diabetes in relatives of people with the disease; and

- uncovering the fundamental cellular and molecular pathways underlying development of diabetes and its complications to develop new approaches to prevention and management.

The NIDDK also administers the Special Statutory Funding Program for Type 1 Diabetes Research, which is a special appropriation dedicated to supporting research on type 1 diabetes and its complications. More information on the Program and the research it supports is available on the Type 1 Diabetes Research Special Statutory Funding Program website.

In addition, the NIDDK's National Diabetes Information Clearinghouse (NDIC) provides information about diabetes to people with diabetes and to their families, health care professionals, and the public.

Ongoing Research in Diabetes Care

The National Diabetes Education Program (NDEP) works with over 200 partners at the federal, state, and local levels to improve the treatment and outcomes for people with diabetes, promote early diagnosis, and prevent or delay the onset of type 2 diabetes.

Recent discoveries from NIDDK research include:

- More than half of Asian Americans with diabetes are undiagnosed

- More than half of Asian Americans and nearly half of Hispanic Americans with diabetes are undiagnosed, according to researchers from the National Institutes of Health and the Centers for Disease Control and Prevention.

- Discovery of naturally occurring fats that may alleviate diabetes and inflammation

- Alefacept helps preserve function of insulin-producing cells in type 1 diabetes

- Results from a clinical trial sponsored by the National Institute of Allergy and Infectious Diseases, part of the National Institutes of Health, suggest that the immune-suppressing drug alefacept helps preserve function of insulin-producing beta cells in people "with newly diagnosed type 1 diabetes."

This National Diabetes Month, you have a role in diabetes education and support

During National Diabetes Month, including World Diabetes Day on Nov. 14, the National Institutes of Health urges you to think about the important role you play in diabetes education and support.

Section 58.3

Pancreatic Islet Transplantation

Text in this section is excerpted from "Pancreatic Islet Transplantation," National Institute of Diabetes and Digestive and Kidney Diseases (NIDDK), National Institutes of Health (NIH), September 2013.

What are pancreatic islets?

Pancreatic islets, also called islets of Langerhans, are tiny clusters of cells scattered throughout the pancreas. The pancreas is an organ about the size of a hand located behind the lower part of the stomach.

Pancreatic islets contain several types of cells, including beta cells that produce the hormone insulin. The pancreas also makes enzymes that help the body digest and use food.

When the level of blood glucose, also called blood sugar, rises after a meal, the pancreas responds by releasing insulin into the bloodstream. Insulin helps cells throughout the body absorb glucose from the bloodstream and use it for energy.

Diabetes develops when the pancreas does not make enough insulin, the body's cells do not use insulin effectively, or both. As a result, glucose builds up in the blood instead of being absorbed by cells in the body.

In type 1 diabetes, the beta cells of the pancreas no longer make insulin because the body's immune system has attacked and destroyed them. The immune system protects people from infection by identifying and destroying bacteria, viruses, and other potentially harmful foreign substances. A person who has type 1 diabetes must take insulin daily to live. Type 2 diabetes usually begins with a condition called insulin resistance, in which the body has trouble using insulin effectively. Over time, insulin production declines as well, so many people with type 2 diabetes eventually need to take insulin.

What is pancreatic islet transplantation?

The two types of pancreatic islet transplantation are:

- Allo-transplantation
- Auto-transplantation

Ongoing Research in Diabetes Care

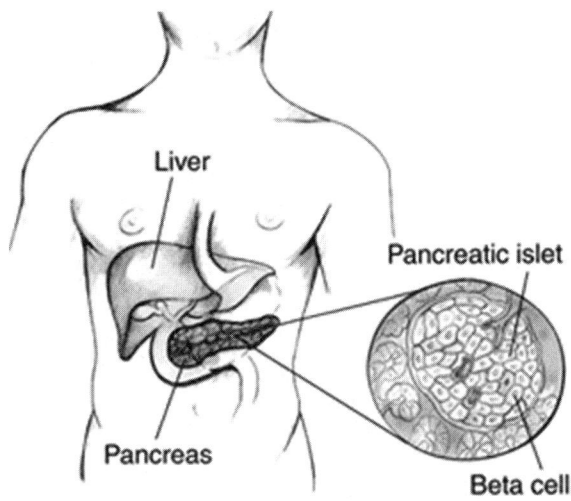

Figure 58.1. *Pancreatic Islet*

Pancreatic islet allo-transplantation is a procedure in which islets from the pancreas of a deceased organ donor are purified, processed, and transferred into another person. Pancreatic islet allo-transplantation is currently labeled an experimental procedure until the transplantation technology is considered successful enough to be labeled therapeutic.

For each pancreatic islet allo-transplant infusion, researchers use specialized enzymes to remove islets from the pancreas of a single, deceased donor. The islets are purified and counted in a lab. Transplant patients typically receive two infusions with an average of 400,000 to 500,000 islets per infusion. Once implanted, the beta cells in these islets begin to make and release insulin.

Pancreatic islet allo-transplantation is performed in certain patients with type 1 diabetes whose blood glucose levels are difficult to control. The goals of the transplant are to help these patients achieve normal blood glucose levels with or without daily injections of insulin and to reduce or eliminate hypoglycemia unawareness—a dangerous condition in which a person with diabetes cannot feel the symptoms of hypoglycemia, or low blood glucose. When a person feels the symptoms of hypoglycemia, steps can be taken to bring blood glucose levels back to normal.

Pancreatic islet allo-transplants are only performed at hospitals that have received permission from the United States. Food and Drug Administration (FDA) for clinical research on islet transplantation.

The transplants are often performed by a radiologist—a doctor who specializes in medical imaging. The radiologist uses x rays and ultrasound to guide the placement of a thin, flexible tube called a catheter through a small incision in the upper abdomen—the area between the chest and hips—and into the portal vein of the liver. The portal vein is the major vein that supplies blood to the liver. The islets are then infused, or pushed, slowly into the liver through the catheter. Usually, the patient receives a local anesthetic and a sedative. In some cases, a surgeon performs the transplant using general anesthesia.

Patients often need two or more transplants to get enough functioning islets to stop or reduce their need for insulin injections.

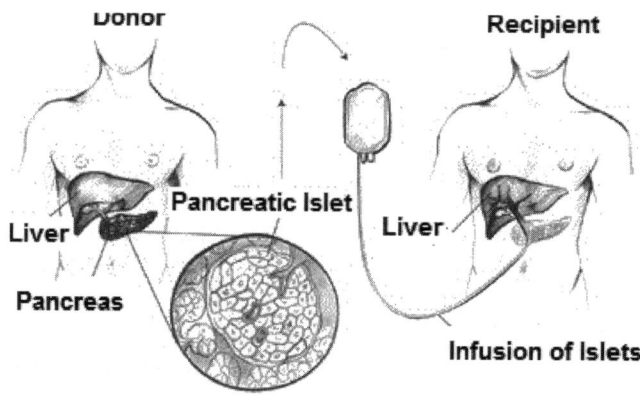

Figure 58.2. *Pancreatic islet allo-transplantation*

Pancreatic islet auto-transplantation is performed following total pancreatectomy—the surgical removal of the whole pancreas—in patients with severe and chronic, or long lasting, pancreatitis that cannot be managed by other treatments. This procedure is not considered experimental. Patients with type 1 diabetes cannot receive pancreatic islet auto-transplantation. The procedure is performed in a hospital, and the patient receives general anesthesia. The surgeon first removes the pancreas and then extracts and purifies islets from the pancreas. Within hours, the islets are infused through a catheter into the patient's liver. The goal is to give the body enough healthy islets to make insulin.

What happens after pancreatic islet transplantation?

Pancreatic islets begin to release insulin soon after transplantation. However, full islet function and new blood vessel growth from the new islets take time. Transplant recipients usually take insulin injections until the islets are fully functional. They may also receive various medications before and after transplantation to promote successful implantation and long-term functioning of the islets. However, the autoimmune response that destroyed transplant recipients' own islets in the first place can happen again and attack the transplanted islets. Although the liver has been the traditional site for infusing the donor islets, researchers are investigating alternative sites, such as muscle tissue or another organ.

What are the benefits and risks of pancreatic islet allo-transplantation?

The benefits of pancreatic islet allo-transplantation include improved blood glucose control, reducing or eliminating the need for insulin injections to control diabetes, and preventing hypoglycemia. An alternative to islet transplantation is whole organ pancreas transplantation that is performed most often with kidney transplantation. The advantages of whole organ pancreas transplantation are less dependence on insulin and longer duration of organ function. The main disadvantage is that a whole organ transplant is a major surgery that involves a greater risk of complications and even death.

Pancreatic islet allo-transplantation can also help reverse hypoglycemia unawareness. Research has shown that even partial islet function after a transplant can eliminate hypoglycemia unawareness.

Improved blood glucose control from a successful allo-transplant may also slow or prevent the progression of diabetes problems, such as heart disease, kidney disease, and nerve or eye damage. Research to evaluate this possibility is ongoing.

The risks of pancreatic islet allo-transplantation include the risks associated with the transplant procedure—particularly bleeding and blood clots. The transplanted islets may not function well or may stop functioning entirely. Other risks are the side effects from the immunosuppressive medications that transplant recipients must take to stop the immune system from rejecting the transplanted islets. When a patient has received a kidney transplant and is already taking immunosuppressive medications, the only additional risks are the islet infusion and the side effects from the immunosuppressive medications given at the time of allo-transplantation. Immunosuppressive medications are not needed in the case of an auto-transplant because the infused cells come from the patient's own body.

What is the role of immunosuppressive medications?

Immunosuppressive medications are needed to prevent rejection—a common problem with any transplant.

Scientists have made many advances in islet transplantation in recent years. In 2000, islet transplantation researchers at the University of Alberta in Edmonton, Canada, reported their findings in the New England Journal of Medicine. Their transplant protocol, known as the Edmonton protocol, has since been adapted by transplant centers around the world and continues to be refined.

The Edmonton protocol introduced the use of a new combination of immunosuppressive medications, also called anti-rejection medications, including daclizumab (Zenapax), sirolimus (Rapamune), and tacrolimus (Prograf). Researchers continue to develop and study modifications to the Edmonton protocol, including improved medication regimens that promote successful transplants. Medication regimens vary from one transplant center to another. Examples of other immunosuppressive medications used in islet transplantation include antithymocyte globulin (Thymoglobulin), alemtuzumab (Campath), basiliximab (Simulect), belatacept (Nulojix), etanercept (Enbrel), everolimus (Zortress), and mycophenolate mofetil (CellCept, Myfortic). Researchers are also evaluating nonimmunosuppresive medications, such as exenatide (Byetta) and sitagliptin (Januvia).

Immunosuppressive medications have significant side effects, and their long-term effects are still not fully known. Immediate side effects may include mouth sores and gastrointestinal problems, such as upset stomach and diarrhea.

Patients may also have:

- increased blood cholesterol, or blood fat, levels
- high blood pressure
- anemia, a condition in which red blood cells are fewer or smaller than normal, which prevents the body's cells from getting enough oxygen
- fatigue
- decreased white blood cell counts
- decreased kidney function
- increased susceptibility to bacterial and viral infections

Taking immunosuppressive medications also increases the risk of developing certain tumors and cancers.

Scientists are seeking ways to achieve immune tolerance of the transplanted islets, in which the patient's immune system no longer recognizes the islets as foreign. Immune tolerance would allow patients to maintain transplanted islets without long-term use of immunosuppressive medications. For example, one approach is to transplant islets encapsulated with a special coating, which may help to prevent rejection.

What are the obstacles to pancreatic islet allo-transplantation?

The shortage of islets from donors is a significant obstacle to widespread use of pancreatic islet allo-transplantation. According to the Organ Procurement and Transplantation Network, in 2011 there were about 8,000 deceased organ donors available in the United States.2 However, only 1,562 pancreases were recovered from donors in 2011.2 Also, many donated pancreases are not suitable for extracting islets for transplants because they do not meet the selection criteria, and islets are often damaged or destroyed during processing. Therefore, only a small number of islet transplants can be performed each year.

Researchers are pursuing various approaches to solve this shortage of islets, such as transplanting islets from a single, donated pancreas, using only a portion of the pancreas from a living donor, or using islets from pigs. Researchers have transplanted pig islets into other animals, including monkeys, by encapsulating the islets with a special coating or by using medications to prevent rejection. Another approach is creating islets from other types of cells, such as stem cells. New technologies could then be employed to grow islets in the lab.

Financial barriers also prevent the widespread use of islet allo-transplantation. Until the transplantation technology is considered successful enough to be labeled therapeutic rather than experimental, the costs of islet allo-transplants must be covered by research funds. Health insurance companies and Medicare generally do not cover experimental procedures. Federal law also does not allow health care providers or hospitals to charge patients or health insurance companies for research procedures.

Some patient advocates and islet researchers feel that islet allo-transplantation is close to having a therapeutic label. The National Institutes of Health (NIH) currently supports studies that are working toward obtaining FDA licensure to reclassify islet allo-transplantation as therapeutic. In other countries, such as Canada and Scandinavia, islet allo-transplantation is no longer considered experimental and is an accepted therapy in certain patients.

Eating, diet, and nutrition

A person who receives a pancreatic islet transplant should follow a meal plan worked out with a health care provider and dietitian. Immunosuppressive medications taken after the transplant can cause changes in a person's body, such as weight gain. A healthy diet after the transplant is important to control weight gain, blood pressure, blood cholesterol, and blood glucose levels.

Section 58.4

Stem Cell Research

Text in this section is excerpted from "Stem Cell Basics," National Institutes of Health (NIH), March 5, 2015

What are the potential uses of human stem cells and the obstacles that must be overcome before these potential uses will be realized?

There are many ways in which human stem cells can be used in research and the clinic. Studies of human embryonic stem cells will yield information about the complex events that occur during human development. A primary goal of this work is to identify how undifferentiated stem cells become the differentiated cells that form the tissues and organs. Scientists know that turning genes on and off is central to this process. Some of the most serious medical conditions, such as cancer and birth defects, are due to abnormal cell division and differentiation.

A more complete understanding of the genetic and molecular controls of these processes may yield information about how such diseases arise and suggest new strategies for therapy. Predictably controlling cell proliferation and differentiation requires additional basic research on the molecular and genetic signals that regulate cell division and specialization. While recent developments with iPS cells suggest some of the specific factors that may be involved, techniques must be devised to introduce these factors safely into the cells and control the processes that are induced by these factors.

Human stem cells are currently being used to test new drugs. New medications are tested for safety on differentiated cells generated from human pluripotent cell lines. Other kinds of cell lines have a long history of being used in this way. Cancer cell lines, for example, are used to screen potential anti-tumor drugs. The availability of pluripotent stem cells would allow drug testing in a wider range of cell types. However, to screen drugs effectively, the conditions must be identical when comparing different drugs. Therefore, scientists must be able to precisely control the differentiation of stem cells into the specific cell type on which drugs will be tested.

For some cell types and tissues, current knowledge of the signals controlling differentiation falls short of being able to mimic these conditions precisely to generate pure populations of differentiated cells for each drug being tested.

Perhaps the most important potential application of human stem cells is the generation of cells and tissues that could be used for cell-based therapies. Today, donated organs and tissues are often used to replace ailing or destroyed tissue, but the need for transplantable tissues and organs far outweighs the available supply. Stem cells, directed to differentiate into specific cell types, offer the possibility of a renewable source of replacement cells and tissues to treat diseases including macular degeneration, spinal cord injury, stroke, burns, heart disease, diabetes, osteoarthritis, and rheumatoid arthritis.

For example, it may become possible to generate healthy heart muscle cells in the laboratory and then transplant those cells into patients with chronic heart disease. Preliminary research in mice and other animals indicates that bone marrow stromal cells, transplanted into a damaged heart, can have beneficial effects. Whether these cells can generate heart muscle cells or stimulate the growth of new blood vessels that repopulate the heart tissue, or help via some other mechanism is actively under investigation.

For example, injected cells may accomplish repair by secreting growth factors, rather than actually incorporating into the heart. Promising results from animal studies have served as the basis for a small number of exploratory studies in humans (for discussion, see call-out box, "Can Stem Cells Mend a Broken Heart?"). Other recent studies in cell culture systems indicate that it may be possible to direct the differentiation of embryonic stem cells or adult bone marrow cells into heart muscle cells).

In people who suffer from type 1 diabetes, the cells of the pancreas that normally produce insulin are destroyed by the patient's own immune system. New studies indicate that it may be possible to direct the differentiation of human embryonic stem cells in cell culture to form insulin-producing cells that eventually could be used in transplantation therapy for persons with diabetes.

To realize the promise of novel cell-based therapies for such pervasive and debilitating diseases, scientists must be able to manipulate

Can Stem Cells Mend a Broken Heart? Stem Cells for the Future Treatment of Heart Disease

Cardiovascular disease (CVD), which includes hypertension, coronary heart disease, stroke, and congestive heart failure, has ranked as the number one cause of death in the United States every year since 1900 except 1918, when the nation struggled with an influenza epidemic. Nearly 2,600 Americans die of CVD each day, roughly one person every 34 seconds. Given the aging of the population and the relatively dramatic recent increases in the prevalence of cardiovascular risk factors such as obesity and type 2 diabetes, CVD will be a significant health concern well into the 21st century.

Cardiovascular disease can deprive heart tissue of oxygen, thereby killing cardiac muscle cells (cardiomyocytes). This loss triggers a cascade of detrimental events, including formation of scar tissue, an overload of blood flow and pressure capacity, the overstretching of viable cardiac cells attempting to sustain cardiac output, leading to heart failure, and eventual death. Restoring damaged heart muscle tissue, through repair or regeneration, is therefore a potentially new strategy to treat heart failure.

The use of embryonic and adult-derived stem cells for cardiac repair is an active area of research. A number of stem cell types, including embryonic stem (ES) cells, cardiac stem cells that naturally reside within the heart, myoblasts (muscle stem cells), adult bone marrow-derived cells including mesenchymal cells (bone marrow-derived cells that give rise to tissues such

> as muscle, bone, tendons, ligaments, and adipose tissue), endothelial progenitor cells (cells that give rise to the endothelium, the interior lining of blood vessels), and umbilical cord blood cells, have been investigated as possible sources for regenerating damaged heart tissue. All have been explored in mouse or rat models, and some have been tested in larger animal models, such as pigs.
>
> A few small studies have also been carried out in humans, usually in patients who are undergoing open-heart surgery. Several of these have demonstrated that stem cells that are injected into the circulation or directly into the injured heart tissue appear to improve cardiac function and/or induce the formation of new capillaries. The mechanism for this repair remains controversial, and the stem cells likely regenerate heart tissue through several pathways. However, the stem cell populations that have been tested in these experiments vary widely, as do the conditions of their purification and application. Although much more research is needed to assess the safety and improve the efficacy of this approach, these preliminary clinical experiments show how stem cells may one day be used to repair damaged heart tissue, thereby reducing the burden of cardiovascular disease.

stem cells so that they possess the necessary characteristics for successful differentiation, transplantation, and engraftment. The following is a list of steps in successful cell-based treatments that scientists will have to learn to control to bring such treatments to the clinic. To be useful for transplant purposes, stem cells must be reproducibly made to:

- Proliferate extensively and generate sufficient quantities of cells for making tissue.
- Differentiate into the desired cell type(s).
- Survive in the recipient after transplant.
- Integrate into the surrounding tissue after transplant.
- Function appropriately for the duration of the recipient's life.

- Avoid harming the recipient in any way.

Also, to avoid the problem of immune rejection, scientists are experimenting with different research strategies to generate tissues that will not be rejected.

To summarize, stem cells offer exciting promise for future therapies, but significant technical hurdles remain that will only be overcome through years of intensive research.

Chapter 59

Targeted Drug Development: Why Is Diabetes Lagging Behind?

Through the efforts of Congress and the U.S. Food and Drug Administration (FDA), FDA's drug approval process has become the fastest in the world—and Americans have first access to new drugs more often than anywhere else in the world. While FDA has worked to transform the landscape for the final stage of drug development, progress in the discovery and testing stages of drug development has not kept pace. As a result, too many diseases are still awaiting treatments and cures.

More than a decade ago, FDA recognized that although scientists were mapping the human genome and making revolutionary discoveries in basic science, translating these discoveries into treatments had not kept pace. In response, FDA has for many years been building collaborations with industry and academia to modernize the "translational" science of drug development. FDA's goal is to improve the efficiency and predictability of clinical drug development through

---

Text in this chapter is excerpted from "Targeted Drug Development: Why Are Many Diseases Lagging Behind?" U.S. Food and Drug Administration (FDA), July 16, 2015.

the development and use of such tools as genomic data, biomarkers and surrogate endpoints, modernized clinical trial designs, disease modeling and clinical trial simulation (bioinformatics), and advanced imaging technology. These tools have the potential to dramatically reduce the length and cost of drug development, for example, by predicting drug efficacy and toxicity earlier and avoiding wasteful late-stage failures. In addition, these tools can help target drugs to specific patient populations who can benefit most without facing unacceptable side effects, thereby limiting the number and size of clinical trials.

The speed with which the scientific community can develop and use these tools to shorten drug development in particular disease areas is highly variable. For example, the ability to use genetic data to identify useful biomarkers and surrogate endpoints in a specific disease is dependent on how well we understand the molecular and genetic bases for the disease. In some disease areas, we have made tremendous progress in our understanding of the causes of the disease and the interventions that can treat or cure it. FDA's success in getting effective drugs for cancer, HIV/AIDS, and other viral infections to market quickly has been widely noted.

This achievement is based on decades of intensive research on cancer and HIV/AIDS that has given us critical insights into the pathways through which these (and related) diseases can be attacked. Such research has also led to the discovery of biomarkers that have provided insight on the genetic and metabolic characteristics that alter patients' responsiveness to particular drugs, and predict whether drug candidates are likely to work. This knowledge has resulted in important breakthroughs, rapid drug development, and a robust pipeline of new therapies for these particular diseases.

For other diseases, however, like Alzheimer's, we still lack basic information about the causes of the disease and the pathways for slowing its progress. As a result, we have witnessed a series of failed attempts to find biomarkers or surrogate endpoints that can predict disease progression or drug activity, and available treatments are limited.

In the middle are many other diseases such as diabetes. For these diseases, our understanding of disease causation and progression is sufficient to permit our use of certain tools such as surrogate endpoints. But it is insufficient to develop others such as biomarkers to help target specific subset of patients who are less likely to suffer side effects from specific drugs. Even where scientific research has not yet identified the molecular and genetic bases for a disease and its treatment, FDA is using tools other than targeting and biomarkers to reduce the length and cost of clinical trials, including flexible trial designs, expedited development pathways, public-private research collaborations, and intensive engagement with drug sponsors.

In addition, these tools can support the development of one of the most promising avenues for accelerating drug development: targeted, or precision, medicine—the ability to target the right drug to the right patient based on understanding of the genetic and biochemical basis of a disease in patient subgroups.

State of Drug Discovery and Development: Diabetes

In patients with diabetes, the pancreas stops making sufficient quantities of insulin to control the amount of sugar in the blood, or the body becomes resistant to insulin, or both. As a result, blood sugar becomes elevated. Over time, uncontrolled blood sugar can lead to major health problems, including heart attack, stroke, kidney disease, amputation of toes or feet, and blindness. There are two main types of diabetes: type 1 (5% of cases) and type 2 (more than 90% of cases).

Type 1 diabetes (formerly known as juvenile diabetes) usually begins in childhood or adolescence and is an auto-immune disease: The immune system attacks the cells that produce insulin and patients become completely dependent on insulin injections. Type 2 diabetes, in which the pancreas produces some insulin but the body can't use it well, typically begins in adulthood, but is increasingly diagnosed in younger people, mainly as a result of childhood obesity. As obesity rates rise, we are facing a dramatic increase of diabetes in this country and worldwide, heightening the need for effective, safe new treatments.

Scientific understanding of the disease

How well do scientists understand the genetic and molecular basis of diabetes? Although the major abnormalities that lead to the development of diabetes are generally understood, the exact genetic, molecular, and even environmental causes of type 1 and type 2 diabetes remain to be discovered. Research has identified some of the genes that influence the onset of diabetes, but multiple genes are thought to play a role, and the influence of each single gene on disease causation is thought to be small. Type 2 diabetes tends to run in families, and there continues to be extensive research aimed at identifying specific susceptibility genes. However, with rare exceptions, scientists have not yet discovered specific genetic markers that are capable of predicting risk of type 2 diabetes.

In addition, diabetes patients vary in their rate of progression, in the signs and symptoms of their disease, and in responses to treatment—but for many patients we do not yet understand why. Triggers other than genes, such as diet, infection, certain metabolic disorders, obesity, and some drugs can also be involved and likely interact with an individual's genetic susceptibilities.

Nevertheless, there have been great advances in identifying genetic and immune biomarkers of susceptibility for type 1 diabetes. Although we do not yet have biomarkers that can predict response to treatment, we are nearing the point at which these biomarkers will be able to predict at-risk patients (usually children or adolescents) for the more limited purpose of deciding which patients may qualify for clinical trials of new drugs and biologics aimed at prevention.

Can scientists target drugs to prevent or treat diabetes in specific patients?

No. Specific genetic defects and abnormalities in patients with type 1 and type 2 diabetes and abnormalities in the regulation of the immune system in type 1 diabetes have been identified. But scientists do not yet understand the multiple genetic, immunologic, and metabolic differences among subsets of patients that would allow them to accurately predict which patients will develop diabetes, which diabetics will respond to specific drugs, the degree of beta cell reserve (for type 2 diabetics) or which patients will be susceptible to serious drug side effects.

Without this information, it is not yet possible to develop drugs targeted to prevent or treat diabetes in particular patients and it remains necessary to test new diabetes drugs in a broader patient population. The major goal of therapy is to normalize blood sugar levels and thereby reduce the risk of short and long-term complications.

What research is needed to allow us to target drugs in diabetes?

More basic research is needed to increase scientists' understanding of the interaction between genetic, immunologic, metabolic, and environmental factors that cause specific subsets of patients to develop the disease and why the progress, signs, and symptoms of the disease are variable from patient to patient. Scientists still need to understand much more about why and how the immune system attacks the pancreas, to allow development of treatments that target the specific auto-immune process rather than suppressing the entire immune system, which carries serious risks. Further research is also needed to find biomarkers for susceptibility to specific complications of diabetes (as opposed to the disease itself).

FDA actions to accelerate diabetes drug development

Use of surrogate endpoints

Despite the incomplete understanding of diabetes and its causes, FDA has long allowed manufacturers to show that a diabetes drug works by using a simple surrogate endpoint—lowering blood sugar. FDA does not require long, expensive clinical trials showing that a drug reduces the long-term health problems caused by diabetes, such as heart disease and limb amputations. In fact, no drug for type 2 diabetes has ever been approved based on demonstrating effectiveness in preventing these complications. There have been longstanding concerns that some drugs for type 2 diabetes that successfully lower blood sugar may nevertheless increase rather than decrease the risk of heart attack. This has resulted in external calls to stop approving diabetes drugs on the basis of a surrogate endpoint.

FDA continues to believe that lowering blood sugar levels is a valid surrogate for diabetes drug efficacy. FDA also recognizes the public health concerns raised by drugs to treat diabetes in a large and growing population of people with diabetes if such drugs have the potential to cause a significant increase in the risk of heart attacks. (More than 20 million people have been diagnosed with diabetes in the United States.)

Because biomarkers are not available to identify patients at greater risk of drug-related heart attacks or strokes, FDA issued a guidance in 2008 recommending testing of the effect of new diabetes drugs on the cardiovascular (CV) system. To minimize the impact on innovation while ensuring acceptable cardiovascular safety, FDA asks for preliminary CV safety data before approval and for detailed additional data to characterize CV effects after the product is on the market.

Use and development of biomarkers

Because patients in early clinical trials of type 1 diabetes drugs may be receiving insulin via an insulin pump, it is difficult to determine how much insulin their own pancreas is secreting. In such cases, FDA allows use of a biomarker of insulin secretion, known as C-peptide, which is secreted along with insulin. C-peptide is universally recognized as a marker of insulin production though it has no established major role in metabolic control and FDA permits its use to establish "proof-of- concept" and to select an appropriate dose. FDA is also participating in the development of biomarkers for measuring the function of insulin-producing cells in type 2 diabetes, through the Biomarker Consortium managed by the Foundation for the National Institutes of Health. Researchers hope this will lead to improved techniques for tracking progression of the disease, stratifying patients by severity for entry into clinical trials, and developing more effective treatments. Research is also ongoing to find biomarkers for susceptibility to specific complications of diabetes.

Working with drug sponsors

Because many drug sponsors (particularly those working on type 1 diabetes) are small companies, and because studying the interventions is challenging, FDA is working intensively with them to help them navigate the regulatory process and design clinical trials.

Designing efficient, flexible clinical trials

FDA scientists are working closely with drug sponsors (particularly small companies and academic investigators) to design clinical trials of promising experimental treatments for type 1 diabetes, including transplantation of insulin-producing islet cells to replace cells destroyed by the immune system. In clinical trials of the effectiveness of allogeneic islets, a randomized, concurrent-control trial design may not be feasible or even necessary.

FDA noted emerging data from phase 2 trials showing that the effects of islet cell transplantation (i.e., insulin independence, prolonged absence of hypoglycemic events, ease of blood sugar control with small amounts of insulin in subjects who still required some insulin) virtually never occur in type 1 diabetes spontaneously, that is without treatment. Based on these considerations, FDA issued a guidance7 stating that a single-arm, open label trial without a concurrent control group may be able to provide adequate evidence of effectiveness of allogeneic islet cells. This guidance also identified endpoints that could be used in such trials. Using these principles, FDA worked with NIH in designing phase 3 islet transplantation trials that are currently being conducted by a consortium of investigators and funded by NIH.

Targeted Drug Development: Why Is Diabetes Lagging Behind

FDA is also helping sponsors develop flexible trial designs for other innovative therapies for type 1 diabetes, including stem cell therapy and therapy to interfere with the auto-immune process that destroys the body's ability to make insulin. FDA also participates in a multidisciplinary group of scientists, in partnership with NIH, to help accelerate the development of the "artificial pancreas." This effort has resulted in an FDA guidance, and clinical trials of an artificial pancreas are underway.

Chapter 60

Clinical Trials and Their Role in Diabetes Treatment

What are clinical trials?

Clinical trials are a part of clinical research and at the heart of all medical advances. Clinical trials look at new ways to prevent, detect, or treat disease. Treatments might be new drugs or new combinations of drugs, new surgical procedures or devices, or new ways to use existing treatments. The goal of clinical trials is to determine if a new test or treatment works and is safe. Clinical trials can also look at other aspects of care, such as improving the quality of life for people with chronic illnesses. Doctors and other health professionals conduct clinical trials according to strict rules that are set by the U.S. Food and Drug Administration (FDA). These rules make sure that people who agree to be in clinical trials are treated safely.

This chapter includes excerpts from "Health Information Frequently Asked Questions," National Institute of Diabetes and Digestive and Kidney Diseases (NIDDK), December 14, 2013; text from "Learn About Clinical Studies," National Institutes of Health (NIH), December 2014; text from "Effect of Short-Term Beta-Cell Rest in Adolescents and Young Adults with Type 2 Diabetes Mellitus," ClinicalTrials.gov, December 15, 2015; text from "Metabolic Effects of Non-Nutritive Sweeteners," ClinicalTrials.gov, December 15, 2015; and text from "Young With Diabetes Type 1 - Test of an mHealth App," ClinicalTrials.gov, December 15, 2015.

Where can I find information about current clinical trials?

Information about clinical trials conducted by the National Institutes of Health (NIH), the National Institute of Diabetes and Digestive and Kidney Diseases (NIDDK), and other federal and private organizations can be found at ClinicalTrials.gov. This site offers information about the location of clinical trials, their design and purpose, participation criteria, and additional information about the disease and treatment under study.

How can I participate in a clinical trial?

Find a clinical trial that's right for you by searching ClinicalTrials.gov. If you are a healthy volunteer, contact the study coordinator listed for the clinical trial. If you are a patient volunteer talk with your doctor. You may need a referral to participate in a study.

Considerations for Participation

Participating in a clinical study contributes to medical knowledge. The results of these studies can make a difference in the care of future patients by providing information about the benefits and risks of therapeutic, preventative, or diagnostic products or interventions.

Clinical trials provide the basis for the development and marketing of new drugs, biological products, and medical devices. Sometimes, the safety and the effectiveness of the experimental approach or use may not be fully known at the time of the trial. Some trials may provide participants with the prospect of receiving direct medical benefits, while others do not.

Most trials involve some risk of harm or injury to the participant, although it may not be greater than the risks related to routine medical care or disease progression. (For trials approved by IRBs, the IRB has decided that the risks of participation have been minimized and are reasonable in relation to anticipated benefits.) Many trials require participants to undergo additional procedures, tests, and assessments based on the study protocol. These will be described in the informed consent document for a particular trial. A potential participant should also discuss these issues with members of the research team and with his or her usual health care provider.

Clinical Trials and Their Role in Diabetes Treatment

Questions to Ask the Research Team

Anyone interested in participating in a clinical study should know as much as possible about the study and feel comfortable asking the research team questions about the study, the related procedures, and any expenses. The following questions might be helpful during such a discussion. Answers to some of these questions are provided in the informed consent document. Many of these questions are specific to clinical trials, but some also apply to observational studies.

- What is being studied?
- Why do researchers believe the intervention being tested might be effective? Why might it not be effective? Has it been tested before?
- What are the possible interventions that I might receive during the trial?
- How will it be determined which interventions I receive (for example, by chance)?
- Who will know which intervention I receive during the trial? Will I know? Will members of the research team know?
- How do the possible risks, side effects, and benefits of this trial compare with those of my current treatment?
- What will I have to do?
- What tests and procedures are involved?
- How often will I have to visit the hospital or clinic?
- Will hospitalization be required?
- How long will the study last?
- Who will pay for my participation?
- Will I be reimbursed for other expenses?
- What type of long-term follow-up care is part of this trial?
- If I benefit from the intervention, will I be allowed to continue receiving it after the trial ends?
- Will results of the study be provided to me?
- Who will oversee my medical care while I am participating in the trial?
- What are my options if I am injured during the study?

Current Clinical Trials on Diabetes

Effect of Short-Term Beta-Cell Rest in Adolescents and Young Adults with Type 2 Diabetes Mellitus

This study is currently recruiting participants.

Sponsor: National Institute of Diabetes and Digestive and Kidney Diseases (NIDDK)

Purpose: This study will determine whether resting beta cells (cells in the pancreas that produce insulin) for 2 weeks will improve the ability of patients with Type 2 diabetes mellitus (T2DM) to make insulin. Beta cells can rest by giving patients insulin shots. The study will also examine how teenagers with T2DM feel about having diabetes and explore differences between young people with and without T2DM.

This study includes patients 12 to 25 years of age with T2DM who are overweight and who were diagnosed within 2 years of enrolling in the study. Healthy individuals of normal weight or who are overweight are also eligible. Candidates are screened with a medical history, physical examination and laboratory tests.

Participants with T2DM are assigned to one of two groups. Group 1 takes an anti-diabetes medicine called metformin and follows a diet prescribed by a study staff dietitian for 2 weeks. Group 2 takes metformin, follows the prescribed diet, and receives insulin through a pump under the skin for 2 weeks. During these two weeks, all participants have the following tests:

- Frequent blood sugar checks.

- Oral glucose tolerance test (routine diabetes test in which blood samples are drawn before and several times after the subject drinks a sugary solution).

- Arginine stimulation to test the response of the body to arginine, a normal ingredient of food that stimulates the release of insulin. Two catheters are placed into veins in the arms, one to administer a liquid containing arginine, the other to draw the blood samples.

- Ultrasound of the blood vessels in the neck to check for hardening of the arteries.

- Metabolism test to measure the amount of oxygen used during rest. The subject breathes normally during rest while wearing a canopy over his or her head for about 20 minutes.

Clinical Trials and Their Role in Diabetes Treatment

- MRI scans of the abdomen to examine the amount of fat in the belly (at the beginning and end of the study)
- DEXA scan to determine percent body fat.
- Tests to explore quality of life and feelings about health, work or school, friends and family.
- Exercise testing on a treadmill or stationary bicycle.
- Genetic studies for information on diabetes and obesity.
- Normal volunteers have blood draws, oral glucose tolerance testing, MRI scan, DEXA scan, psychological testing, exercise testing, and genetic testing.

Metabolic Effects of Non-Nutritive Sweeteners

This study is currently recruiting participants.

Sponsor: National Institute of Diabetes and Digestive and Kidney Diseases (NIDDK)

Purpose: Artificial sweeteners, such as sucralose (brand name Splenda), are very commonly found in products such as diet soft drinks. Recently, researchers learned that these sweeteners may affect hormones in the body, especially when they are consumed in combination with real sugar. Changes in hormone levels may, in turn, result in changes in blood sugar, appetite, and weight. Researchers are interested in studying the effects of artificial sweeteners on the metabolism and hormonal levels of healthy volunteers.

Objectives:

- To study the effects that artificial sweeteners have on hormone levels, blood sugar, and appetite.
- To evaluate whether artificial sweeteners change the rate at which food passes out of the stomach into the gut, or the rate at which the body absorbs sugar from the gut.
- To evaluate the effects that different amounts of artificial sweeteners have on hormone levels.

Eligibility: Healthy volunteers between 18 and 45 years of age.

Design:

- This study will require one screening visit and four testing visits, scheduled on different days.

- At the screening visit, eligible participants will be screened with a physical examination, medical history, blood samples, and body measurements (including height, weight, body circumferences, and skin folds). Participants will also be asked about how much artificial sweetener they typically consume and will have taste tests, in which a small amount of flavored liquid is placed on the tongue and participants will name the flavor and rate its intensity.

- Participants will have four glucose tolerance tests on four different days. In preparation for the test, participants will not eat or drink anything but water for 12 hours prior to the test. Blood will be drawn before the test, and participants will drink one of the following study liquids, selected at random:

- Plain water

- Water mixed with sucralose (the amount found in one 12 oz diet soft drink)

- Water mixed with sucralose (the amount found in 2.5 12 oz diet soft drinks)

- Water mixed with sucralose (the amount found in 3.7 12 oz diet soft drinks)

- Ten minutes after drinking the study liquid, participants will have a sugary drink that will allow researchers to measure sugar absorption and the speed with which food leaves the stomach.

- In addition, participants will complete questionnaires about hunger levels before drinking the sugar solution and at regular intervals for 2 hours afterward. Blood samples will be taken at regular intervals as well

The Role of Non-Alcoholic Fatty Liver Disease in Gestational Diabetes

This study is currently recruiting participants.

Sponsor: University of Florida

Clinical Trials and Their Role in Diabetes Treatment

Purpose: The thought is that Non-Alcoholic Fatty Liver Disease (NAFLD) plays a key role in the progression to prediabetes/T2DM in those with a history of Gestational Diabetes (GDM). The investigators want to know if having a fatty liver will be connected with more glucose abnormalities (higher fasting/oral glucose tolerance test glucose, more insulin resistance) and that a history of GDM will be common in those with NAFLD.

Detailed Description: A liver ultrasound will be completed during the last trimester of pregnancy along with a questionnaire. The questionnaire includes baseline maternal characteristics, age, race, ethnicity, parity, blood pressure, medications, activity level, sociodemographic and behavioral risk factors, pregravid BMI, previous obstetric history, medical and family history.

The subject will come in person to clinic two to three times after the subject has had their baby (at 6 weeks postpartum [clinic visit], 6 months postpartum [clinic visit, or via phone if subject cannot come to clinic], and 12 months postpartum [clinic visit]).

The Subject will give blood samples during the 6 weeks postpartum visit and 12 months postpartum visit in clinic, and an Oral Glucose Tolerance Test will be done at these visits. The blood will be drawn by putting a small needle or IV catheter (a small plastic tube) into a vein in the subject's arm. Blood samples will be obtained at timed intervals both before and after the subject is given a glucose beverage to drink, to see how well the subject's body deals with sugar in the blood over time. The total amount of blood to be drawn for each Oral Glucose Tolerance Test and research blood work will be approximately 90 ml (about 6 tablespoons). The total volume of blood taken over the course of the study for each subject will be approximately 180 ml (about 12 tablespoons).

The subject will have their blood pressure measured with a blood pressure cuff during each clinic visit. The height, weight and pulse rate will also be measured. This will take about five minutes.

The subject will have an ultrasound of her liver at the 6 week postpartum visit and 12 month postpartum visit. This will take about 30 to 60 minutes.

The investigator's study coordinator will call the subject to do a questionnaire over the phone at 3 months and 9 months after the subject has had the baby. If the subject cannot come to clinic at 6 months postpartum, then the study coordinator will call the subject at that time to do a questionnaire as well. During each phone call, the study coordinator will ask the subject how the baby is being fed. The investigators will also update information about development of any new medical problems and medications the subject's doctor might have started, activity levels, and health habits. Subjects will be asked questionnaires to update this information during their 6 week postpartum and 12 month postpartum clinic visits.

The subject's understanding and approval of these procedures is required if they are to participate in this study.

Eligibility

- Ages Eligible for Study: 18 Years to 50 Years
- Genders Eligible for Study: Female
- Accepts Healthy Volunteers: No
- Sampling Method: Probability Sample
- Study Population
  - a pregnant female
  - age between 18-50 years

Inclusion Criteria

- a pregnant female
- age between 18-50 years

Young With Diabetes Type 1 – Test of an mHealth App

This study is currently recruiting participants.

Sponsor: Nordsjaellands Hospital

Purpose: Young people with diabetes type 1, their parents and health care providers have participated in developing the mHealth app "Young with Diabetes."

The aim of the app is to support young people to self-manage their diabetes type 1.

A test group of 70 young people with diabetes type 1 test the app for 12 months as a supplement to standard care and the control group receives standard care only.

At baseline and after 2, 7, and 12 months HbA1c, problem areas in diabetes, perceived competences in diabetes and health care climate are measured.

Clinical Trials and Their Role in Diabetes Treatment

Eligibility

- Ages Eligible for Study:15 Years to 22 Years
- Genders Eligible for Study: Both
- Accepts Healthy Volunteers: No

Inclusion Criteria:

- Type 1 Diabetes
- 15 to 22 years old
- Followed at one of the six diabetes departments/centers
- Pediatric and Adolescent Department, Nordsjællands Hospital, Hillerød
- Department of Cardiology, Nephrology and Endocrinology, Nordsjællands Hospital, Hillerød
- Pediatric and Adolescent Department, Herlev Hospital
- Steno Diabetes Center, Gentofte
- Pediatric Department, Roskilde Hospital
- Department of Endocrinology, Køge Hospital
- have an iOS or android smartphone

Part Nine

Additional Help and Information

Chapter 61

Financial Help for Diabetes Care

How costly is diabetes management and treatment?

Diabetes management and treatment is expensive. According to the American Diabetes Association (ADA), the average cost of health care for a person with diabetes is $13,741 a year—more than twice the cost of health care for a person without diabetes.

Many people who have diabetes need help paying for their care. For those who qualify, a variety of government and nongovernment programs can help cover health care expenses. This publication is meant to help people with diabetes and their family members find and access such resources.

What is health insurance?

Health insurance helps pay for medical care, including the cost of diabetes care. Health insurance options include the following:

- private health insurance, which includes group and individual health insurance

---

Text in this chapter is excerpted from "Financial Help for Diabetes Care," National Institute of Diabetes and Digestive and Kidney Diseases (NIDDK), National Institutes of Health (NIH), May 2014.

- government health insurance, such as Medicare, Medicaid, the Children's Health Insurance Program (CHIP), TRICARE, and veterans' health care programs

Starting in 2014, the Affordable Care Act (ACA) prevents insurers from denying coverage or charging higher premiums to people with preexisting conditions, such as diabetes. The ACA also requires most people to have health insurance or pay a fee. Some people may be exempt from this fee. Read more about the ACA at HealthCare.gov or call 1-800-318-2596, TTY 1-855-889-4325.

Does Medicare cover diabetes services and supplies?

Medicare helps pay for the diabetes services, supplies, and equipment listed below and for some preventive services for people who are at risk for diabetes. However, coinsurance or deductibles may apply. A person must have Medicare Part B or Medicare Part D to receive these covered services and supplies.

Medicare Part B helps pay for:

- diabetes screening tests for people at risk of developing diabetes
- diabetes self-management training
- diabetes supplies such as glucose monitors, test strips, and lancets
- insulin pumps and insulin if used with an insulin pump
- counseling to help people who are obese lose weight
- flu and pneumonia shots
- foot exams and treatment for people with diabetes
- eye exams to check for glaucoma and diabetic retinopathy
- medical nutrition therapy services for people with diabetes or kidney disease, when referred by a health care provider
- therapeutic shoes or inserts, in some cases

Medicare Part D helps pay for:

- diabetes medications
- insulin, excluding insulin used with an insulin pump

Financial Help for Diabetes Care

- diabetes supplies such as needles and syringes for injecting insulin

People who are in a Medicare Advantage Plan or other Medicare health plan should check their plan's membership materials and call for details about how the plan provides the diabetes services, supplies, and medications covered by Medicare.

What other federal programs can help people with diabetes?

The following federal programs can provide more resources for people with diabetes:

- Department of Veterans Affairs (VA)
- TRICARE
- The Indian Health Service
- The Hill-Burton Free and Reduced-Cost Health Care Program
- Bureau of Primary Health Care
- Social Security Administration
- Social Security Disability Insurance (SSDI)
- Supplemental Security Income (SSI)
- Women, Infants, and Children (WIC)

What other state programs can help people with diabetes?

The following state programs can provide more resources for people with diabetes:

- Medicare Savings Programs
- State Health Insurance Assistance Programs (SHIPs)
- State Pharmaceutical Assistance Programs (SPAPs)

Local resources such as the following charitable groups may offer financial help for some expenses related to diabetes:

- Lions Clubs International can help with vision care. Visit www.lionsclubs.org

- Rotary International clubs provide humanitarian and educational assistance. Visit www.rotary.org

- Elks clubs provide charitable activities that benefit youth and veterans. Visit www.elks.org Shriners of North America offer free treatment for children at Shriners hospitals throughout the country. Visit www.shrinershq.org

- Kiwanis International clubs conduct service projects to help children and communities. Visit www.kiwanis.org

In many areas, nonprofit or special-interest groups, such as those listed above, can sometimes provide financial assistance or help with fundraising. Religious organizations also may offer assistance. In addition, some local governments may have special trusts set up to help people in need. The local library or local city or county government's health and human services office may provide more information about such groups.

How can a person save money on diabetes medications and medical supplies?

People should talk with their health care providers if they have problems paying for diabetes medications. Some people do not fill prescriptions or take less medication than what a provider prescribes in order to save money; however, health care providers advise against taking less than the prescribed amount of medication. Less expensive generic medications for diabetes, blood pressure, and cholesterol are available. If a health care provider prescribes medications that a person cannot afford, the person should ask the health care provider about cheaper alternatives.

Health care providers may also be able to assist people who need help paying for their medications and diabetes testing supplies, such as glucose test strips, by providing free samples or referring them to local programs. Drug companies that sell insulin or diabetes medications often have patient assistance programs. Each patient assistance program has its own eligibility criteria.

The websites below provide links to programs that can help patients determine if they qualify for the different types of assistance and find free or low-cost health care. People can also search these websites for needed diabetes testing supplies by using keywords such as "glucose test strips" or the names of specific diabetes medications.

Financial Help for Diabetes Care

- The Partnership for Prescription Assistance website at www.PPARx.org lists more than 475 programs that help pay for medications. The drug companies that produce medications provide many of these programs. People can find programs and apply for help by calling 1-888-477-2669.

- NeedyMeds is a nonprofit group that helps people find programs that help pay for medications. The NeedyMeds website at www.NeedyMeds.org allows the user to search a list of programs by medication or manufacturer name. Some of the forms to apply are online.

- RxAssist has a website at www.rxassist.org that provides information about drug company programs, state programs, discount drug cards, copay help, and more.

- Rx Outreach is a nonprofit pharmacy that provides affordable medications to people in need. The Rx Outreach website at www.rxoutreach.org provides information about the medications offered and how to apply.

- The National Council on Aging provides benefit information for seniors with limited income and resources at www.benefitscheckup.org

Also, some programs for the homeless may be able to provide help. A person can contact a local homeless shelter for more information about how to obtain free medications and medical supplies. People can access the number or location of the nearest homeless shelter online or in the phone book under "Human Service Organizations" or "Social Service Organizations."

Where can a person find help paying for prosthetic care?

People who have had an amputation may need assistance in paying their rehabilitation expenses and the cost of a prosthesis. The following organizations provide financial assistance or information about finding resources for people who need prosthetic care:

Amputee Coalition
900 East Hill Avenue, Suite 290
Knoxville, TN 37915
Phone: 1-888-AMP-KNOW (1-888-267-5669)

TTY: 865-525-4512
Website: www.amputee-coalition.org

Limbs for Life Foundation
218 East Main Street
Oklahoma City, OK 73104
Phone: 1-888-235-5462 or 405-605-5462
Fax: 405-843-5123
E-mail: admin@limbsforlife.org
Website: www.limbsforlife.org

Where can a person find help paying for kidney dialysis and transplantation?

Kidney failure, also called end-stage renal disease, is a complication of diabetes. People of any age with kidney failure can get Medicare if they meet certain criteria.

What is assistive technology and what organizations might provide assistance?

Assistive technology is any device that assists, adapts, or helps to rehabilitate someone with a disability so he or she may function more safely, effectively, and independently at home, at work, and in the community. Assistive technology may include:

- computers with features that make them accessible to people with disabilities
- adaptive equipment, such as wheelchairs
- bathroom modifications, such as grab bars or shower seats

The following organizations may be able to provide information, awareness, and training in the use of technology to assist people with disabilities:

Alliance for Technology Access
1119 Old Humboldt Road
Jackson, TN 38305
Phone: 1-800-914-3017 or 731-554-5ATA (731-554-5282)
TTY: 731-554-5284
Fax: 731-554-5283
E-mail: atainfo@ataccess.org
Website: www.ataccess.org

Financial Help for Diabetes Care

National Assistive Technology Technical Assistance Partnership
1700 North Moore Street, Suite 1540
Arlington, VA 22209-1903
Phone: 703-524-6686
Fax: 703-524-6630
TTY: 703-524-6639
E-mail: resnaTA@resna.org
Website: www.resnaprojects.org/nattap

United Cerebral Palsy
1825 K Street NW, Suite 600
Washington, DC 20006
Phone: 1-800-872-5827 or 202-776-0406
Website: www.ucp.org/resources/assistive-technology

Chapter 62

Recipes for People with Diabetes and Their Families

What Is Diabetes?

Diabetes means that your blood glucose (blood sugar) is too high. Glucose comes from the food we eat. An organ called the pancreas makes insulin. Insulin helps glucose get from your blood into your cells. Cells take the glucose and turn it into energy.

When you have diabetes, your body has a problem making or properly using insulin. As a result, glucose builds up in your blood and cannot get into your cells. If the blood glucose stays too high, it can damage your body.

What Are the Symptoms of Diabetes?

Common symptoms of diabetes include the following:

- Having to urinate often
- Being very thirsty
- Feeling very hungry or tired
- Losing weight without trying

Text in this chapter is excerpted from "Recipes for People with Diabetes and Their Families," Centers for Disease Control and Prevention (CDC), July 22, 2015.

But many people with diabetes have no symptoms at all.

Why Should I Be Concerned about Diabetes?

Diabetes is a very serious disease. Do not be misled by phrases that suggest diabetes is not a serious disease, such as "a touch of sugar," "borderline diabetes," or "my blood glucose is a little bit high."

Diabetes can lead to other serious health problems. When high levels of glucose in the blood are not controlled, they can slowly damage your eyes, heart, kidneys, nerves, and feet.

What Are the Types of Diabetes?

There are three main types of diabetes:

- **Type 1 diabetes:** In this type of diabetes, the body does not make insulin. People with type 1 diabetes need to take insulin every day.

- **Type 2 diabetes:** In this type of diabetes, the body does not make enough insulin or use insulin well. Some people with type 2 diabetes have to take diabetes pills, insulin, or both. Type 2 diabetes is the most common form of diabetes.

- **Gestational diabetes:** This type of diabetes can occur when a woman is pregnant. It raises the risk that both she and her child might develop diabetes later in life.

You Can Control Diabetes

Diabetes can be managed. You can successfully manage diabetes and avoid the serious health problems it can cause if you follow these steps:

- Ask your doctor how you can learn more about your diabetes to help you feel better today and in the future.

- Make healthy food choices and be physically active most days. Following this advice will help you keep off extra pounds and will also help keep your blood glucose under control.

- Check your blood glucose as your doctor tells you to.

- If you are taking diabetes medications, take them even if you feel well.

Recipes for People with Diabetes and Their Families

- To avoid problems with your diabetes, see your healthcare team at least twice a year. Finding and treating any problems early will prevent them from getting worse. Ask how diabetes can affect your eyes, heart, kidneys, nerves, legs, and feet.

- Be actively involved in your diabetes care. Work with your healthcare team to come up with a plan for making healthy food choices and being active—a plan that you can stick to.

Good news! You can control diabetes

Diabetes can be managed. You can successfully manage diabetes and avoid the serious health problems it can cause if you follow these steps:

- Ask your doctor how you can learn more about your diabetes to help you feel better today and in the future.

- Know your diabetes "ABCs"

- Make healthy food choices and be physically active most days. Following this advice will help you keep off extra pounds and will also help keep your blood glucose under control.

- Check your blood glucose as your doctor tells you to.

- If you are taking diabetes medications, take them even if you feel well.

- To avoid problems with your diabetes, see your health care team at least twice a year. Finding and treating any problems early will prevent them from getting worse. Ask how diabetes can affect your eyes, heart, kidneys, nerves, legs, and feet.

- Be actively involved in your diabetes care. Work with your health care team to come up with a plan for making healthy food choices and being active—a plan that you can stick to.

Creating a healthy meal plan

This chapter is a place to start creating healthy meals. Ask your doctor to refer you to a registered dietitian or a diabetes educator who can help you create a meal plan for you and your family. The dietitian will work with you to come up with a meal plan tailored to your needs.

Your meal plan will take into account things like:

- Your blood glucose levels.
- Your weight.
- Medicines you take.
- Other health problems you have.
- How physically active you are.

Making healthy food choices

- Eat smaller portions. Learn what a serving size is for different foods and how many servings you need in a meal.
- Eat less fat. Choose fewer high-fat foods and use less fat for cooking. You especially want to limit foods that are high in saturated fats or trans fat, such as:
- Fatty cuts of meat.
- Whole milk and dairy products made from whole milk.
- Cakes, candy, cookies, crackers, and pies.
- Fried foods.
- Salad dressings.
- Lard, shortening, stick margarine, and nondairy creamers.
- Eat more fiber by eating more whole-grain foods. Whole grains can be found in:
- Breakfast cereals made with 100% whole grains.
- Oatmeal.
- Whole grain rice.
- Whole-wheat bread, bagels, pita bread, and tortillas.
- Eat a variety of fruits and vegetables every day. Choose fresh, frozen, canned, or dried fruit and 100% fruit juices most of the time. Eat plenty of veggies like these:
- Dark green veggies (e.g., broccoli, spinach, brussel sprouts).
- Orange veggies (e.g., carrots, sweet potatoes, pumpkin, winter squash).
- Beans and peas (e.g., black beans, garbanzo beans, kidney beans, pinto beans, split peas, lentils).
- Eat fewer foods that are high in sugar, such as:

Recipes for People with Diabetes and Their Families

- Fruit-flavored drinks.
- Sodas.
- Tea or coffee sweetened with sugar.
- Use less salt in cooking and at the table. Eat fewer foods that are high in salt, such as:
- Canned and package soups.
- Canned vegetables. Pickles. Processed meats.
- Never skip meals. Stick to your meal plan as best you can.
- Limit the amount of alcohol you drink.
- Make changes slowly. It takes time to achieve lasting goals.

Following a meal plan that is made for you will help you feel better, keep your blood glucose levels in your target range, take in the right amount of calories, and get enough nutrients.

Where can you learn more about making a diabetes meal plan?

- Contact a registered dietitian to make a meal plan just for you.
- Visit the American Dietetic Association Web site to find a nutrition professional that can help you develop a healthy meal plan (www.eatright.org).
- Visit the American Association of Diabetes Educators to find a diabetes educator (www.diabeteseducator.org).
- Visit the American Diabetes Association Web site for more information on carbohydrate counting and the exchange method (www.diabetes.org).
- Visit http://www.diabetes. org/food-and-fitness/ food/planning-meals/ carb-counting/ to get more information on carbohydrate counting.

Where can you learn how to read food labels?

You can learn a lot about foods by reading food labels. Visit these Web sites to learn more about reading food labels:

- U.S. Food and Drug Administration (www. cfsan.fda.gov/~dms/foodlab.html)

- U.S. Department of Agriculture (www.fns. usda.gov/tn/ Resources/ Nibbles/healthful_labels. pdf)
- American Diabetes Association (http://www. diabetes.org/ food-andfitness/food/what-can-i-eat/ taking-a-closer-look-atla-bels.html).

Recipes

Spanish Omelet / Tortilla española

This tasty dish provides a healthy array of vegetables and can be used for breakfast, brunch, or any meal! Serve with fresh fruit salad and a whole grain dinner roll.

Ingredients:

- 5 small potatoes, peeled and sliced Vegetable cooking spray
- ½ medium onion, minced
- 1 small zucchini, sliced
- 1½ cups green/red peppers, sliced thin
- 5 medium mushrooms, sliced
- 3 whole eggs, beaten
- 5 egg whites, beaten Pepper and garlic salt with herbs, to taste
- 3 ounces shredded part-skim mozzarella cheese
- 1 Tbsp. low-fat parmesan cheese

Directions:

- Preheat oven to 375 °F.
- Cook potatoes in boiling water until tender.
- In a nonstick pan, add vegetable spray and warm at medium heat.
- Add onion and sauté until brown. Add vegetables and sauté until tender but not brown.
- In a medium mixing bowl, slightly beat eggs and egg whites, pepper, garlic salt, and low-fat mozzarella cheese. Stir egg-cheese mixture into the cooked vegetables.
- In a 10-inch pie pan or ovenproof skillet, add vegetable spray and transfer potatoes and egg mixture to pan. Sprinkle with

low-fat parmesan cheese and bake until firm and brown on top, about 20–30 minutes.

- Remove omelet from oven, cool for 10 minutes, and cut into five pieces.

Exchanges:

Meat	2
Bread	2
Vegetable	2/3
Fat	2

Note: Diabetic exchanges are calculated based on the American Diabetes Association Exchange System.

Nutrition Facts	
Spanish Omelet	
Serving Size 1/5 of omelet	
Amount Per Serving	
Calories 260	Calories from Fat 90
	% Daily Value (DV)*
Total Fat 10g	**15%**
Saturated Fat 3.5g	**18%**
Trans Fat 0g	
Cholesterol 135mg	**45%**
Sodium 240mg	**10%**
Total Carbohydrate 30g	**10%**
Dietary Fiber 3g	**12%**
Sugars 3g	
Protein 16g	
Vitamin A	8%
Vitamin C	60%
Calcium	15%
Iron	8%
* Percent Daily Values are based on a 2,000 calorie diet.	

Figure 62.1. *Nutrition Facts Label, Spanish Omelet*

Beef or Turkey Stew

This dish goes nicely with a green leaf lettuce and cucumber salad and a dinner roll. Plantains or corn can be used in place of the potatoes.

Ingredients:

- 1 pound lean beef or turkey breast, cut into cubes
- 2 Tbsp. whole wheat flour
- ¼ tsp. salt (optional)
- ¼ tsp. pepper
- ¼ tsp. cumin
- 1½ Tbsp. olive oil 2 cloves garlic, minced
- 2 medium onions, sliced
- 2 stalks celery, sliced
- 1 medium red/green bell pepper, sliced
- 1 medium tomato, finely minced
- 5 cups beef or turkey broth, fat removed
- 5 small potatoes, peeled and cubed
- 12 small carrots, cut into large chunks
- 1¼ cups green peas

Directions:

- Preheat oven to 375 °F.
- Mix the whole wheat flour with salt, pepper, and cumin. Roll the beef or turkey cubes in the mixture. Shake off excess flour.
- In a large skillet, heat olive oil over medium-high heat. Add beef or turkey cubes and sauté until nicely brown, about 7–10 minutes.
- Place beef or turkey in an ovenproof casserole dish.
- Add minced garlic, onions, celery, and peppers to skillet and cook until vegetables are tender, about 5 minutes.

Recipes for People with Diabetes and Their Families

- Stir in tomato and broth. Bring to a boil and pour over turkey or beef in casserole dish. Cover dish tightly and bake for 1 hour at 375 °F.
- Remove from oven and stir in potatoes, carrots, and peas. Bake for another 20–25 minutes or until tender.

Exchanges:

Lean Meat	3
Vegetable	2 1/3
Bread	2 2/3
Fat	1

Note: Diabetic exchanges are calculated based on the American Diabetes Association Exchange System.

Caribbean Red Snapper

This fish can be served on top of vegetables along with whole grain rice and garnished with parsley. Salmon or chicken breast can be used in place of red snapper.

Ingredients:

- 2 Tbsp. olive oil
- 1 medium onion, chopped
- ½ cup red pepper, chopped
- ½ cup carrots, cut into strips
- 1 clove garlic, minced
- ½ cup dry white wine

Nutrition Facts	
Beef or Turkey Stew	
Serving Size 1½ cup	
Amount Per Serving	
Calories 320	Calories from Fat 60
	% Daily Value (DV)*
Total Fat 7g	11%
Saturated Fat 1.5g	8%
Trans Fat 0g	
Cholesterol 40mg	13%
Sodium 520mg	22%
Total Carbohydrate 41g	14%
Dietary Fiber 8g	32%
Sugars 9g	
Protein 24g	
Vitamin A	340%
Vitamin C	80%
Calcium	6%
Iron	15%
* Percent Daily Values are based on a 2,000 calorie diet.	

Figure 62.2. *Nutrition Facts Label, Beef or Turkey Stew*

- ¾ pound red snapper fillet
- 1 large tomato, chopped
- 2 Tbsp. pitted ripe olives, chopped
- 2 Tbsp. crumbled low-fat feta or low-fat ricotta cheese

Directions:

- In a large skillet, heat olive oil over medium heat. Add onion, red pepper, carrots, and garlic. Sauté mixture for 10 minutes. Add wine and bring to boil. Push vegetables to one side of the pan.
- Arrange fillets in a single layer in center of skillet. Cover and cook for 5 minutes.
- Add tomato and olives. Top with cheese. Cover and cook for 3 minutes or until fish is firm but moist.
- Transfer fish to serving platter. Garnish with vegetables and pan juices.

Exchanges:

Meat	2
Vegetable	1 ¼
Bread	½
Fat	2

Note: Diabetic exchanges are calculated based on the American Diabetes Association Exchange System. Total Servings 4 Serving

Nutrition Facts	
Caribbean Red Snapper	
Serving Size ¼ red snapper with ½ cup vegetables (233g)	
Amount Per Serving	
Calories 220	Calories from Fat 80
	% Daily Value (DV)*
Total Fat 10g	**15%**
Saturated Fat 2g	**10%**
Trans Fat 0g	
Cholesterol 35mg	**12%**
Sodium 160mg	**7%**
Total Carbohydrate 8g	**3%**
Dietary Fiber 2g	**8%**
Sugars 4g	
Protein 19g	
Vitamin A	80%
Vitamin C	70%
Calcium	8%
Iron	4%
* Percent Daily Values are based on a 2,000 calorie diet.	

Figure 62.3. *Nutrition Facts Label, Caribbean Red Snapper*

Suggestion: Serve with whole grain rice. ½ cup cooked rice = 1 serving of rice.

Two Cheese Pizza

Serve your pizza with fresh fruit and a mixed green salad garnished with red beans to balance your meal.

Ingredients:

- 2 Tbsp. whole wheat flour
- 1 can (10 ounces) refrigerated pizza crust Vegetable cooking spray
- 2 Tbsp. olive oil
- ½ cup low-fat ricotta cheese
- ½ tsp. dried basil 1 small onion, minced
- 2 cloves garlic, minced
- ¼ tsp. salt (optional)
- 4 ounces shredded part-skim mozzarella cheese
- 2 cups mushrooms, chopped
- 1 large red pepper, cut into strips

Directions:

- Preheat oven to 425 °F.
- Spread whole wheat flour over working surface. Roll out dough with rolling pin to desired crust thickness.
- Coat cookie sheet with vegetable cooking spray. Transfer pizza crust to cookie sheet. Brush olive oil over crust.
- Mix low-fat ricotta cheese with dried basil, onion, garlic, and salt. Spread this mixture over crust.
- Sprinkle crust with part-skim mozzarella cheese. Top cheese with mushrooms and red pepper.
- Bake at 425 °F for 13–15 minutes or until cheese melts and crust is deep golden brown.
- Cut into 8 slices.

Exchanges:

Meat	2 ½
Bread	3
egetable	1
Fat	3 ¾

Note: Diabetic exchanges are calculated based on the American Diabetes Association Exchange System.

Rice with Chicken, Spanish Style

This is a good way to get vegetables into the meal plan. Serve with a mixed green salad and some whole wheat bread.

Ingredients:

- 2 Tbsp. olive oil
- 2 medium onions, chopped
- 6 cloves garlic, minced
- 2 stalks celery, diced
- 2 medium red/green peppers, cut into strips
- 1 cup mushrooms, chopped
- 2 cups uncooked whole grain rice
- 3 pounds boneless chicken breast, cut into bite-sized pieces, skin removed
- 1½ tsp. salt (optional)
- 2½ cups low-fat chicken broth Saffron or SazónTM for color
- 3 medium tomatoes, chopped
- 1 cup frozen peas
- 1 cup frozen corn

Nutrition Facts	
Two Cheese Pizza	
Serving Size 2 slices (¼ of pie)	
Amount Per Serving	
Calories 420	Calories from Fat 170
% Daily Value (DV)*	
Total Fat 19g	**29%**
Saturated Fat 7g	**35%**
Trans Fat 0g	
Cholesterol 25mg	**8%**
Sodium 580mg	**24%**
Total Carbohydrate 44g	**15%**
Dietary Fiber 3g	**12%**
Sugars 5g	
Protein 20g	
Vitamin A	30%
Vitamin C	90%
Calcium	40%
Iron	15%
* Percent Daily Values are based on a 2,000 calorie diet.	

Figure 62.4. *Nutrition Facts Label, Two Cheese Pizza*

Recipes for People with Diabetes and Their Families

- 1 cup frozen green beans
  Olives or capers for garnish (optional)

Directions:

- Heat olive oil over medium heat in a non-stick pot. Add onion, garlic, celery, red/green pepper, and mushrooms. Cook over medium heat, stirring often, for 3 minutes or until tender.

- Add whole grain rice and sauté for 2–3 minutes, stirring constantly to mix all ingredients.

- Add chicken, salt, chicken broth, water, Saffron/SazónTM, and tomatoes. Bring water to a boil.

- Reduce heat to medium-low, cover, and let the casserole simmer until water is absorbed and rice is tender, about 20 minutes.

- Stir in peas, corn, and beans and cook for 8–10 minutes. When everything is hot, the casserole is ready to serve. Garnish with olives or capers, if desired.

Exchanges:

Meat	5
Bread	3
Vegetable	1
Fat	1

Nutrition Facts	
Rice with Chicken, Spanish Style	
Serving Size 1½ cup	
Amount Per Serving	
Calories 400	Calories from Fat 60
	% Daily Value (DV)*
Total Fat 7g	**11%**
Saturated Fat 1.5g	**8%**
Trans Fat 0g	
Cholesterol 85mg	**28%**
Sodium 530mg	**22%**
Total Carbohydrate 46g	**15%**
Dietary Fiber 3g	**12%**
Sugars 5g	
Protein 37g	
Vitamin A	30%
Vitamin C	70%
Calcium	4%
Iron	20%
* Percent Daily Values are based on a 2,000 calorie diet.	

Figure 62.5. *Nutrition Facts Label, Rice with Chicken, Spanish Style*

Note: Diabetic exchanges are calculated based on the American Diabetes Association Exchange System.

Pozole

Only a small amount of oil is needed to sauté meat.

Ingredients:

- 2 pounds lean beef, cubed
- 1 Tbsp. olive oil
- 1 large onion, chopped
- 1 clove garlic, finely chopped
- ¼ tsp. salt tsp. pepper
- ¼ cup fresh cilantro, chopped
- 1 can (15 ounces) stewed tomatoes
- 2 ounces tomato paste
- 1 can (1 pound 13 ounces) hominy

Directions:

- In a large pot, heat olive oil. Add beef and sauté.
- Add onion, garlic, salt, pepper, cilantro, and enough water to cover meat. Stir to mix ingredients evenly. Cover pot and cook over low heat until meat is tender.
- Add tomatoes and tomato paste. Continue cooking for about 20 minutes.
- Add hominy and continue cooking another 15 minutes, stirring occasionally. If too thick, add water for desired consistency. Option: Skinless, boneless chicken breasts can be used instead of beef cubes.

Exchanges:

Meat	3
Bread	1
Vegetable	½
Fat	1

Note: Diabetic exchanges are calculated based on the American Diabetes Association Exchange System.

Nutrition Facts	
Pozole	
Serving Size 1 cup	
Amount Per Serving	
Calories 220	Calories from Fat 70
	% Daily Value (DV)*
Total Fat 7g	11%
Saturated Fat 2g	10%
Trans Fat 0g	
Cholesterol 70mg	23%
Sodium 390mg	16%
Total Carbohydrate 17g	6%
Dietary Fiber 3g	12%
Sugars 5g	
Protein 21g	
Vitamin A	4%
Vitamin C	10%
Calcium	4%
Iron	15%
* Percent Daily Values are based on a 2,000 calorie diet.	

Figure 62.6. *Nutrition Facts Label, Pozole*

References

American Diabetes Association. Reading Food Labels. American Diabetes Association Website. Available at www.diabetes.org/food-and-fitness/food/what-can-i-eat/taking-a-closer-look-at-labels.html.

American Diabetes Association. Virtual Grocery Store. American Diabetes Association Website. Available at www.diabetes.org/food-and-fitness.

Bestfoods CPC International, Inc. *Live Healthy America, A Guide from Mazola*. Coventry, CT: Mazola; 1991.

Centers for Disease Control and Prevention. *Take Charge of Your Diabetes,3rd edition*. Atlanta: U.S. Department of Health and Human Services; 2003. Available at www.cdc.gov/diabetes/pubs/pdf/tctd.pdf.

Centers for Disease Control and Prevention. Fruits & Veggies— More Matters. Centers for Disease Control and Prevention Website. Available at www.fruitsandveggiesmatter.gov.

Gardner L. *Health and the Hispanic Kitchen/La Salud y la Cocina Latina*. Potomac, MD: Precepts, Inc.; 1996.

National Cattlemen's Beef Association. *Eating Smart Even When You Are Pressed for Time*. Chicago: National Cattleman's Beef Association; 1996.

National Cancer Institute. *Celebre la Cocina Hispana, Healthy Hispanic Recipes*. Washington, DC: U.S. Department of Health and Human Services; 1995. NIH Publication Number 95-3906(s).

Pockenpaugh N, Poleman C. *Nutrition: Essential and Diet Therapy, 8th edition*. Philadelphia: WB Saunders; 1996.

Sizer F, Whitney E. *Nutrition: Concepts and Controversies, 8th edition*. Belmont, CA: Wadsworth Publishing; 2000.

U.S. Department of Agriculture. Nutrition Value of Foods. *Home and Garden Bulletin* Number 72. Department of Agriculture Website. Available at www.nal.usda.gov/fnic/foodcomp/Data/HG72/hg72_2002.pdf.

U.S. Department of Health and Human Services. A Healthier You. Department of Health and Human Services Website. Available at www.health.gov/dietaryguidelines/dga2005/healthieryou/contents.htm.

U.S. Department of Health and Human Services and U.S. Department of Agriculture. *Dietary Guidelines for Americans, 6th edition*. Washington, DC: U.S. Government Printing Office; 2005. Available at www.health.gov/dietaryguidelines.

U.S. Food and Drug Administration. How to Understand and Use the Nutrition Facts Label. Food and Drug Administration Website. Available at www.cfsan.fda.gov/~dms/foodlab.html.

Warshaw H. *Diabetes Meal Planning Made Easy: How to Put the Food Pyramid to Work for Your Busy Lifestyle*. Alexandria, VA: American Diabetes Association; 2000.

Chapter 63

Glossary of Terms Related to Diabetes

A1C: A test that measures a person's average blood glucose level over the past two to three months.

acanthosis nigricans: A skin condition characterized by darkened skin patches; common in those with insulin resistance.

albumin: The main protein in blood. People who are developing diabetic kidney disease leak small amounts of albumin into the urine. As the amount of albumin in the urine increases, the kidneys' ability to filter the blood decreases.

albuminuria: A condition in which the urine has more than normal amounts of a protein called albumin.

alpha cell: A type of cell in the pancreas that makes and releases a hormone called glucagons, which tells the liver to release glucose into the blood for energy.

alpha-glucosidase inhibitor: A class of oral medicine for type 2 diabetes that slows down the digestion of foods high in carbohydrate. The result is a slower and lower rise in blood glucose after meals.

amylin: A hormone formed by beta cells in the pancreas that regulates the timing of glucose release into the bloodstream after eating by slowing the emptying of the stomach.

This glossary contains terms excerpted from documents produced by several sources deemed reliable.

angiotensin receptor blocker (ARB): An oral medicine that lowers blood pressure. It also helps slow down kidney damage in diabetics.

angiotensin-converting enzyme (ACE) inhibitor: An oral medicine that lowers blood pressure. It also helps slow down kidney damage in diabetics.

autoimmune disease: A disorder of the body's immune system in which the immune system mistakenly attacks and destroys body tissue that it believes to be foreign.

autonomic neuropathy: A type of neuropathy affecting the lungs, heart, stomach, intestines, bladder, or genitals.

beta cell: A cell that makes insulin. Beta cells are located in the islets of the pancreas.

biguanide: A class of oral medicine used to treat type 2 diabetes that lowers blood glucose by reducing the amount of glucose produced by the liver. Also used to treat insulin resistance.

blood glucose level: The amount of glucose in a given amount of blood. In the United States, blood glucose levels are noted in milligrams per deciliter, or mg/dL.

blood glucose meter: A small, portable machine used by people with diabetes to check their blood glucose levels.

blood glucose: The main sugar found in the blood and the body's main source of energy. Also called blood sugar.

body mass index (BMI): A measure used to evaluate body weight relative to a person's height. BMI is used to find out if a person is underweight, normal weight, overweight, or obese.

calorie: A unit of energy in food. Carbohydrates, fats, protein, and alcohol in the foods and drinks we eat provide food energy or "calories."

carbohydrate counting: A method of meal planning for people with diabetes based on counting the number of grams of carbohydrate in food.

carbohydrate: One of the three main nutrients in food. Foods that provide carbohydrate are starches, vegetables, fruits, dairy products, and sugars.

cholesterol: Cholesterol is a fat-like substance that is made by your body and found naturally in animal foods such as dairy products, eggs, meat, poultry, and seafood.

Glossary of Terms Related to Diabetes

creatinine: A waste product from meat protein in the diet and from the muscles of the body. As kidney disease progresses, the level of creatinine in the blood increases.

dextrose: Simple sugar found in blood that serves as the body's main source of energy. Also called glucose.

diabetic ketoacidosis: An emergency condition in which extremely high blood glucose levels, along with a severe lack of insulin, result in the breakdown of body fat for energy and an accumulation of ketones in the blood and urine.

diabetic retinopathy: Damage to the small blood vessels in the retina. Loss of vision may result. Also called diabetic eye disease.

dialysis: The process of cleaning wastes from the blood artificially. The two major forms of dialysis are hemodialysis and peritoneal dialysis.

fasting blood glucose test: A check of a person's blood glucose level after the person has not eaten for eight to twelve hours; usually overnight.

gastroparesis: A form of neuropathy that affects the stomach. Digestion of food may be incomplete or delayed, resulting in nausea, vomiting, or bloating, making blood glucose control difficult.

glaucoma: An increase in fluid pressure inside the eye that may lead to vision loss.

glomerular filtration rate (GFR): The rate at which the kidneys filter wastes and extra fluid from the blood, measured in milliliters per minute.

glucagon: A hormone produced by the alpha cells in the pancreas that raises blood glucose.

glucose gel: Pure glucose in gel form used for treating hypoglycemia.

glucose tablets: Chewable tablets made of pure glucose used for treating hypoglycemia.

glucose: One of the simplest forms of sugar.

glycogen: The form of glucose found in the liver and muscles; the main source of stored fuel in the body.

haplotype: A haplotype is a set of DNA variations, or polymorphisms, that tend to be inherited together. A haplotype can refer to a combination of alleles or to a set of single nucleotide polymorphisms (SNPs) found on the same chromosome.

healthy weight: Healthy weight status is often based on having a body mass index (BMI) that falls in the normal (or healthy) range. A healthy body weight may lower the chances of developing health problems such as type 2 diabetes and heart disease.

high-density lipoprotein (HDL): HDL is a compound made up of fat and protein that carries cholesterol in the blood to the liver, where it is broken down and excreted. Commonly called "good" cholesterol, high levels of HDL cholesterol are linked to a lower risk of heart disease.

hyperglycemia: Higher than normal blood glucose.

hypertension: A condition present when blood flows through the blood vessels with a force greater than normal. Also called high blood pressure.

hypoglycemia unawareness: A state in which a person does not feel or recognize the symptoms of hypoglycemia.

hypoglycemia: Also called low blood glucose, a condition that occurs when one's blood glucose is lower than normal, usually below 70 mg/dL. If left untreated, hypoglycemia may lead to unconsciousness.

impaired fasting glucose (IFG): A condition in which a fasting blood glucose test shows a level of glucose higher than normal but not high enough for a diagnosis of diabetes. IFG, also called Prediabetes, is a level of 100 to 125 mg/dL.

impaired glucose tolerance (IGT): A condition in which blood glucose levels are higher than normal but are not high enough for a diagnosis of diabetes. IGT, also called Prediabetes, is a level of 140 to 199 mg/dL two hours after the start of an oral glucose tolerance test.

incidence: The number of new cases of a given disease during a given period in a specified population. It also is used for the rate at which new events occur in a defined population.

inhaled insulin: A type of insulin under development taken with a special device that enables the user to breathe in insulin through the mouth.

insulin: A hormone that helps the body use glucose for energy. The beta cells of the pancreas make insulin. When the body cannot make enough insulin, insulin is taken by injection or other means.

insulin infuser: A device for taking insulin in which a small tube is inserted just below the skin and remains in place for several days. Insulin is injected into the end of the tube.

Glossary of Terms Related to Diabetes

insulin pen: A device for injecting insulin that looks like a fountain pen and holds replaceable cartridges of insulin.

insulin pump: An insulin-delivering device about the size of a deck of cards that can be worn on a belt or kept in a pocket.

insulin resistance: The body's inability to respond to and use the insulin it produces.

islet transplantation: Moving the islets from a donor pancreas into a person whose pancreas has stopped producing insulin.

islets: Groups of cells located in the pancreas that make hormones that help the body break down and use food.

jet injector: A device that uses high pressure instead of a needle to propel insulin through the skin and into the body.

ketone: A chemical produced when there is a shortage of insulin in the blood and the body breaks down body fat for energy.

ketosis: A ketone buildup in the body that may lead to diabetic ketoacidosis.

lactic acidosis: A serious condition in which there is a buildup of lactic acid in the body.

lancet: A spring-loaded device used to prick the skin with a small needle to obtain a drop of blood for blood glucose monitoring.

leukocyte: White blood cell. Refers to a blood cell that does not contain hemoglobin. White blood cells include lymphocytes, neutrophils, eosinophils, macrophages, and mast cells.

lipoprotein: A compound made up of fat and protein that carries fats and fat-like substances, such as cholesterol, in the blood.

low-density lipoprotein (LDL): LDL is a compound made up of fat and protein that carries cholesterol in the blood from the liver to other parts of the body.

maturity-onset diabetes of the young (MODY): A monogenic form of diabetes that usually first occurs during adolescence or early adult- hood.

metabolic syndrome: A grouping of health conditions associated with an increased risk for heart disease and type 2 diabetes.

metabolism: The process that occurs in the body to turn the food you eat into energy your body can use.

nephropathy: Disease of the kidneys.

neuropathy: Disease of the nervous system. The three major forms in people with diabetes are peripheral neuropathy, autonomic neuropathy, and mononeuropathy.

oral glucose tolerance test (OGTT): A test to diagnose prediabetes and diabetes, given after an overnight fast. Test results show how the body uses glucose over time.

pancreas transplantation: A surgical procedure to take a healthy whole or partial pancreas from a donor and place it into a person with diabetes.

pancreas: An organ that makes insulin and enzymes for digestion. The pancreas is located behind the lower part of the stomach and is about the size of a hand.

peripheral neuropathy: Nerve damage that affects the feet, legs, or hands. Peripheral neuropathy causes pain, numbness, or a tingling feeling.

physical activity: Any form of exercise or movement.

polydipsia: Excessive thirst; may be a sign of diabetes.

polyuria: Excessive urination; may be a sign of diabetes.

portion size: The amount of a food served or eaten in one occasion. A portion is not a standard amount. The amount of food it includes may vary by person and occasion.

prediabetes: A condition in which blood glucose levels are higher than normal but are not high enough for a diagnosis of diabetes.

proteinuria: A condition in which the urine contains large amounts of protein, a sign that the kidneys are not working properly.

rapid-acting insulin: A type of insulin with an onset of fifteen minutes, a peak at thirty to ninety minutes, and a duration of three to five hours.

saturated fat: This type of fat is solid at room temperature. Saturated fat is found in full-fat dairy products (like butter, cheese, cream, regular ice cream, and whole milk), coconut oil, lard, palm oil, ready-to-eat meats, and the skin and fat of chicken and turkey, among other foods.

sulfonylurea: A class of oral medicine for type 2 diabetes that lowers blood glucose by helping the pancreas make more insulin and by helping the body better use the insulin it makes.

Glossary of Terms Related to Diabetes

triglycerides: A type of fat in your blood, triglycerides can contribute to the hardening and narrowing of your arteries if levels are too high.

type 1 diabetes: A condition characterized by high blood glucose levels caused by a total lack of insulin. Occurs when the body's immune system attacks the insulin-producing beta cells in the pancreas and destroys them.

type 2 diabetes: A condition characterized by high blood glucose levels caused by either a lack of insulin or the body's inability to use insulin efficiently.

Chapter 64

Directory of Diabetes-Related Resources

American Association of Clinical Endocrinologists
245 Riverside Ave.
Ste. 200
Jacksonville, FL 32202
Phone: 904-353-7878
Website: www.aace.com

American Association of Diabetes Educators
200 W. Madison St.
Ste. 800
Chicago, IL 60606
Toll-Free: 800-338-3633
E-mail: aade@aadenet.org
Website: www.diabeteseducator.org

American Diabetes Association National Service Center
1701 N. Beauregard St.
Alexandria, VA 22311
Toll-Free: 800-DIABETES (342-2383)
E-mail: AskADA@diabetes.org
Website: www.diabetes.org

Canadian Diabetes Association
1400-522 University Ave.
Toronto, ON M5G 2R5
Canada
Toll-Free: 800-BANTING (226-8464)
E-mail: info@diabetes.ca
Website: www.diabetes.ca

Resources in this chapter were compiled from several sources deemed reliable; all contact information was verified and updated in December 2015.

Centers for Disease Control and Prevention
1600 Clifton Rd.
Atlanta, GA 30333
Toll-Free: 800-CDC-INFO (232-4636)
TTY: 888-232-6348
E-mail: cdcinfo@cdc.gov
Website: www.cdc.gov

Diabetes Action Research and Education Foundation
6701 Democracy Blvd.
Bethesda, MD 20827
Phone: 202-333-4520
Fax: 202-558-5240
E-mail: info@diabetesaction.org
Website: www.diabetesaction.org

Diabetes Insipidus Foundation
Website: www.diabetesinsipidus.org

Johns Hopkins Diabetes Center
1800 Orleans St.
Baltimore, MD 21287
Phone: 1-410-955-5000
Website: www.hopkinsmedicine.org/diabetes

Joslin Diabetes Center
One Joslin Pl.
Boston, MA 02215
Website: www.joslin.org

National Center for Complementary and Alternative Medicine (NCCAM)
National Institutes of Health
9000 Rockville Pike
Bethesda, MD 20892
Toll-Free: 888-644-6226
TTY: 866-464-3615
Fax: 866-464-3616
E-mail: info@nccam.nih.gov
Website: nccam.nih.gov

National Diabetes Education Program
1 Diabetes Way
Bethesda, MD 20814-9692
Toll-Free: 888-693-NDEP (6337)
TTY: 866-569-1162
E-mail: ndep@mail.nih.gov
Website: www.ndep.nih.gov

National Diabetes Information Clearinghouse
1 Information Way
Bethesda, MD 20892-2560
Phone: 301-654-3327
Toll-Free: 800-860-8747
E-mail: ndic@info.niddk.nih.gov
Website: www.diabetes.niddk.nih.gov

National Institute on Aging
Bldg. 31, Rm. 5C27 MSC 2292
Bethesda, MD 20892
Phone: 301-496-1752
TTY: 800-222-4225
Fax: 301-496-1072
E-mail: niaic@nia.nih.gov
Website: www.nia.nih.gov

Directory of Diabetes-Related Resources

Office of Minority Health Resource Center (OMH-RC)
P.O. Box 37337
Washington, DC 20013-7337
Phone: 1-800-444-6472
Fax: 301-251-2160
E-mail: info@minorityhealth.hhs.gov
Website: www.minorityhealth.hhs.gov

UCSF Diabetes Teaching Center
University of California, San Francisco
400 Parnassus Ave.
5th Fl. Box 1222
San Francisco, CA 94143-1222
Phone: 415-353-2266
Fax: 415-353-2392
E-mail: diabetesteachingcenter@ucsfmedctr.org
Website: www.diabetes.ucsf.edu

Diabetes-Related Bone Diseases

Juvenile Diabetes Research Foundation (JDRF)
26 Broadway 14th Fl.
New York, NY 10004
Phone: 1-800-533-2873
Fax: 212-785-9595
E-mail: info@jdrf.org
Website: www.jdrf.org

NIH Osteoporosis and Related Bone Diseases National Resource Center
2 AMS Cir.
Bethesda, MD 20892-3676
Phone: 800-624-2663
Fax: 202-293-2356
E-mail: NIHBoneInfo@mail.nih.gov
Website: www.niams.nih.gov/Health_Info/Bone/default.asp

Diabetic Eye Disease

American Academy of Ophthalmology
P.O. Box 7424
San Francisco, CA 94120-7424
Phone: 415-561-8500
Fax: 415-561-8533
E-mail: eyesmart@aao.org
Website: www.geteyesmart.org

Eye Care America
P.O. Box 429098
San Francisco, CA 94142
Phone: 877-887-6327
Fax: 415-561-8567
E-mail: aaoe@aao.org
Website: www.eyecareamerica.org

National Eye Institute (NEI)
31 Center Dr. MSC 2510
Bethesda, MD 20892-2510
Phone: 301-496-5248
E-mail: 2020@nei.nih.gov
Website: www.nei.nih.gov

Prevent Blindness America
211 W. Wacker Dr. #1700
Chicago, IL 60606
Phone: 312-363-6001
Toll-Free: 800-331-2020
E-mail: info@preventblindness.org
Website: www.preventblindness.org

Diabetes-Related Foot Problems

National Institute of Arthritis and Musculoskeletal and Skin Diseases
1 AMS Cir.
Bethesda, MD 20892-3675
Phone: 1-877-22-64267
TTY: 301-565-2966
Fax: 301-718-6366
E-mail: NIAMSinfo@mail.nih.gov
Website: www.niams.nih.gov

Diabetes-Related Heart Disease

American Heart Association
7272 Greenville Ave.
Dallas, TX 75231-4596
Phone: 1-800-242-8721
E-mail: Review.personal.info@heart.org
Website: www.americanheart.org

National Heart, Lung, and Blood Institute
P.O. Box 30105
Bethesda, MD 20824-0105
Phone: 301-592-8573
Fax: 240-629-3246
E-mail: nhlbiinfo@nhlbi.nih.gov
Website: www.nhlbi.nih.gov

Diabetic Kidney Disease

American Association of Kidney Patients
3505 E. Frontage Rd.
Ste. 315
Tampa, FL 33607
Toll-Free: 800-749-2257
Fax: 813-636-8122
E-mail: info@aakp.org
Website: www.aakp.org

National Kidney Disease Education Program
3 Kidney Information Way
Bethesda, MD 20892
Toll-Free: 866-4-KIDNEY (454-3639)
Fax: 301-402-8182
E-mail: nkdep@info.niddk.nih.gov
Website: www.nkdep.nih.gov

National Kidney Foundation
30 E. 33rd St.
New York, NY 10016
Toll-Free: 800-622-9010
Fax: 212-689-9261
E-mail: info@kidney.org
Website: www.kidney.org

Directory of Diabetes-Related Resources

Diabetes-Related Mouth Problems

National Institute of Dental and Craniofacial Research
1 NOHIC Way
Bethesda, MD 20892-3500
Phone: 1-866-232-4528
Fax: 301-480-4098
E-mail: nidcrinfo@mail.nih.gov
Website: www.nidcr.nih.gov/OralHealth

Juvenile Diabetes

Barbara Davis Center for Childhood Diabetes
1775 Aurora Ct.
Aurora, CO 80045
Phone: 303-724-6836 (research)
Phone: 303-724-2323 (clinic)
Fax: 303-724-6839
Website: www.ucdenver.edu/academics/colleges/medicalschool/centers/BarbaraDavis/Pages/barbaradaviscenter.aspx

Children With Diabetes
Website: www.childrenwithdiabetes.com

Diabetes and Endocrinology Service
Office of Specialty Care Services, Department of Veterans Affairs
810 Vermont Ave. N.W.
Washington, DC 20420
Website: www.va.gov/diabetes/#veterans

IHS Division of Diabetes Treatment and Prevention
5300 Homestead Rd. N.E.
Albuquerque, NM 87110
Phone: 505-248-4549
E-mail: diabetesprogram@ihs.gov
Website: www.ihs.gov/medicalprograms/diabetes

Juvenile Diabetes Research Foundation International
26 Broadway 14th Fl.
New York, NY 10004
Toll-Free: 800-533-CURE (2873)
E-mail: info@jdrf.org
Website: www.jdrf.org

National Digestive Diseases Information Clearinghouse (NDDIC)
2 Information Way
Bethesda, MD 20892-3570
Phone: 1-800-891-5389
TTY: 1-866-569-1162
Fax: 703-738-4929
E-mail: nddic@info.niddk.nih.gov
Website: www.digestive.niddk.nih.gov

Nemours Foundation
10140 Centurion Pkwy N.
Jacksonville
Florida, FL 32256
Phone: 1-904-697-4100
Website: www.nemours.org

***University of Chicago
Diabetes Research and
Training Center (DRTC)***
5841 S. Maryland Ave. AMB
N237 MC1207
Chicago, IL 60637
Phone: 773-702-9116
Fax: 773-702-9237
E-mail: g-bell@uchicago.edu
Website: drtc.bsd.uchicago.edu

***Vanderbilt University
Diabetes Center***
2215 Garland Ave.
802 Light Hall
Nashville, TN 37232-0202
Phone: 615-936-7678
Fax: 615-936-0063
E-mail: al.powers@vanderbilt.edu
Website: www.mc.vanderbilt.edu/diabetes/drtc

Index

Index

Page numbers followed by 'n' indicate a footnote. Page numbers in italics indicate a table or illustration.

A

A1C test
  blood glucose level 102
  blood tests 21
  described 310
  diagnostic testing 134
  heart disease 50
  overview 149–55
  prediabetes 133
  pregnancy 138
"The A1C Test and Diabetes" (NIDDK) 149n
acanthosis nigricans, defined 445
acarbose, Alpha-glucosidase Inhibitors 170
ACE Inhibitors *see* angiotensin-converting enzyme inhibitors
acromegaly, endocrine diseases 43
Actoplus Met (pioglitazone and metformin), combination medicines 174
adolescents
  overweight 300
  physical activity 230
  type 1 diabetes 299
adult-onset diabetes
  medicines 162
  type 2 diabetes 320
aerobic exercise, physical activity 231
affordable medications, Rx Outreach 425
albumin
  creatine measurement 107
  defined 445
  proteinuria 293
albuminuria
  defined 445
  see also proteinuria
alcohol
  blood pressure 63
  osteoporosis 240
allergy, Ryzodeg 194
alpha cell, defined 445
alpha-glucosidase inhibitors, described 170
alpha-lipoic acid, described 211
"Alzheimer's Disease: Unraveling the Mystery" (NIA) 55n
Amaryl, sulfonyureas 171
"Am I at Risk for Gestational Diabetes?" (OHPHP) 71n
"Am I at Risk for Type 2 Diabetes? Taking Steps to Lower Your Risk of Getting Diabetes" (NIDDK) 61n

461

American Association of Clinical Endocrinologists, contact 453
American Association of Diabetes Educators, contact 453
American Association of Kidney Patients, contact 456
American Diabetes Association, contact 453
amputations
  carbohydrate counting 206
  complications 7
  type 2 diabetes 19
Amputee Coalition, contact 425
Amylin, defined 445
Amylin Analog, described 175
anaphylaxis, Ryzodeg 194
androgens, polycystic ovary syndrome 291
angina *see also* chest pain
angiotensin converting enzyme (ACE) inhibitors, proteinuria 295
angiotensin receptor blockers (ARB)
  blood pressure medications 276
  defined 446
  proteinuria 295
antibodies, autoimmune disorders 43
anti-VEGF injection therapy, described 247
appetite, gastroparesis 237
ARB *see* angiotensin receptor blockers
arginine, clinical trials 412
arginine stimulation, type 2 diabetes mellitus 412
artificial sweeteners, non-nutritive sweeteners 413
aspart, insulin 193
atherosclerosis
  blood vessels 268
  defined 112
athlete's foot
  described 255
  tabulated *255*
autoimmune disease
  defined 446
  type 1 diabetes 299
autoimmune disorder, described 11
autonomic neuropathy
  defined 446
  described 285

Avandamet, tabulated *174*
Avandaryl (rosiglitazone + glimepiride), tabulated *174*

B

bacteremia, vaccines 186
Barbara Davis Center for Childhood Diabetes, contact 457
Bariatric surgery, obesity 222
"Be Active" (CDC) 347n
beta blockers, blood pressure medications 276
beta cells
  autoimmune process 34
  defined 446
  insulin 412
  pancreatic islet 390
  risk factors 300
  toxins 44
  type 1 diabetes 299
beta cell impairment, beta cell dysfunction 40
beverage, glucose 415
bezoars, gastroparesis 264
biguanide, defined 446
biomarkers, surrogate endpoints 402
biopsy, estimated glomerular filtration rate 108
blindness
  A1C tests 155
  blood vessel damage 305
  diabetic eye disease 118
  glaucoma 121
  retinopathy 218
  type 2 diabetes 320
blisters
  depicted *253*
  feet 93
  nerve damage 237
  tabulated *253*
blood clots, healthy routines 367
blood draws, diabetes treatment 413
blood flow
  blood pressure 12
  cardiovascular disease 398
  feet 115
  smoking 218

Index

blood glucose
  beta cell dysfunction 41
  defined 446
  diagnosis 21
  endocrine diseases 43
  family history 42
  gestational diabetes 41
  healthy food choices 430
  hypoglycemia 88
  insulin 429
  insulin resistance 18
  nervous system 284
  physical activity 309
  plasma glucose test 151
  prediabetes 14
  targets 86
  type 2 diabetes 7
  types of diabetes 4
  see also blood sugar
blood glucose control *see* glucose control
blood glucose levels
  A1C test 151
  carbohydrates 205
  carbohydrate counting 209
  diabetes medicines 162
  diabetic kidney disease 275
  foodborne illness 198
  gestational diabetes 163
  insulin 164
  ketones 310
  labor and delivery 314
  meal planning 164
  nutrition 330
  onset 389
  prediabetes 14
  retina damage 118
  strokes 206
  type 2 diabetes 159
  see also hyperglycemia; hypoglycemia
blood glucose meter, defined 446
blood glucose monitoring
  hepatitis B 185
  research 388
  vaccines 185
"Blood Glucose Monitoring Devices" (FDA) 144n

blood glucose records
  pregnancy 310
  tabulated *342*
blood pressure control
  nerve disease 353
  proteinuria 295
  systolic blood pressure 353
blood pressure cuff
  blood pressure test 107
  diabetes treatment 415
blood sugar
  gestational diabetes 29
  glucose 4
  hypoglycemic events 406
  insulin guide 178
  Medicare 51
  prediabetes 56
  type 1 diabetes 9
blood sugar test, overview 142–4
blood tests
  prediabetes 20
  pregnant women 138
  type 2 diabetes 320
blurred vision
  symptoms 320
  type 1 diabetes 9
BMI *see* body mass index
body mass index (BMI)
  defined 446
  described 139
  obesity 221
bone density test, described 241
breastfeeding, meglitindes 31
bruises
  infections 322
  symptoms 320
brunch, recipes 434
bunions
  depicted *254*
  described 354
Byetta (exenatide)
  nonimmunosuppresive medications 394
  tabulated *175*

C

caffeine, xerostomia 281

calcium
　herbal supplements 212
　osteoporosis 239
　vitamins 214
calcium channel blockers, blood pressure medications 276
calluses
　depicted *253*
　nerve damage 285
　podiatrist 116
calorie
　carbohydrate intake 206
　defined 446
　diabetes prevention program 140
　prediabetes 22
　type 2 diabetes 63
CAM *see* complementary and alternative medicine
Canadian Diabetes Association, contact 453
canned vegetables, recipes 130
carbohydrate counting
　defined 446
　overview 204–10
carbohydrate
　insulin 332
　pregnant 210
cardiovascular disease (CVD)
　chronic kidney disease 155
　physical activity 352
　triglycerides 91
　type 2 diabetes 37
caregivers, monitor blood glucose 194
cataracts, diabetic eye disease 236
"Causes of Diabetes" (NIDDK) 33n
CDC *see* Centers for Disease Control and Prevention
cell lines, human stem cells 397
Centers for Disease Control and Prevention (CDC)
　contact 454
　publications
　　be active 347n
　　diabetes 6n
　　diabetes and adult vaccines 185n
　　diabetes and hepatitis B 185n

Centers for Disease Control and Prevention (CDC)
　publications, *continued*
　　family history 75n
　　flu season 259n
　　gestational diabetes and pregnancy 315n
　　manage diabetes 125n
　　prevent complications 235n
　　recipes 429n
　　research projects 386n
　　sick days 355n
　　smoking and diabetes 217n
　　stay healthy 351n
Charcot's foot
　depicted *256*
　described 252
chemicals
　arsenic 44
　inflammation 217
　ketones 312
　physical activity 232
　test strip 16
chest pain, diabetic kidney disease 275
Children With Diabetes, contact 457
children
　body mass index 139
　gestational diabetes 68
　insulin-dependent diabetes 162
　hepatitis B vaccine 187
　polycystic ovarian syndrome 69
　prediabetes 137
　type 2 diabetes 7
Chlorpropamide, tabulated *171*
cholesterol
　alpha-lipoic acid 211
　central obesity 268
　defined 50
　metabolic syndrome 39
　nutrition 49
　pancreatic islet transplant 396
　triglyceride 57
cholesterol levels
　alpha-lipoic acid 211
　blood pressure numbers 94
　Medicare 330
　type 1 diabetes 12

Index

"Choose More than 50 Ways to Prevent Type 2 Diabetes" (NDEP) 129n
chromium, described 212
chronic kidney disease
  A1C test 155
  dietary supplements 216
  metabolic syndrome 20
  proteinuria 293
cilantro, Pozole 442
CKD *see* chronic kidney disease
clinical trials
  Asian ginseng 212
  biomarkers 403
  magnesium 213
  overview 409–17
  relatives 388
  Tresiba 193
  type 1 diabetes 388
ClinicalTrials.gov
  publications
    mHealth app 409n
    non-nutritive sweeteners 409n
    short-term beta-cell rest 409n
combination medicines, tabulated *174*
complementary and alternative medicine (CAM), dietary supplements 24
control group, clinical trials 417
corns, podiatrist 116
counseling
  employee rights 381
  vision loss 122
creatinine
  defined 447
  diabetic kidney disease 109
  proteinuria 295
"Creating a Family Health History" (NIH) 75n
cuts
  exercise 349
  healthy food 432
  symptoms 320
Cushing's syndrome, hormonal disorders 43

D

daclizumab, immunosuppressive medications 394
dairy products, healthy eating plan 330
Dapagliflozin, tabulated *174*
dark green veggies, healthy food 432
DASH *see* dietary approaches to stop hypertension
DCCT *see* diabetes control and complications trial
dehydration
  blood glucose 301
  gastroparesis 264
delayed gastric emptying *see also* gastroparesis
depression, pregnancy 31
DEXA scan, body fat 413
dextrose, defined 447
DiaBeta (glyburide), tabulated *171*
"Diabetes" (NIA) 159n
"Diabetes" (CDC) 6n
"Diabetes" (OWH) 303n
"Diabetes" (NIDDK) 388n
Diabetes Action Research and Education Foundation, contact 454
"Diabetes and African Americans" (OMH) 323n
"Diabetes and American Indians/Alaska Natives" (OMH) 323n
"Diabetes and Asians and Pacific Islanders" (OMH) 323n
"Diabetes and Dietary Supplements" (NCCIH) 210n
"Diabetes and Hepatitis B Vaccination" (CDC) 271n
"Diabetes and Hispanic Americans" (OMH) 323n
"Diabetes and Native Hawaiians/Pacific Islanders" (OMH) 323n
"Diabetes and You: All Medicines Matter!" (NDEP) 166n
"Diabetes and You: Healthy Feet Matter!" (NDEP) 115n
"Diabetes and You: Healthy Teeth Matter!" (NDEP) 102n
diabetes complications, physical activity 348
diabetes control and complications trial (DCCT)
  home monitors 145
  retinopathy 247

diabetes educators, health care team 126
"Diabetes, Heart Disease, and Stroke" (NIDDK) 267n
Diabetes Insipidus Foundation, contact 454
"Diabetes Latest" (NCCDPHP) 45n
diabetes meal plan, recipes 444
diabetes medicines
  action steps 361
  overview 162–5
diabetes mellitus, Ryzodeg 70/30 194
diabetes prevention program (DPP), insulin resistance 22
diabetes prevention program outcomes study (DPPOS), metformin 23
diabetes-related bone disease, overview 239–42
diabetes-related mouth disease, overview 279–82
Diabetes Teaching Center, contact 436
diabetes-related eye disease, overview 243–49
diabetic ketoacidosis
  defined 447
  ketones 194
  type 1 diabetes 9
diabetic kidney disease
  diabetic nephropathy 273
  overview 273–8
  symptoms 107
"Diabetic Kidney Disease" (NIDDK) 273n
diabetic nephropathy, kidney damage 10
diabetic neuropathy, described 237
diabetic retinopathy
  described 243
  macular edema 119
Diabinese, tabulated *171*
diagnosis
  autoimmune destruction 34
  overview 133–40
  prediabetes 21
  type 2 diabetes 150
"Diagnosis of Diabetes and Prediabetes" (NIDDK) 133n

dialysis
  defined 447
  diabetic nephropathy 236
  kidney failure 277
  see also hemodialysis; peritoneal dialysis
dietary approaches to stop hypertension (DASH), blood pressure 277
diet
  blood glucose 144
  kidney disease 277
  pancreatic islet transplant 396
  physical activity 19
  type 2 diabetes 213
dietary supplements *see also* supplements
differentiated cells, human stem cells 396
digestive system, autonomic neuropathy 285
diuretic
  blood pressure medications 276
  human immunodeficiency virus 44
dopamine receptor agonists, tabulated *173*
"Do You Know Some of the Health Risks of Being Overweight?" (NIDDK) 220n
DPP *see* Diabetes Prevention Program
DPPOS *see* Diabetes Prevention Program Outcomes Study
dry and cracked skin, depicted *255*
dual-energy X-ray absorptiometry (DXA) test, bone density 242
Duetact, tabulated *174*
DXA test *see* dual-energy X-ray absorptiometry

E

eAG *see* estimated average glucose
EEOC *see* Equal Employment Opportunity Commission
eGFR *see* estimated glomerular filtration rate
electronic blood glucose tracking system, internet 87
embryonic stem (ES) cells, human development 396

Index

employee rights, overview 369–81
end-stage renal disease (ESRD)
  dialysis 293
  Medicare 426
endocrinology, clinical trials 417
endothelial progenitor cells, heart tissue 399
engraftment, cell-based treatments 399
environmental factors
  described 35
  risk factors 300
  type 1 diabetes 7
Equal Employment Opportunity Commission (EEOC), Americans with Disabilities Act 369
erectile dysfunction, sex organs 286
ES *see* embryonic stem
ESRD *see* end-stage renal disease
estimated glomerular filtration rate (eGFR), described 108
estimated average glucose (eAG), A1C test 154
euglycemic clamp, insulin resistance 20
exenatide
  immunosuppressive medications 394
  tabulated *175*
exercise
  angina 112
  blood test 152
  diet 159
  physical activity program 228
  proteinuria 295
  type 1 diabetes 9
Eye Care America, contact 455
eye examinations, Medicare 51
eyes
  A1C 76
  cataracts 236
  diabetes problems 85
  eye exams 122
  optic nerve 118
  pregnancy 31
  tabulated *86*

F

"Facts about Diabetic Eye Disease" (NEI) 243n

"Family History" (CDC) 75n
family history
  osteoporosis 239
  overview 75–7
  prediabetes 14
  proteinuria 294
  type 2 diabetes 320
fasting blood glucose test, defined 447
FDA *see* U.S. Food and Drug Administration
federal poverty level (FPL), healthy eating 70
financial help, overview 421–7
"Financial Help for Diabetes Care" (NIDDK) 421n
fish
  healthy foods 81
  prevent type 2 diabetes 129
  protein 200
flu
  blood sugars 51
  overview 259–61
  pneumonia vaccine 321
flu vaccine, tabulated *345*
focal/grid macular laser surgery, described 248
food labels, meal plan 433
"Food Safety for Diabetes Patients" (HHS) 198n
foot problems
  exercise 353
  infections 252
  podiatrist 115
FPL *see* federal poverty level
fruit-flavored drinks, healthy food choices 432
fungal Infection
  mouth problems 238
  smoking 100
  tabulated *255*
future therapies, technical hurdles 400

G

gangrene, blood flow 252
gastrointestinal problems, immunosuppressive medications 394
"Gastroparesis" (NIDDK) 263n

gastroparesis
  defined 447
  digestion 237
  overview 263–6
genes
  genetic susceptibility 34
  type 1 diabetes 303
  type 2 diabetes 403
Genetics Home Reference (GHR) publication
    type 1 diabetes 9n
genetic syndromes, diabetes 43
gestational diabetes
  blood glucose levels 41
  carbohydrate counting 210
  diabetes pills 164
  diabetic retinopathy 121
  overview 29–32
  pregnancy 5
  type 2 diabetes 62
"Gestational Diabetes and Pregnancy" (CDC) 315n
"Gestational Diabetes Screening: Questions for the doctor" (ODPHP) 123n
GFR *see* glomerular filtration rate
gingivitis
  oral health 237
  tabulated *280*
glaucoma
  defined 447
  eye problems 121
  Medicare 422
  optic nerve damage 236
glimepiride, tabulated *171*
glipizide, tabulated *174*
glomerular filtration rate (GFR), defined 447
glomeruli, kidney disease 274
GLP-1 Receptor Agonists, described 174
glucagon
  defined 447
  endocrine diseases 43
  hypoglycemia 287
  low blood glucose 311
glucagon emergency kit, insulin 367
glucometer, diabetes 8
Glucophage (metformin), tabulated *172*

glucose
  A1C test 50
  blood sugar 4
  exercise regimen 349
  defined 447
  insulin resistance 37
  natural disaster 362
  nerve damage 121
  retina 118
glucose beverage, blood samples 415
glucose gel
  defined 447
  hypoglycemia 89
  medication 367
glucose meter
  health care provider 147
  pregnancy 309
glucose screening test, gestational diabetes 71
glucose tablets, defined 447
glucose toxicity, beta cell dysfunction 40
Glucotrol (glipizide), tabulated *171*
Glucovance, tabulated *174*
Glulisine, tabulated *179*
Glyburide, tabulated *171*
glycogen, defined 447
glycohemoglobin test, diabetes management 149
Glynase (glyburide), tabulated *171*
Glyset (miglitol), tabulated *170*
gum disease, plaque 279

H

hair growth, polycystic ovary syndrome 291
hammertoe, depicted *254*
haplotype
  defined 447
  HLA genes 11
HAPO study *see* Hyperglycemia and Adverse Pregnancy Outcome study
HbA1C
  A1C test 336
  prediabetes 133
  see also hemoglobin A1C
health care team, medications 159
healthy weight, defined 448

Index

heart attack
  blood fat 143
  carbohydrate counting 206
  described 113
  health problems 177
  high blood pressure 50
  smoking 100
  type 2 diabetes 15
heart disease
  cholesterol 110
  health problems 220
heart healthy fats, described 202
hemoglobin A1C test
  blood glucose level 351
  see also glycohemoglobin test
hemodialysis, kidney 109
hepatic impairment, glucose-lowering medications 194
herbal supplements, described 212
high blood pressure *see also* hypertension
high-density lipoprotein (HDL), defined 448
high-fat diet, cholesterol 110
high-fat foods, healthy food choices 432
HLA complex *see* human leukocyte antigen
hormones, obesity 37
"How to Help Your Children Stay Healthy" (NDEP) 223n
human leukocyte antigen (HLA) complex, type 1 diabetes 11
human pluripotent cell lines, medications 397
human stem cells, pluripotent cell 397
hyperglycemia
  defined 448
  high blood glucose 88
hyperglycemia and adverse pregnancy outcome (HAPO) study, pregnancy complications 136
hypertension
  defined 448
  proteinuria 294
hypoglycemia
  A1C level 155
  defined 448
  low blood glucose 30

Meglitinides 170
nerve damage 287
Ryzodeg 70/30 194

I

Ibuprofen, painkillers 109
IDDM *see* insulin-dependent diabetes
IFG *see* impaired fasting glucose
IGT *see* impaired glucose tolerance
IHS Division of Diabetes, contact 457
impaired fasting glucose (IFG)
  A1C level 62
  defined 448
  fasting plasma glucose test 134
  type 2 diabetes 7
impaired glucose tolerance (IGT)
  defined 448
  type 2 diabetes 7
  see also impaired fasting glucose
incidence
  defined 448
  diabetes mellitus 386
  type 1 diabetes 10
  type 2 diabetes 300
infections
  bladder 286
  feet 237
  hyperglycemia 88
  nerve problems 4
  SGLT2 Inhibitors 173
inflammation
  congenital rubella syndrome 35
  insulin resistance 20
  oxidative stress 218
  proteinuria 293
informed consent document, trials 411
ingrown toenails, tabulated *253*
inhaled insulin, defined 448
"Insulin" (FDA) 177n
insulin
  beta cell dysfunction 40
  blood sugar 143
  defined 448
  described 163
  glucose 4
  high blood glucose 312
  overview 177–83
  pancreatic islet transplantation 392

469

physical activity 349
   type 1 diabetes 299
   type 2 diabetes 221
insulin aspart injection, blood sugar 193
insulin degludec injection, Tresiba 193
insulin-dependent diabetes (IDDM)
   type 1 diabetes 12
   type 2 diabetes 48
insulin detemir, tabulated *179*
insulin glargine, tabulated *179*
insulin infuser
   defined 448
   diabetes medicines 164
insulin pens
   described 180
   hepatitis B virus 272
insulin pumps
   cartridge 160
   described 181
   Medicare 422
   X-ray machines 361
insulin replacement therapy, type 1 diabetes 9
insulin resistance
   blood glucose levels 301
   body mass index 138
   defined 449
   described 37
   endocrine diseases 43
   gestational diabetes 73
   overview 17–26
   type 2 diabetes 162
"Insulin Resistance and Prediabetes" (NIDDK) 17n
insulin resistance syndrome, type 2 diabetes 39
interference
   A1C test 153
   glucose meter 146
   harassment 379
interventions
   health policies 387
   kidney failure 126
iPS cells, genetic signals 397
islet transplantation
   clinical trials 406
   defined 449
   immunosuppressive medications 394
   overview 390–6

islets
   defined 449
   enzymes 391
islets of Langerhans
   beta cells 390
   see also pancreatic islets
"It's Not Too Late to Prevent Type 2 Diabetes" (NDEP) 80n

J

Janumet (sitagliptin + metformin), tabulated *174*
Januvia (sitagliptin), nonimmunosuppresive medications 394
jet injector
   defined 449
   insulin devices 180
Johns Hopkins Diabetes Center, contact 454
Joslin Diabetes Center, contact 454
juvenile diabetes
   diabetes medicines 162
   type 1 diabetes 33
Juvenile Diabetes Research Foundation International, contact 457
juvenile-onset diabetes *see also* type 1 diabetes mellitus

K

ketoacidosis
   ketones 337
   Ryzodeg 194
   type 1 diabetes 299
ketones
   defined 449
   hyperglycemia 312
   insulin deficiency 300
   ketoacidosis 194
   physical activity 232
   type 1 diabetes 10
ketosis
   defined 449
   ketone Levels 312
kidneys
   depicted *105*

Index

kidneys, *continued*
  described 198
  diabetes problems 85
  diabetic nephropathy 236
  health care team 431
  high blood pressure 352
  kidney disease 274
  overview 104–11
  pregnancy 309
kidney disease
  angiotensin receptor blockers 276
  blood pressure 106
  carbohydrate counting 206
  incurable diseases 189
  metabolic syndrome 20
  smoking 218
  see also nephropathy
kidney failure
  behavioral approaches 388
  blood vessels 236
  chronic kidney disease 273
  dietary supplements 216
  end-stage renal disease 426
  estimated glomerular filtration rate test 108
  false A1C results 154
  proteinuria 294
  type 2 diabetes 15
kidney transplantation, pancreatic islet allo-transplantation 393
"Know Your Blood Sugar Numbers" (NDEP) 142n

L

labor
  blood glucose control 314
  gestational diabetes 72
lactic acidosis
  biguanides 172
  defined 449
LADA *see* latent autoimmune diabetes in adults
lancets
  Medicare 422
  natural disaster 362
latent autoimmune diabetes in adults (LADA)
  genetic conditions 302
  type 1 diabetes 33

LDL *see* low-density lipoprotein
lifestyle
  A1C blood test 151
  diabetes medicines 332
  kidney disease 274
  metabolic syndrome 39
  osteoporosis 240
Limbs for Life Foundation, contact 426
lipodystrophy
  adverse reactions 194
  defined 44
lipoprotein
  blood fat 352
  defined 449
  triglyceride level 14
lispro, tabulated *179*
liver
  abnormal blood fat 268
  gestational diabetes 415
  insulin resistance 20
  obesity 220
  pancreatic islet transplantation 392
long-term complications
  A1C test 154
  smoking 269
  target drugs 404
  type 1 diabetes 300
low blood glucose
  autonomic neuropathy 285
  breathing problems 31
  described 311
  insulin 332
  see also hypoglycemia
low-density lipoprotein (LDL), defined 449
lower-extremity amputation, cardiovascular risk profiles 126

M

macrovascular complications, diabetes management 125
macular degeneration
  cells and tissues 397
  sexually transmitted disease 190
macular edema
  alpha-lipoic acid 211
  diabetic eye disease 243
  diabetic retinopathy 119

magnesium, described 213
"Managing Your Diabetes during the Holidays" (CDC) 365n
maturity-onset diabetes of young (MODY)
  beta cell dysfunction 40
  defined 449
  latent autoimmune diabetes 302
meal plan
  blood pressure 106
  carbohydrate counting 204
  cholesterol 91
  gestational diabetes 163
  nutrition 396
meat
  diet and nutrition 277
  food choices 432
  high-fat diet 110
  pozole 442
  protein 200
Medicaid, health insurance 422
medical conditions
  kidney disease 274
  metabolic syndrome 19
medications
  anti-seizure drugs 44
  exercise 348
  gastroparesis 264
  hypoglycemia 316
  Medicare 422
  osteoporosis 239
  overview 161–76
  pancreatic islet transplantation 393
  see also insulin; prescription drugs
meglitinides, described 170
menopause
  heart disease 267
  osteoporosis 239
metabolic syndrome
  defined 449
  described 19
  triglycerides 236
  see also insulin resistance syndrome
metabolism
  chronic diseases 210
  defined 449
  insulin resistance 20
  thrifty gene 37
Metaglip, tabulated *174*

metformin
  gestational diabetes 26
  prediabetes 140
  tabulated *174*
  type 2 diabetes 63
mHealth app, diabetes type 1 - test 416
microalbuminuria, insulin resistance 302
microvascular complications, eye disease 125
miglitol, tabulated *170*
MODY *see* maturity-onset diabetes of young
"Monitor Your Diabetes" (NIDDK) 335n
monogenic diabetes
  diabetes medicines 163
  genetic mutations 42
mouth problems
  bleeding gums 99
  overview 279–82
  post-surgery healing 238

N

NAFLD *see* non-alcoholic fatty liver disease
Nateglinide, tabulated *170*
National Center for Chronic Disease Prevention and Health Promotion (NCCDPHP)
  publications
    diabetes 45n
    type 2 diabetes 68n
National Center for Complementary and Alternative Medicine (NCCAM), contact 454
National Center for Complementary and Integrative Health (NCCIH)
  publication
    diabetes and dietary 210n
The National Council on Aging, affordable medications 425
National Diabetes Education Program (NDEP)
  publications
    blood sugar 142n
    children and adolescents 299n
    diabetes medicines 166n

Index

National Diabetes Education Program (NDEP)
  publications, *continued*
    healthy children 223n
    healthy feet 115n
    healthy food 198n
    healthy teeth 102n
    prevent diabetes 80n
    prevent type 2 diabetes 129n
National Diabetes Information Clearinghouse (NDIC)
  contact 454
  publications
    prediabetes 13n
    type 2 diabetes 27n
National Eye Institute (NEI)
  contact 455
  publication
    diabetic eye disease 243n
National Heart, Lung, and Blood Institute, contact 456
National Institute on Aging (NIA)
  contact 454
  publications
    Alzheimer's disease 55n
    diabetes 159n
    frequently asked questions 47n
National Institute of Arthritis and Musculoskeletal and Skin Diseases, contact 456
National Institute of Child Health and Human Development (NICHD)
  publication
    gestational diabetes 71n
National Institute of Diabetes and Kidney Diseases (NIDDK)
  publications
    A1C test 149n
    being overweight 220n
    carbohydrate counting 204n
    care records 335n
    causes of diabetes 33n
    diabetes 388n
    diabetes care 329n, 421n
    diabetes medicines 162n
    diabetes, heart disease, and stroke 267n
    diagnosis 133n
National Institute of Diabetes and Kidney Diseases (NIDDK)
  publications, *continued*
    gastroparesis 263n
    gestational diabetes 29n
    healthy eyes 117n
    healthy feet 251n
    healthy heart and blood vessels 111n
    healthy kidneys 104n
    healthy mouth 279n
    healthy nervous system 283n
    insulin resistance 17n
    kidney disease 273n
    monitor your diabetes 334n
    pancreatic islet transplantation 390n
    physical activity 227n
    pregnancy 308n
    prevent diabetes 85n
    proteinuria 293n
    type 1 and type 2 9n
    type 2 diabetes 27n
National Kidney Disease Education Program, contact 456
National Kidney Foundation, contact 456
NCCAM *see* National Center for Complementary and Alternative Medicine
NDEP *see* National Diabetes Education Program
NDM *see* neonatal diabetes mellitus
NeedyMeds, nonprofit group 425
NEI *see* National Eye Institute
Nemours Foundation, contact 457
neonatal diabetes mellitus (NDM), genetic mutations 42
nephropathy
  defined 449
  kidney disease 273
  type 1 diabetes 10
nerve damage
  carbohydrate counting 206
  described 251
  diabetes medicines 162
  gestational diabetes 315
  see also neuropathy

nervous system disease, gastroparesis 264
neuropathy
  defined 450
  described 121
  end-stage renal disease 10
  nervous system 284
  smoking 218
NIA *see* National Institute on Aging
NIAMS *see* National Institute of Arthritis and Musculoskeletal and Skin Diseases
National Institute of Arthritis and Musculoskeletal and Skin Diseases (NIAMS)
  publication
    osteoporosis 239n
NIDDK *see* National Institute of Diabetes and Digestive and Kidney Diseases
NIH *see* National Institutes of Health
NIH Osteoporosis and Related Bone Diseases, contact 455
non-alcoholic fatty liver disease (NAFLD), Gestational Diabetes 414
nondairy creamers, healthy food 432
nonsteroidal anti-inflammatory drugs, omega-3 supplements 214
NSAID *see* nonsteroidal anti-inflammatory drugs

O

OB *see* obstetrician
obesity
  body mass index 221
  metabolic syndrome 20
  physical inactivity 37
obstetrician (OB)
  blood glucose levels 136
  gestational diabetes 29
obstetric history, gestational diabetes 415
OCT *see* optical coherence tomography
Office of Disease Prevention and Health Promotion (ODPHP)
  publications
    gestational diabetes 123n
    preventing diabetes 123n
Office of Minority Health (OMH)
  publications
    African Americans 323n
    American Indians/Alaska Natives 323n
    Asians and Pacific Islanders 323n
    Hispanic Americans 323n
    Native Hawaiians/Pacific Islanders 323n
Office of Specialty Care Services Department of Veterans Affairs, contact 457
Office on Women's Health (OWH)
  publications
    diabetes 303n
    polycystic ovary syndrome 291n
OGTT *see* oral glucose tolerance test
older adults
  body mass index 139
  diabetes 49
  proteinuria 294
omega-3s, described 213
online pharmacy, prescription drugs 190
ophthalmologists, macular edema 119
optical coherence tomography (OCT), described 246
oral glucose tolerance test (OGTT)
  defined 450
  gestational diabetes 71
  prediabetes 21
orange veggies, food choices 432
osteoporosis, overview 239–42
"Overview of Diabetes in Children and Adolescents" (NDEP) 299n
overweight
  body mass index 221
  type 2 diabetes 27
  metabolic syndrome 19
  nervous system 284
  prediabetes 13

P

PAD *see* peripheral artery disease
pancreas transplantation, defined 450

Index

pancreatic Islet
  depicted *391*
  described 390
pancreatic islet auto-transplantation, described 392
"Pancreatic Islet Transplantation" (NIDDK) 390n
PCOS *see* polycystic ovary syndrome
pediatricians, diabetic kidney disease 275
periodontitis
  oral health 237
  tabulated *280*
peripheral artery disease (PAD), poor blood flow 252
peripheral neuropathy
  defined 450
  described 284
  smoking 218
PG test *see* post glucola test
pharmacists, health care team 126
phase 2, clinical trials 406
physical activity
  blood glucose levels 88
  defined 450
  described 24
  diabetes medicines 162
  gestational diabetes 73
  tabulated *92*
  insulin resistance 22
pioglitazone, tabulated *174*
plaque
  described 279
  saliva 99
pneumococcal vaccine, vaccines 186
pneumonia vaccine, managing diabetes 321
polycystic ovary syndrome (PCOS)
  overview 291–2
  prediabetes 13
"Polycystic Ovary Syndrome (PCOS) Fact Sheet" (OWH) 291n
polydipsia
  defined 450
  type 1 diabetes 9
polyphenols, supplements 215
polyuria, defined 450
portion sizes, described 129

post glucola (PG) test, gestational diabetes 71
potassium, kidneys 109
PPOD providers, diabetes management 126
pramlintide acetate, tabulated *175*
Prandin (repaglinide), tabulated *170*
Precose (acarbose), tabulated *170*
prediabetes
  defined 450
  endocrine diseases 43
  insulin resistance 18
  overview 13–5
  plasma glucose test 134
  see also impaired fasting glucose; impaired glucose tolerance
"Prediabetes What You Need to Know" (NDIC) 13n
pregnancy
  A1C test 151
  blood glucose levels 136
  carbohydrate counting 210
  diabetes 308
  diabetic retinopathy 245
  gestational diabetes 29
  gestational diabetes 5
  medicines 313
  preeclampsia 31
  see also gestational diabetes
pregnant woman
  blood glucose levels 136
  high blood pressure 316
pregravid BMI, gestational diabetes 415
pre-mixed insulin, tabulated *179*
prescription drugs, diabetes treatment 190
Prevent Blindness America, contact 456
"Prevent Complications" (CDC) 235n
"Prevent Diabetes Problems: Keep Your diabetes under Control" (NIDDK) 85n
"Prevent Diabetes Problems: Keep Your Eyes Healthy" (NIDDK) 117n
"Prevent Diabetes Problems: Keep Your Feet healthy" (NIDDK) 115n

"Prevent Diabetes Problems: Keep Your Heart and Blood Vessels Healthy" (NIDDK) 111n
"Prevent Diabetes Problems: Keep Your Kidneys Healthy" (NIDDK) 104n
"Prevent Diabetes Problems: Keep Your Mouth Healthy" (NIDDK) 98n
"Prevent Diabetes Problems: Keep Your Nervous System Healthy" (NIDDK) 283n
"Preventing Diabetes: Questions for the doctor" (ODPHP) 123n
Prograf (tacrolimus), immunosuppressive medications 394
protein
  carbohydrate 206
  food 199
  tabulated *86*
  type 1 diabetes 10
"Proteinuria" (NIDDK) 293n
proteinuria
  defined 450
  overview 293–5
  see also albuminuria
PVD *see* peripheral vascular disease

Q

"Questions & Answers about Diabetes in the Workplace and the Americans with Disabilities Act (ADA)" (EEOC) 369n
"Questions and Answers: FDA Alerts- Companies to Stop the Illegal Sale of Products Claiming to Treat Diabetes" (FDA) 189n

R

race
  diabetes 69
  diabetes statistics 45
  physical activity 70
  diabetes mellitus 386
random plasma glucose (RPG) test
  blood test 134
  type 2 diabetes 151

Rapamune (sirolimus) 394
rapid-acting insulin, defined 450
reasonable accommodation, employment 375
recipes, overview 429–44
red patches, feet 322
renal disease
  kidney failure 426
  proteinuria 293
  type 1 diabetes 9
Repaglinide, tabulated *170*
"Research Projects" (CDC) 386n
respiratory distress syndrome, gestational diabetes 31
resting beta cells, clinical trials 412
Riomet (metformin), tabulated *172*
risk factors
  diabetes 56
  insulin resistance 19
  physical activity 24
  gestational diabetes mellitus
  osteoporosis 239
  obesity 37
  prediabetes 19
  pregnant women 138
  type 2 diabetes 301
Rosiglitazone, tabulated *174*
RPG test *see* random plasma glucose test
RxAssist, affordable medications 425
Rx Outreach, affordable medications 425
Ryzodeg, diabetes drugs 194

S

safety considerations, exercise 348
salt
  food choices 225
  high-sodium foods 114
  diabetic kidney disease 275
saturated fat, defined 450
saxagliptin, tabulated *174*
sedentary lifestyle, osteoporosis 240
self-tests
  blood glucose 88
  described 142
seniors *see also* older adults

Index

sex organs, autonomic neuropathy 285
sexual problems, nerve damage 288
SGLT2 inhibitors, described 173
SHIP *see* state health insurance assistance program
shoes
 foot exam 256
 podiatrist 115
 tabulated *253*
 walking 82
short-acting, insulin 178
"Sick Days" (CDC) 355n
sick days
 managing diabetes 355
signs
 diabetes 5
 ketones 337
 mouth problems 279
 proteinuria 294
sirolimus (rapamune), immunosuppressive medications 394
sitagliptin
 immunosuppressive medications 394
 tabulated *174*
skin infections, type 2 diabetes 320
sleep apnea, obesity 220
sleep problems, kidney disease 107
smoking
 mouth 100
 osteoporosis 239
 tabulated *93*
 type 2 diabetes 217
"Smoking and Diabetes" (CDC) 217n
Social Security Disability Insurance (SSDI), federal programs 423
social worker, employment discrimination 380
sores
 clogged blood vessels 114
 nerve damage 251
 tabulated *86*
soy, fiber 200
SPAP *see* state pharmacy assistance programs
Splenda, metabolic effects 413
SSDI *see* Social Security Disability Insurance
SSI *see* Supplemental Security Income
Starlix (nateglinide), tabulated *170*

state health insurance assistance programs (SHIPs), state programs 423
state pharmaceutical assistance programs (SPAPs), state programs 423
statistics, diabetes 324
"Stay Healthy" (CDC) 351n
"Stay Well in Flu Season" (CDC) 259n
stick margarine, healthy food 432
strength training, physical activity 348
stretching
 physical activity 348
 strength training 231
stroke
 cholesterol 91
 heart disease 267
 high blood pressure 316
 type 1 diabetes 9
sucralose, artificial sweeteners 413
sugar disease *see also* diabetes mellitus
sulfonylurea
 defined 450
 described 171
sugary solution, oral glucose tolerance test 412
supplements
 alpha-lipoic acid 211
 herbal 212
 magnesium 213
sweat glands, autonomic neuropathy 285
Symlin (pramlintide acetate), Amylin analog 175
syndrome X *see also* metabolic syndrome
systolic blood pressure, diabetes 352

T

tacrolimus, immunosuppressive medications 394
"Take Care of Your Diabetes during Special Times or Events" (NIDDK) 359n
"Take Care of Your Diabetes Each Day" (NIDDK) 329n

"Targeted Drug Development: Why Are Many Diseases Lagging Behind?" (FDA) 401n
T cells, autoimmune destruction 34
tests
  A1C test 155
  blood sugar 143
  gastroparesis 263
  insulin resistance 20
  insurance coverage 84
  kidney disease 107
  oral glucose tolerance test 133
  proteinuria 294
test strips
  blood glucose levels 335
  glucose meter 147
tetanus, vaccines 186
thrifty gene, genetic susceptibility 37
"Tips for Teens with Diabetes: Make Healthy Food Choices" (NDEP) 198n
tobacco use
  cardiovascular disease 46
  nerve damage 125
Tolazamide, tabulated *171*
Tolbutamide, tabulated *171*
tonometry, diabetic retinopathy 246
transplant
  end-stage kidney disease 278
  risks 393
transplantation therapy, embryonic stem cells 398
Tresiba, described 193
triggers
  heart disease 398
  type 2 diabetes 36
triglycerides, defined 451
"Type 1 Diabetes" (GHR) 9n
type 1 diabetes
  defined 451
  described 4
  ketones 194
  overview 9–12
  pancreatic islets 390
  vitamin D supplements 35
"Type 2 Diabetes – What You Need to Know" (NDIC) 27n
type 2 diabetes
  carbohydrate counting 204
  defined 451

type 2 diabetes, *continued*
  described 221
  diagnostic testing 134
  herbal supplements 212
  overview 27–8
  pregnancy 72
  target drugs 404

U

UCSF Diabetes Teaching Center University of California, contact 455
ultrasound
  optical coherence tomography 246
  pregnancy 415
umbilical cord blood cells, broken heart 399
University of Chicago Diabetes Research and Training Center (DRTC), contact 458
urinary tract infections, common side effects 173
urine albumin, kidney disease 108
urine test, tabulated *344*
U.S. Department of Health and Human Services (HHS)
  publication
    food safety 198n
U.S. Equal Employment Opportunity Commission (EEOC)
  publication
    frequently asked questions 369n
U.S. Food and Drug Administration (FDA)
  publications
    blood glucose 144n
    diabetes drugs 193n
    drug development 401n
    illegal sale of drugs 189n
    insulin 177n
    women and diabetes 169n
UTI *see* urinary tract infections

V

vaccination, diabetes 187

Index

vaginal
  delivery 315
  nerve damage 305
  symptoms 306
vagus nerve, gastroparesis 263
Vanderbilt University Diabetes Center, contact 458
veterans, health insurance 422
visual acuity testing, diabetic retinopathy 246
vitamins, diabetes medicines 214

W

"We Have the Power to Prevent Diabetes" (NDEP) 80n
weight loss
  bariatric surgery 222
  diabetes in children 300–1
  diabetic kidney disease 107, 275
  diabetic problem 7
  gastroparesis 237
  genetic susceptibility 36
  hyperglycemia 312
  insulin resistance 22
  insurance coverage 84
  physical activity 227, 349
  type 1 diabetes 9
  type 2 diabetes 61
"What I need to Know about Carbohydrate Counting and Diabetes" (NIDDK) 204n
"What I Need to Know about Diabetes Medicines" (NIDDK) 162n
"What I Need to Know about Gestational Diabetes" (NIDDK) 29n
"What I Need to Know about Physical Activity and Diabetes" (NIDDK) 227n
"What I Need to Know about Preparing for Pregnancy if I Have Diabetes" (NIDDK) 308n
"What You Need to Know about Diabetes and Adult Vaccines" (CDC) 185n
whole grains, carbohydrates 204
WIC program *see* women infants and children program
"Will Diabetes Be Part of Your Story?" (CDC) 55n
women
  A1C Test 310
  cholesterol 353
  diabetic kidney disease 273
  diabetic retinopathy 245
  gastroparesis 264
  gestational diabetes 5
  hypoglycemia 316
  insulin resistance 41
  polycystic ovary syndrome 291
  preeclampsia 316
  sexual response 238
  statistics 56
  type 2 diabetes 42, 68
  weight loss
"Women and Diabetes – Diabetes Medicines" (FDA) 169n
women infants and children (WIC) program 423
workplace, vaccines 186
"Working Together to Manage Diabetes: A Guide for Pharmacy, Podiatry, Optometry, and Dentistry" (CDC) 125n

X

xerostomia, tabulated *281*

Y

yoga, nerve damage 289

Z

zinc, herbal supplements 212
zucchini
  nonstarchy vegetables 205
  Spanish omelet 434